Perceptual Neuroscience

THE CEREBRAL CORTEX

For my beloved granddaughter Julia Bainbridge [Vernon!] with love & affection [from]

Vernon B. Mountcastle

Harvard University Press

Cambridge, Massachusetts, and London, England   1998

Library of Congress Cataloging-in-Publication Data

Mountcastle, Vernon B.
Perceptual neuroscience : the cerebral cortex /
Vernon B. Mountcastle.
    p.   cm.
Includes bibliographical references and index.
ISBN 0-674-66188-5 (alk. paper)
1. Neocortex.   2. Perception.   I. Title.
QP383.12.M68   1998
612.8'25—dc21   98-15241

Designed by Gwen Nefsky Frankfeldt

To the students, staff, and faculty of the Johns Hopkins University School of Medicine, where for more than half a century I have been immersed in that warm collegiality most conducive to scientific research and intellectual endeavor

Contents

Expanded Contents

Preface

The advance in our understanding of the function of the brain over the last few decades is widely recognized as one of the triumphs of modern biology, still in part promissory in nature. This increment in knowledge has been generated by anatomical, physiological, and biochemical investigations combined with theoretical studies, carried out by neuroscientists using many methods of modern technology. Advances with considerable promise have been made in studies of the cerebral cortex, the part of the brain which shows the most rapid increase in absolute size in phylogeny. The cortex comprises about 60–65 percent of the volume of the human brain; if spread flat, it would occupy about 2,600 cm^2; it contains between 20 and 30 billion cells, called neurons, and as many as twice that number of nonneural cells, the glia. Cortical nerve cells are organized in highly specific patterns into many systems, which are heavily connected with one another; the number of interconnections between nerve cells in the neocortex reaches an astronomical figure. Neurons communicate with one another by passing signals over connections both between cortical elements and between the cortex and other parts of the brain. They are so numerous that it is unlikely that any portion of the brain ever functions in complete isolation from other parts; the signal processing systems of the brain are distributed in nature.

Research has provided detailed information about how the external world is represented in the cerebral neocortex. These representations include the geographic maps of the external world in afferent systems and their cortical projection areas, as well as the dynamic and time-varying patterns of activity in their neuronal populations that compose continually updated pictures of external events. Parallel studies on the output side have revealed how it is that brain systems generate the patterns of neuronal activity that lead to and control the execution of movements, both those initiated at will and those emitted in direct response to sensory stimuli. Moreover, neuroscientists now probe the even more difficult problems of the brain operations that intervene between sensory representations of the external world and motor operations upon it. Rather suddenly it has become possible to study with a variety of methods, in waking humans, even the most complex of brain functions, including thinking, learning, remembering, attending, and the like. No aspect of the inner life of man can now arbitrarily be excluded from scientific study. I do not imply that we yet understand these higher functions of the human brain very well, but that they are now in the field of play.

A major unknown lurks at the center of this accumulation of knowledge about brain function. We know very little of the *operations* of local circuits in cortical modules, nor of the *operations* in the distributed systems of the cortex formed by the linking together of many modules. We have learned a great deal about the functional properties of individual cortical neurons and of their synaptic interactions, much less of operations executed by groups of those neurons linked in processing chains. Areas of the cerebral cortex are frequently labeled in terms of their extrinsic connections, as they have been since the dawn of neurological science. Yet it is obvious that there is nothing intrinsically motor about the motor cortex, nor sensory about the sensory. How similar or different the intrinsic operations may be in cortical areas with such different patterns of extrinsic connections is presently unknown, certain to be a subject of intensive study in the future.

My objective in writing this book has been to bring together knowledge that bears upon the central problem of intrinsic cortical operations, in the context of the brain operations in perception. I do not provide a systematic overview of the vast field of perception, but rather highlight certain aspects of perceptual studies in experimental psychology and neurophysiology that are essential for the objects in view. Prominent among these are psychophysical measures of perceptual performances both in humans and in nonhuman primates, for it is the combination of these data with new methods for simultaneous recording of the relevant brain activity that has created the present revolution in the field of what I shall call *perceptual neuroscience*. These combinations now dominate perceptual research, and the continuation of such combined experiments and of microneuro-physiological studies of local cortical circuits will eventually lead to a unified theory of the brain mechanisms in perception based upon knowledge of intrinsic cortical operations.

Knowledge about the cerebral cortex grows at such a pace, and information about it comes from so many different fields, that I found it necessary to delve into several disciplines as I worked on the present volume. I am now preparing a second volume on subjects of my primary interest, somesthesis and spatial perception. I have expanded the scope of that volume to include some aspects of the sensory-motor interface, because although somesthesis stands as an independent field of enquiry (especially as it concerns the perceptual capacities of the primate hand), it is the somesthetic perhaps more than any other sensory system that is closely linked to the motor system. Those terms of engagement are strong and effective at every level of the nervous system. They are of particular importance at the level of the neocortex, the part of the cortex that is most complex in structure (with six layers) and most recent in phylogenetic development. In the neocortex (also known as the "isocortex"), population interfaces execute coordinate transforms and generate patterns of activity driving movement.

This volume is filled with descriptions—of anatomical structure, connectivity, systems organization, and experimental observations of all sorts. A major criticism of this field is that it is data-rich and theory-poor. This is of course better than the reverse! There is now developing a significant theoretical effort in relation to cortical function, however, and I have referred to some of the new models in this volume. Surely the future will see a rapid synthesis between theory and experiment in perceptual neuroscience, with a gradual evolution toward new and better theories of the cerebral operations in perception, and new and better experiments to test them. It is important to emphasize the relatively primitive state of this field: both theories and (most) experimental results are of a transient nature, fated to flash across the neuroscience sky, only to fade and be replaced by new "facts" and new theoretical ideas; but some, by the greatest of fortune, will remain as small bricks in the construction of a scientific base for perception. Anyone who doubts the rapid turnover of ideas in an emerging science has only to look at the monographs and textbooks of physiology immediately after World War II. Can we ever forget the era of the cortical suppressor strips—confirmed by cytoarchitectural descriptions? Or the idea that worms who eat other worms absorb their memories? I hope we shall avoid such aberrations in the future, but there is absolutely no assurance that we shall do so.

Chapter 1 introduces the reader to the field of perceptual neuroscience. Chapters 2–4 describe the phylogenetic development of the neocortex, of the cells and local circuits of the neocortex, and of cortical organization at the systems level of areas and connectivity. The mechanisms of synaptic transmission in the neocortex are described in Chapter 5, and Chapter 6 contains an account of the activity-dependent changes in synaptic transmission in the hippocampus and in the neocortex thought to be the essential cellular mechanisms of learning and memory in cortical circuits. I then insert in Chapter 7 a description of the columnar organization of the neocortex. Chapter 8 deals with a subject for which advances have been rapid in recent years, the ontogenesis of the neocortex, followed in Chapter 9 by a discussion of the secondary events in cortical histogenesis; I have tried to strike some balance between the evidence for genetic and that for epigenetic influences regulating development. Chapter 10 turns back again to organization, with a brief description of the concept of distributed systems in the neocortex and the evidence supporting it.

Chapters 11 and 12 deal with dynamic actions in neocortical systems. I selected for Chapter 11 information from many sources that might bear upon the question of the intrinsic neocortical operations. I chose as a model the example of an invertebrate circuit from the gastropod. Knowledge of this circuit and others in invertebrates is probably more complete from the view of neurophysiology than for any others. Sorrowfully, at the end of this effort I cannot provide a simple and direct answer to the question, What is the intrinsic function of the neocortex?

In Chapter 12 I take up subjects with long histories in neuroscience and of great current interest: rhythmicity and synchronization in cortical networks. I provide there a brief history and current description of the electroencephalogram in humans. A major portion of the chapter contains a review of the evidence concerning the role in perceptual integration of temporal correlation between populations of neurons in neocortical circuits. I conclude that the new discoveries upon which the hypothesis is based are valid and real, but that we are still short of understanding how synchronization in a distributed system highlights the dynamic neural representation of one sensory event versus others, and how this synchronization is recognized and leads to further processing in circuits leading to perception itself. In Chapter 13 I offer my commentary on what has gone before.

It is my hope that this monograph and the one to follow will provide a knowledge base for students and fellows in neuroscience, as well as for investigators from other areas of neuroscience who set about studying the cerebral cortex. Perhaps it will also be useful for the many talented scientists in related fields who now wish to turn to study of the neocortex.

I owe thanks to my colleagues at the Krieger Mind-Brain Institute for their tolerance of many discussions of the matters treated in this book; to its director, Guy M. McKhann, for allowing me freedom from other responsibilities; to C. Edward Connor and Ernst Niebur, each of whom read the manuscript and made important observations and suggestions; and to Chris Lukasik of the Department of English of the Johns Hopkins University for his many suggestions that improved form and clarity.

The good company of people at Harvard University Press have been especially helpful, and ignored long delays. I owe thanks to its editors Michael G. Fisher and Christine Thorsteinsson. Finally, I thank Kathryn Schmit for her uncanny eye and remarkable attention to detail in editing.

Perceptual Neuroscience

Perception and the Cerebral Cortex

The mere outward sense, being passive in responding to the
impression of the objects that come in its way and strike upon it,
perhaps cannot help entertaining and taking notice of everything that
addresses it, be it useful or unuseful; but in the exercise of his mental
perception, every man, if he chooses, has a natural power to turn
himself upon all occasions, and to change and shift with the greatest of
ease to what he shall himself judge desirable.

—Plutarch, *Life of Pericles*

How we apprehend objects and events in the world around us and
how they are represented in our brains are continuing themes in
man's endeavor to understand himself. They have occupied the
thoughts of philosophers for more than two thousand years, and
perhaps nowhere with more insight and poetic description than in
the quotation given above. Plutarch infers that the central signals of
external events are always available, we would say at the level of the
neocortex, and are brought to consciousness by the act of attention.
Asking what the nature of central representations may be is a rich
and rewarding enterprise in brain research. The general aim is to
determine the relation between the material order and the sensory-
perceptual order, and how the former is transformed into the latter.

The long history of the development of ideas about perception
extends from the time of Democritus, about 400 B.C. Democritus
postulated that *eidola,* small images of external objects, were transmitted by atomic movements to the sense organs and from these to
sensation. These bear an uncanny resemblance to what we call "representations," which I define below. Intensive studies of perception,
particularly of vision, continued through the golden period of Greek
philosophy and science, from the time of Euclid and Aristotle (300
B.C.). The concepts that emerged in this early period survived the

many intervening centuries largely through the scholarship and discoveries of Arabic scientists, and flowered again in the early Renaissance with the discovery of many properties of visual perception, especially visual perspective. (This has been a frequent subject for the historians of science; for relevant monographs, see Boring, 1952; Crombie, 1952; Finger, 1994; Wolman, 1968; for briefer scholarly reviews, see Jung, 1984; or no. 10, vol. 25 of *Perception,* ed. R. A. Gregory.) The scientific, that is to say, the objective study of perception evolved through the lines of thought of Descartes (1965) and Hobbes (1651) to the psychological theory of association derived from Locke (1690) and Hume (1748). It was Hartley (1749) who proposed that, borrowing Newton's phrase, it is the "corresponding vibrations of the nerves" that leads to mental association. These general ideas reached an experimentally based formulation a century later in the work of the great German polymath, Hermann von Helmholtz (1962), in the period 1850–1870.

Crombie (1952) has pointed out that the success of seventeenth-century scientists and of those who followed after them in studies of hearing and vision depended upon their separation of the problem of perception into three parts: (a) the physical and physiological, the mechanisms of peripheral transduction and central representation; (b) the link between physiology and psychology; and (c) the purely psychological problem of perception. What has happened since then, at first slowly and now at an accelerating rate, is the fusion of these previously isolated fields of research into perceptual neuroscience.

The Neural Mechanisms in Perception: A Brief Résumé

The neural processes leading to perception are outlined briefly as follows. The primary features of the stimuli that impinge upon us—the "distal" stimuli of heat, force, light, sound, and chemical substances—are selectively transduced at the peripheral ends of sets of sensory (afferent) nerve fibers. Different groups of those sensory fibers respond selectively at lower thresholds than do others to different forms of impinging energy. This tuning, sometimes called "feature detection," is accomplished in evolution by the development of specific transducer mechanisms for different forms of energy, either in the nerve endings themselves or in complex sensory organs in which the afferent fibers terminate, like the mammalian retina or cochlea or the glabrous skin of the primate hand.

These few million afferent nerve fibers are our only links to reality. We know nothing of the outside world directly; we face it through our sensory receptors, and they are narrow filters often selectively sensitive only to special features of stimuli. Our perceptual experience is mediate, once removed, slightly delayed in time, an abstracted construction determined by the transducing properties of receptors and their afferent fibers and the processing properties of the central neural networks they engage. The total input picture after receptor transformation is composed of several types of information that vary in precision and detail.

1. The quality of a stimulus is signaled with certainty. This principle of the labeled line derives from Muller's (1838) original doctrine of specific nerve energies.

2. The input signals allow precise estimation of the intensities of stimuli when they can be compared, but our performance is poor when asked to categorize a series of stimuli distributed along an intensive continuum; on average, we can make only about seven such categories (Miller, 1956).

3. For the spatial senses of touch, hearing, and vision, the primary afferent input population signals with accuracy the position of a point in space and the spatial extent and form of more complex stimuli.

4. The afferent input provides a precise signal of the spatial translations of stimuli across a receptor field, of the speed and duration of movements, as well as of serial order in the temporal patterns of stimuli.

Afferent nerve impulses are projected into and relayed through the afferent sensory pathways of the nervous system, susceptible at every synaptic level to transformations imposed by the properties of the genetically determined and experientially modified microstructure within the relevant neuronal populations; they are subject also, from the first synaptic engagement onward, to the regulating and controlling influence of neural systems of central origin. The visual, somesthetic, and auditory systems project into the primary sensory areas of the cerebral cortex in what is usually a topographically intact mapping of the relevant sheet of sensory receptors. The maps of the visual and somesthetic areas are, at the simplest level of analysis, maps with visual space or body location as the initial parameters; other parameters are mapped within them in an intermittently recursive manner. The auditory cortex maps sound frequency (which is a map of position on the cochlear partition) as its initial parameter. These quasi-isomorphic representations in the sensory areas of the cortex are transformed further and divergently for feature processing in the distributed systems of the homotypical areas of the neocortex. The word *representation* has a specific meaning in neuroscience. It conveys the idea of a central neural reflection of the external world, frequently shown in the topographic mapping of sensory sheets at successive levels of the central nervous system. The idea is extended further to include the successive serial/parallel transformations imposed upon the ordered replication of sensory events, transformations which, it is supposed, impose further abstractions and modifications by the genetically determined structures and by complexion with the stored record of past events.

Some afferent channels lead more or less directly to motor output, by execution of the spatial coordinate transforms linking at many levels sensory inputs to motor response. The input representations in these and other channels are surmised to be further combined with stored records of past experience and to lead to perception. Transformations along different channels and in different systems differ qualitatively, but have in common that in the distributed processing systems they become less isomorphic to the input and more abstract. Neural representations in different channels vary along a continuum, from those relatively isomorphic to the physical stimuli that evoke them to those I term "constructions."

Constructions are generated by the titration of transformed and abstracted sensory input with the neural replications of past experience derived from memory, and are conditioned by control signals such as those for attention and cognitive and affective states. The nature of a construction is determined in part by the microconnectivity between neurons in the relevant brain systems, particularly in the distributed systems of the neocortex. Synaptic linkages in the neocortical neuropil are to some degree dynamic and changeable, influenced by epigenetic experiential factors. Thus each human brain is unique at the microstructural level. The images we each create of the world are to a certain degree idiosyncratic; they may resemble or be different from one brain to another, each receiving the same afferent input. Perhaps what is so striking is not that our perceptual images differ from time to time but that in ordinary experiences of life there is a remarkable similarity between perceptions reported by different persons.

The interactions within those neocortical systems are between large populations of neurons; neither grandmother cells nor pontifical modules exist in the brain. To my knowledge no neurophysiologist has ever proposed, nor does any of my acquaintance believe, that a single neuron or even a small group of neurons anywhere in the mammalian central nervous system is essential for any perceptual operation—absent scotomata produced by a local lesion in an afferent fiber track. Hundreds of neurons in a region of thalamus or cortex relevant for the perceptual operation under study can be destroyed, and the losses produce no obvious changes in the behavior under study. It is the population signal that counts, and the major objective of those using the method of single-neuron analysis has been from its inception to reconstruct population signals. This was initially possible only by retrospective reconstruction of the recordings of the activity of single neurons observed in sequence, and thus with the loss of a major aspect of the population signal, the temporal relation between the discharges of different neurons. This deficiency has now been remedied by the development of the multiple-microelectrode method, in which large numbers of neurons can be observed simultaneously.

The immunity of cerebral function from the loss of significant numbers of neurons in the systems relevant for a particular function is well known in clinical neurology and neuropsychology. It is only when the cell loss reaches some relatively significant proportion of the total that function in a system is degraded. How a certain level of function is maintained with declining numbers prior to that critical point is poorly understood. Moreover, we have no reliable method for detecting what more subtle changes in behavior may occur in humans or in experimental animals after the loss of even small numbers of cortical neurons, and this possibility cannot be dismissed.

The work of recent decades having implications for the problem of whether cortical perceptual systems converge to a highest-order integrating area has exposed a major principle in perceptual neuroscience. That is, the higher-order neuronal processing in perceptual operations in the neocortex is carried out in widely distributed systems, and the neural images of perceptual events are embedded in the dynamic ongoing activity within those systems: they converge nowhere. How then is such a dynamic pattern identified as depicting a particular perceptual event, and discriminated from other patterns evoked by other, perhaps competing, stimuli; and how do those dynamic patterns flow through to conscious awareness? I consider the first of these problems in Chapter 12 of this volume; the second is at least for the present beyond rational explanation. The transition from the information about the world provided by afferent sensory systems to the evaluation and storage of knowledge about the world is a primary function of the cerebral neocortex, a function that is greatly elaborated in hominids—especially in man—and that has been paralleled by an explosive increase in the size of man's cerebral cortex (see Chapter 2). Thus, the study of perception has always been seen as the initial step toward understanding the more complex functions of the brain, especially learning and memory.

Psychological Theories of Perception

It was Helmholtz more than any other scientist of the nineteenth century who placed knowledge of perception at the gateway to more general scientific knowledge. And it was Helmholtz who made the early formulation of what in its modern eclectic form I believe to be the dominant working hypothesis of perception in present-day neuroscience, *the neural-processing hypothesis of perception:* that is, that the perceptions we experience in everyday life are generated directly by patterns of activity in the perceptual systems of the brain, and particularly in their neocortical components. No intervening process of symbolization is deemed necessary or thought to exist.

The aim of neuroscientists is to discover the neural processes that discharge the behavior called perception. Perception is regarded as an emergent property of brain operations in large populations of neurons in the distributed systems of the neocortex. Emergent properties are not regarded as forever irreducible but as produced by some principles controlling the interaction between lower-level events in neural networks. Those principles are poorly understood. A significant corollary forms a major theme in present-day research, that the brain operations involved in perception can now be studied directly in human subjects, as well as in nonhuman primates.

The most famous—and the most controversial—of Helmholtz's ideas about perception is what he called "unconscious inference." He held, correctly I think, that generally we are unaware of the primary qualities of stimuli, like sound frequency *qua* frequency, or the individual patterns of activity in the several afferent channels innervating the hand that after central "integration" lead to perceptions of spatial form (stereognosis). And, I add, that we are equally unaware of the neuronal activity in the distributed perceptual systems of the neocortex that leads in a seemingly effortless transition to conscious perception. Helmholtz contended that this seamless flow is accomplished by referring the central displays of sensory stimuli to "mental constructs" of the world and events within it. These constructs are thought to be generated by past experience and to be stored in and readily recalled from memory. Perceptions are then thought to be produced by the comparison of recalled and evoked neural images, and perceptual identification inferred by the likeness between them, the simplest and most appropriate recalled construction winning the day. On this hypothesis, perhaps what we perceive are patterns of neural activity recalled from memory for the matching operation, rather than the activity evoked directly by sensory stimuli themselves! It will come as no surprise that direct neurophysiological evidence for the processes of unconscious inference has been hard to come by. This set of propositions includes as assumptions several of the major unsolved problems of neuroscience: how are experiences stored in and recalled from memory; how are neural populations matched and compared; how does the chosen match flow through to conscious experience, and so on. Nevertheless, the ideas of unconscious inference and matching identification remained themes in some later psychological theories of perception (Mackay, 1970).

Present-day theoretical formulations in experimental psychology are based in the first instance upon the general idea that perception is to be explained specifically in terms of peripheral and central neural processing. However, the theoretical stance of most practicing psychologists derives also from three major themes in the history of psychology (Rock, 1983). I believe that the dominant neural-processing theme derives from Helmholtz, greatly strengthened by the work of a host of psychologists and neuroscientists since that time. Helmholtz's concept of unconscious inference as a process for identification and categorization has fared less well, perhaps because it is neurologically vague and was never explicitly defined. Nevertheless, no experimentally based alternative hypothesis has been proposed to replace it.

The second is the theory of the gestalt psychologists (*Gestalt* = "configuration") (Koffka, 1935; Rock, 1986; Rock and Palmer, 1990), who more than any other group were concerned with the problem of perceptual organization: how is it that we effortlessly perceive a world in which parts or regions of the field are grouped together? The perceived whole is an emergent phenomenon, for the perceptual experience evoked by any other than the simplest scene is more than the sum of the sensations evoked by the individual stimuli within the scene. The gestaltists generated a number of laws they found to be important in perceptual organization. *Proximity* is the general rule that, other things being equal, elements grouped together will be perceived together. *Similarity* indicates that like objects will be perceived as parts of a whole, depending in part on proximity. *Good continuation* comes from the observation that two or more contours will be grouped together in the perceptual whole on the basis of a smooth continuation from one contour to another; perception requires connectedness. *Common fate* is the rule that the spatial relations between elements are unchanged during movement of the whole. Obviously these rules are important for the general figure-ground problem.

Gestalt psychology was generated by Wertheimer, Koffka, and Kohler, derived from earlier work of Ehrenfus. The gestalt laws have repeatedly been confirmed in laboratory settings; how universal they are in our normal perceptions of the natural world is uncertain. Other than the gestalt ideas of "simplicity" and "goodness" of the perceptual whole, no general underlying principles governing perceptual organization have been discovered with this approach. However, some of the gestalt laws have taken on added interest in view of recent discoveries in cortical neurophysiology that appear to provide a neurological base for them (Chapter 12).

The third theme is the stimulus or psychophysical theory, in the tradition that all the information necessary to account for our perceptual experiences is present in the environment, and that for each perception there is a unique combination of sensory information that accounts wholly for the perception (Gibson, 1966). It was just this direct correlation of subjective sensation with physical stimulus attributes that occupied Fechner and Stevens and all who followed them in the study of psychophysics.

The Rise of Psychophysics

At the time Helmholtz was studying the distal-proximal stimulus transition and formalizing his ideas about perception, Gustav Fechner of Leipzig made an important step in establishing psychology as an experimental science: he created psychophysics. Fechner conceived that the "mental" acts of perception could be measured in terms of quantitative measures of the stimuli that evoke them. Although Fechner was not the first to make quantitative measurements of sensory perceptions, the experimental and mathematical methods he developed for this purpose laid the groundwork for modern methods of measuring human sensory-perceptual performance (Fechner, 1966). Present-day versions of his designs allow measurement of the human capacity to detect and discriminate between stimuli and to classify them. Fechner's additional major contribution was to use statistical methods to analyze experimental results, and the mathematics of normal distributions used by him are one part of those used in modern decision theory and signal detection.

Fechner studied sensation magnitude in an indirect way by measuring the just noticeable differences (JNDs) between stimuli distributed along an intensive continuum. He formalized into a law Weber's contention that just noticeable differences in subjective sensations are related to a constant ratio of the stimulus intensity relative to the base stimulus, over a range of base stimulus intensities. It is now known that Weber's law holds only over the middle range of sensory intensity continua. Nevertheless Fechner assumed that all sensation JNDs are equal, and he integrated Weber's equation to obtain the general relation that sensation magnitude increases as a logarithmic function of stimulus magnitudes. While this law is incorrect, and all JNDs are not equal, the importance of Fechner's contribution is little diminished by that, for his general aim of showing that perceptual experiences could be quantified was important for a future experimental psychology. He devised several psychophysical methods still in use today, and his work inspired continuing efforts of several kinds, among them multidimensional scaling, in which attempts are made to infer perceptual distances between individual elements of complex stimuli. In the succeeding decades after 1860 and into the 1930s Fechner's law reached canonical status.

S. S. Stevens and his colleagues asked subjects to report directly upon the intensities of sensations by assigning numbers to them. The data obtained by Stevens and Galanter (1957) in studies of a dozen sensory continua showed that subjects did this reliably, and that the functions relating subjective magnitude estimations to stimulus intensities are power functions of the general form $S = kI^p + c$, where S is the numerical report of the sensation magnitudes evoked by the stimuli *I, k* is a constant, *p* is the slope parameter of the function plotted in double logarithm coordinates, and *c* the intercept. The exponent *p* varies for different sensory continua, from 0.33 for brightness to 3.5 for electrical shock to the finger (pain) (Stevens, 1957, 1959, 1960, 1961, 1970; Galanter, 1984). These results showed that sensations are phenomenally experienced and introspectable. The concept that equal stimulus ratios produce equal ratios of sensation magnitudes, originated in the studies of visual perception by Plateau (1872), was used to derive what is now usually called Stevens' law. Literally hundreds of papers have been published over the last fifty years providing support for either Fechner's or Stevens' laws, and many describe efforts to reconcile the two (Krueger, 1989; Norwich, 1993).

The psychophysical methods have been elaborated to provide accurate measurements of almost every perceptual experience human subjects describe. Many laws, frequently designated eponymously, have evolved that govern specific stimulus continua and the human perceptions of them. However, no comprehensive theoretical framework has appeared, no general theory with predictive value. Perhaps this is so because the central neural operations in different perceptual continua and different modalities differ too greatly to allow an encompassing generalization.

It has now been shown for a number of sensory continua that the value of the exponent *p* is set by the initial transduction and encoding phase at the peripheral interface, as witness the compressive effect of the retina that sets the low exponent for brightness. This initial transform is especially clear in the somatic afferent system, where the frequency of impulses in primary mechanoreceptive afferents is a power function of stimulus intensity, with an exponent identical to that characterizing the psychophysical relation for identical sets of stimuli. The exponent *p* differs for mechanoreceptive afferents innervating the hairy (0.5) and the glabrous (1.0) skin of the monkey's hand and arm, and these exponents are identical to those of the psychophysical functions for identical stimuli delivered at the same locations.

Observations such as these lead to the general hypothesis that the relations between the physical values of stimuli and our perceptions of them are set at the level of peripheral induction and encoding (Mountcastle, 1967). A comparison of the input, defined as the input in first-order fibers, with the subjective perceptual experience or a behavioral response reveals no nonlinear transformations, at least along a considerable range of stimulus intensities over which the functions relating the two are uniformly consistent. Central neural mechanisms follow their primary afferent drive with considerable fidelity.

The Development of Systems Neurophysiology

It is a major accomplishment of neurophysiology and biophysics that there now exists a sophisticated understanding of the mechanisms of nerve impulse conduction and synaptic transmission (Hodgkin, 1964; Eccles, 1964; Katz, 1969). Major research enterprises now under way are yielding detailed descriptions of the molecular mechanisms of these events. Descriptions of reflex actions produced in the Sherrington era have been extended by electrophysiological studies of the integrative mechanisms of neural circuits at the segmental levels of the nervous system. The study of the brain by electrophysiological methods, particularly of the sensory pathways and their related cerebral cortical areas, dominated systems neurophysiology in the period 1930–1960. These studies were generally made in anesthetized animals and were thus necessarily aimed at answering geographical questions—the *where* questions that occupied both clinical and experimental neuroscience for nearly a century (1870–1960). This period was marked by the union of neurophysiology and neuroanatomy; the methods and concepts of these two disciplines are now often embedded in a single investigator. Detailed descriptions of the topography of and connectivity within the brain were provided for both humans and nonhuman primates. These form the basis of advances made since 1960, and of those one can project for the decades ahead. The method of single-neuron analysis, applied intensively in anesthetized nonhuman primates, produced descriptions of the static properties of the neuronal elements of sensory systems and cerebral cortex. Static properties are those determined by the simple presence of neural connections, as contrasted to dynamic properties determined by the temporal patterns of impulse activity traversing those networks. These studies also produced evidence for some general theories about the macro- and micro-organization of the central nervous system, particularly of the cerebral cortex, described in later chapters. Little research of this period could be concerned with the questions that are now seen to be of central importance; e.g., the dynamic mechanisms by which information is represented, channeled, processed, stored, and accessed within the brain, and how that dynamic neural activity generates perceptual experience.

Perceptual Neuroscience: The Union of Systems Neurophysiology and Psychophysics

Traditionally, the study of the perceptual process and of the neural events evoked in brains by sensory stimuli were separate research programs carried out by different scientists working in different conceptual milieus. A major development of the last decades has been the union of these two disciplines. Simultaneous recording of the behavioral performance of humans or nonhuman primates and of the neural events in their brains by electrophysiological and imaging methods is now the dominant experimental approach to problems of the brain mechanisms in perception. An important first step was the demonstration that the psychophysical paradigm proven so useful in human studies could be adapted by operant conditioning methods to measure the sensory-perceptual-motor performance in nonhuman primates (Stebbins, 1970; Stebbins et al., 1984). The first result was the discovery that humans and nonhuman primates have identical sensory-perceptual capacities when measured over a wide range of stimulus continua in the somesthetic, auditory, and visual domains. The second was the demonstration that the electrical signs of the activity of central neurons could be recorded under stable conditions in waking monkeys. The method was first developed by Herbert Jasper and his colleagues (Jasper et al., 1959) for their studies of postulated mechanisms of closure in the Pavlovian conditioning paradigm. It was soon elaborated with elegance by the late Edward Evarts (Evarts, 1966) for his studies of the motor cortex. This led to the combined experiment described below, which is now the most productive research method in perceptual neuroscience.

Parallel developments had long been under way in the study of human subjects working in sensory-perceptual tasks while electroencephalographic recordings of brain activity were made simultaneously. Later this evolved into the use of evoked and event-related potentials for studies in humans of the perceptual performance and changes in the location of brain activity. These have now been greatly elaborated with the use of new methods of EEG recording and analysis (see Chapter 12) and with a variety of imaging methods for specifying which areas of the brain are selectively activated as human subjects work in sensory-perceptual, motor, or cognitive tasks.

The Combined Experiment in Primates

The experimental method indicated briefly above has become so dominant in studies of the brain mechanisms in perception it warrants further description. Monkeys are most commonly used, although the method has been adapted for rodents and carnivores as well. Animal subjects are trained by operant conditioning methods to emit a particular item of behavior hundreds of times per day. The behaviors studied in this way have included the execution of skilled movements, sensory detections and discriminations, more complex perceptual tasks like the direction of attention, and those involving cognitive tasks such as learning and memory. In effect, any behavior a monkey can be trained to emit can be studied in this way. The behavioral variables of attention and set can be brought under control and manipulated at will. Simultaneously, recordings are made of the electrical signs of the activity of neurons within the brain, and consistent correlations are sought between the two sets of variables observed. Strength for causality beyond simple correlation is evidenced by the consistency of the relation under a variety of conditions, knowledge of the structure and connectivity of the region under study, and the behavioral defects that follow its removal. The use of single microelectrodes has now been followed by several methods for multiple microelectrode recording (Mountcastle et al., 1991) and techniques for their chronic implantation. The experiment can be repeated daily for several weeks. This experimental combination of psychophysical and neurophysiological methods has now become the most widely used and successful experimental paradigm in studies of brain physiology, and particularly in studies of perception. It has yielded information about the initial "representation" of sensory events in primary sensory areas of the neocortex, and how those neural images are transformed further in widely distributed cerebral systems, within which the sensory inflow is multiply represented, and how these higher-order representations can be modulated by changing behavioral contingencies. On the output side, similar descriptions have been made of the neural events that precede and continue during the execution of skilled movements, at least for those brain regions "close" to the output portals. It is clear that the union between neurophysiology and psychophysics has been accomplished, and that it opens for study any class of behavior that can be identified and measured.

The Philosophical Position in Perceptual Neuroscience

Immersed in the problems and impedimenta of his laboratory studies, the perceptual neuroscientist may pursue his research objectives unconcerned with whether or not they have philosophical implications. This agnostic stance has much to recommend it and is strongly urged by many neuroscientists (e.g., Jung, 1984). This is uncommonly good advice. Nevertheless, in the midst of his everyday studies almost every student of brain function is from time to time confronted with these issues.

It is my own belief that no form of dualism will do, whether in classical Cartesian or more recent formulations. The idea that a non-material essence exists that interacts with, controls, or is controlled by the brain is so unlikely as to be outside the realm of scientific discourse. The death of dualism puts a heavy responsibility on those engaged in the study of the brain and how it generates behavior. And it evokes in every neuroscientist a compelling sense of modesty, for he understands how far we are from solving these difficult problems at the level of scientific realism.

The form of physicalism most attractive to neuroscientists is emergent materialism, that form described with elegance and precision by Mario Bunge (Bunge, 1980; Bunge and Artila, 1987). The central idea is that the properties of a system like the brain are emergent and are to be understood in terms of its constituent elements and their couplings. System properties are not the result of summing identical properties over the elements of a population; rather, they emerge from the dynamic and multiplicative interactions between elements of the system that yield new properties not possessed by any single item of the system. On this monistic theme every mental process *is* a brain process, but mind and brain are not identical; the former is an emergent property of the latter. A central concept of emergent materialism is that the brain is not a machine, and above all not like a digital computer: it is a biological system with its own evolutionary and ontogenetic histories and is endowed with properties and laws peculiar to living things, some unique to brains. In Bunge's (1980, p. 219) own words:

Moreover emergent materialism is the only philosophy that enjoys support from all the sciences, has not been concocted *ad hoc* for the mind-body problem, does not promote quixotic reductionism, and defends neuroscience and psychology against obstruction by obsolete and barren philosophy and ideologies. By so doing it defends the freedom and creativity of man: neither machine to be programmed nor pigeon to be conditioned at will, but the only absolutely creative animal, and one capable of creating a science of the mental and of shaping his own life—for better or worse—in the light of his knowledge and prejudice.

While all mental states are brain states, the reverse is not true. Only the *results* of the perceptual operations within our brains that flow through to conscious perception may be considered *mental* states. It is perhaps fortunate that we are unaware of the massive neuronal operations that intervene between the initial representations of peripherally transduced events and our conscious awareness of them; we escape system overload! Yet it is certain that we will achieve little understanding of the brain mechanisms of consciousness itself without a deeper knowledge of preconscious events. A century of research in experimental psychology and psychophysics has yielded detailed descriptions of human perceptual capacities and analyses of these capacities in terms of hypothetical processes thought to produce them. Valuable as they are, these descriptions and speculations offer no solution to what are now the central problems: the brain operations themselves. Their study is the task of perceptual neuroscience. Their solutions will lead to the central problem of brain science, consciousness itself, a problem that is often posed, discussed, and written about voluminously, but one that remains distant from direct empirical study. The questions are easy to put: how are we consciously aware of certain brain states and not others; how does one set of neuronal systems observe and interpret—be aware of—activity in others? These are twenty-first-century questions, and neuroscientists must face them directly, as Crick and Koch have done in their theoretical essays (Crick and Koch, 1990a,b; Koch and Crick, 1994). However, I believe it unlikely, but of course unpredictable, that a new discovery will suddenly reveal to us how brains are conscious. We may hope by successive approximations to come nearer the truth and successively narrow the field of the unknown, which in this area, in the absence of scientific explanations, is susceptible to the hobgoblins of mysticism, of liaison brains, of extrasensory events, and of every other charade of the human imagination. This position is derided in some quarters as promissory materialism. I embrace it.

What we can study in an elegant fashion, in both humans and in nonhuman primates, are those many aspects and levels of intracerebral processing that intervene between the initial cortical display of sensory events and the flow through to conscious awareness. Moreover, a particularly rich line of study will be of the interfaces between the preconscious processing of input and the equally complex, high-level machinery that produces the complex patterns of efferent activity leading to movement, to action.

In sum, the welding concepts of neuroscience are these:

- The fusion of acquired and rational knowledge

- A monistic view of the mind-brain problem, embodied in emergent materialism

- Mechanistic vs. mentalistic concepts of perception and of consciousness

- The use of objective methods in the study of brain and behavior

The neuroscientist has a responsibility not to leave these philosophical problems wholly to the imaginative ratiocinations of those innocent of knowledge of the structure and function of the brain.

Prospects

I have followed several general principles in considering the function of the neocortex in perception; they will be apparent in the following chapters. Perhaps the most important is that internal representations of material reality exists in the brain, and that those representations lie at the heart of the mechanisms of mind. What we call representations are instantiated in dynamic patterns of activity in large populations of central neurons, particularly in those of the distributed systems of the neocortex. This dynamic activity is set in motion by sensory stimuli (and sometimes triggered by internal events), successively transformed through interconnected populations of neurons, complexed against stored information, contributing to and conditioned by those neural locales and activities concerned with set or affect. These neural activities themselves lead to and are in fact the essence of the private act of perception and, at will, its verbal description. Both private and public happenings result from the same chain of neural events. They are now studied directly during controlled perceptual behavior in nonhuman primates. No gulf exists between what were traditionally called sensations (and described in neural terms) and what is a perception (and traditionally described in psychological terms). The inferred dichotomy is a continuum in neural space: *perceptual events are neural events*. Further studies of these phenomena will require recording the activity of large numbers of cortical neurons via numbers of chronically implanted microelectrodes, as well as new methods for data analysis and guiding models and theory.

The sequence of events that leads from willing to moving is a poorly understood aspect of brain function. The motivation to act, the fulfilling of intention, the choice of one movement from alternatives, the regulation of movement during its execution—all these seemingly effortless achievements of everyday life still evade full understanding. Significant advances have been made in the last two decades in knowledge of the cerebral control of movement, from the level of its inception in the neocortex to that of its execution at the motoneurons (Evarts et al., 1984; Georgopoulos, 1991, 1995; Georgopoulos and Pellizer, 1995; Georgopoulos et al., 1993; Porter and Lemon, 1993). These discoveries, combined now with new theoretical concepts and experimental methods, provide a base for further rapid accumulation of knowledge of the brain mechanisms, particularly those of the neocortex, that initiate and control movement. The initiation of movement is an externally experienced act of will; it is one aspect of the mind-brain relation that will eventually be studied directly.

It is for this reason that I combine in a forthcoming volume the subjects of somesthesis and the sensory-motor interface. I do so because the somatic afferent system is powerfully linked to the motor system. This is true at all levels, and the interface at the level of the distributed systems of the neocortex now becomes the subject of focused interest.

For both perception and the willing of movement, we are unaware of the complex and spatially extended cerebral and particularly neocortical operations that intervene between a decision to act and the movement itself, or between a sensory stimulus and our conscious perception of it. It is possible that by pursuing study of these mechanisms inward from the sensory areas, and "backward" from the primary motor areas, we may close in on what lies in between, the brain mechanisms of consciousness itself. This may lie in the distant future, a goal that will be reached after many intermittently recursive corrective movements in neuroscience research.

The Phylogenetic Development of the Cerebral Cortex

This chapter contains an account of the phylogenetic development of the cerebral cortex, with special reference to the evolution of the neocortex (isocortex) in hominids. It is followed by chapters in which I treat general aspects of the structure and function of the neocortex. My specific aim in this group of chapters is to provide a factual base for considerations in a later volume of the neocortical mechanisms in the many varieties of somesthetic experience. My more general aim is to determine what these fields of enquiry can contribute to our understanding of the function of the neocortex.

The neocortices of extant mammals have several properties in common: all possess six layers, all display a modular organization, the constituent neuronal phenotypes of all differ only in detail, and all use widely overlapping sets of synaptic transmitter agents and receptors. Even the smallest of those studied possesses the primary visual, auditory, and somatic sensory areas—and most a motor field as well. Extant mammals of the several radiations elaborate greatly increased areas of neocortex not only by enlarging primary fields but by generating many new areas. The number of identifiable cortical areas varies from 10 to 20 in mammals with the smallest cortices, to perhaps 100 in humans. Living mammals display different combinations of derived and primitive cortical characteristics, and none represents any particular extinct ancestor. It is reasonable to suggest that the enlarging neocortex in ancient and now extinct mammals—e.g., in early hominids—possessed some characteristics we now recognize in living mammals: six layers, modular organization, primary sensory and motor areas, and congeries of other cortical fields differing between taxa, with different patterns of connectivity (Northcutt and Kaas, 1995).

A pervasive aspect of vertebrate phylogeny is the differential increase in brain weight or volume in relation to body weight. Changes in mammals are most marked in primates, and particularly in the hominoid/hominid line leading to man. (See Martin, 1990, for an authoritative monograph on primate evolution.) The brain-body relation has been studied for more than a century by measuring these two variables in living mammals and by measuring the volume of the cranial endocasts of extinct species. Body weights are calculated from evidence in the fossil record, such as lengths of long bones.

The Allometric Equation, Brain-Body Relation, and Encephalization Indices

A regular relation between the growths of brain and body for a series of animals is described by the allometric equation suggested long ago by Snell (1891) and used by many since then. Thus,

$$E = cP^a$$

or, by logarithmic transformation to a linear equation,

$$\log E = \log c + a \log P,$$

where E = brain weight, P = body weight, a is the slope of the line fitted to the data (e.g., the major axis), and c is the intercept of that line at 1 on the y axis. Many early studies indicated that the exponent a is about 2/3, a value predicted by the simple enlargement of a spherical object, without a major change in three-dimensional form between smaller and larger brains. Recent studies in many mammalian species show, however, that the true exponent is about 3/4 (Martin, 1982; Martin and Harvey, 1985; Hofman, 1982; for reviews see Hofman, 1989; Pirlot, 1987). This relation is shown in Fig. 2-1, taken from the analyses of Hofman (1982). The line is the best-fitted major axis for the relation of brain weights to body weights for 249 mammalian species; the values for each set of variables were nor-

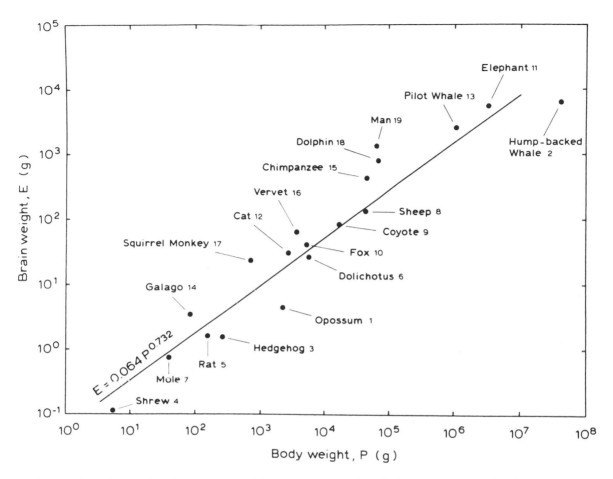

Fig. 2-1 Brain weights as functions of body weights; logarithmic scales. The line is fitted to the data for a set of 249 mammalian species. The numbers refer to a table not shown. (From Hofman, 1982.)

mally distributed. However, the slope of this line varies between taxa, all of which are grouped for the graph as shown here. The slope is 0.58 for pongids and 0.57 for Old World monkeys (Holloway, 1982). The constant $c = 0.064$ is the "average for all mammals." When calculated separately for individual species, c has often been taken as one index of encephalization for that species, where encephalization is defined as that proportion of brain size not determined directly by body size (Jerison, 1991). MacPhail (1982), e.g., calculated an encephalization index as the ratio of c for a given species to the average c

The Phylogenetic Development of the Cerebral Cortex

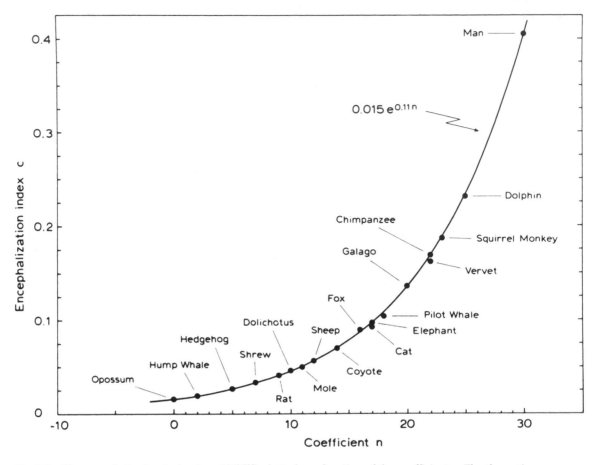

Fig. 2-2   The encephalization index ($c = E/P^{0.732}$) plotted as a function of the coefficient *n*. The theoretic curve $c = 0.015e^{0.11n}$ fits the calculated encephalization indices almost perfectly. (From Hofman, 1982.)

for all mammals. This index varied from 0.4 for the rabbit to 7.44 for man.

The values for the constant *c* form a regular sequence described by the following relation (Hofman, 1982):

$$c = 0.015e^{0.11n}$$

where *n* is taken as a positive integer. Fig. 2-2 shows the range of values for this index in several mammalian species; clearly, this function is a close fit to the calculated values of *c* and the coefficient *n* for those species. The graph illustrates that a rapid encephalization has

The Phylogenetic Development of the Cerebral Cortex

occurred in primates. The measurements shown do not imply a direct line of descent, however, for a salient feature of evolution is its parallel and radiating nature. It is unlikely that any living mammalian species has evolved from any other species still extant.

These differences in the progression indices for different cerebral structures between living species hint that similar differences may have existed between extinct species with different brain sizes. While this is likely, it is unprovable, for the only direct data available for extinct species are intracranial volumes obtained from natural or constructed endocasts of fossil crania; the gross geometry of the brains obtained from those endocasts; and surface markings on endocasts that suggest the location of sulci and gyri. *A widely accepted generalization is that a comparative series of living mammals is not equivalent to an evolutional series of extinct mammals.*

The Enlargement of the Brain in Mammalian Phylogeny Is Produced by an Increase in the Cerebral Cortex

The contribution of the cortex to increase in brain size is suggested by inspection of the brains of a series of mammals like that shown in Fig. 2-3. Fig. 2-4 shows the relation between increasing cortical volume and brain volume. The slope of the fitted major axis is slightly above 1. The order of neurogenesis of different structures in nervous systems is conserved over a wide range in mammals. Peak neurogenesis is shortest for cranial motor nuclei and lengthens from brain stem to thalamic to cortical structures. This pattern correlates with the disproportionate increase in the size of late-generated structures like the cerebral cortex. Finlay and Darlington (1995) found in a meta-analysis of published data that about 96 percent of the total variance in the sizes of individual brain structures in mammals can be accounted for by the single factor of brain size, rather than body size, per se.

Stephan and his colleagues sought a quantitative measure of the enlargement of different brain parts in phylogeny. They assumed that living basal insectivores have evolved very little from their ancestral insectivores (but see above), from which man's line also arose. They used this idea of a "living fossil" to establish an index of phyletic enlargement of different brain structures, for which they studied the brains of many species and made measurements of all major brain parts (Stephan et al., 1988, 1991). The progression index of Stephan is the ratio of a brain structure in a prosimian or simian to

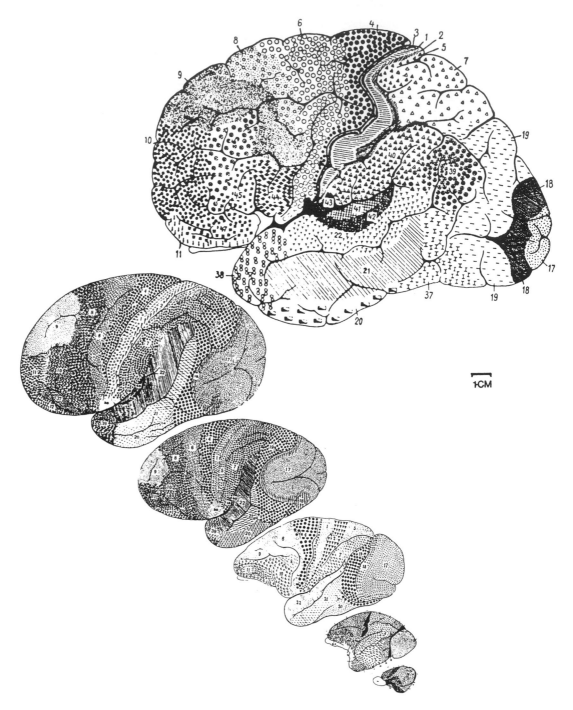

1CM

Fig. 2-3 Cytoarchitectural studies of the lateral surfaces of the cerebral cortices of a series of primates and an insectivore, arranged by E. G. Jones in descending order of size by reference to the magnifications given by each of the authors in their original papers. At the top is the map for man, by Brodmann (1912); the sequence from above left to below right, in order: orangutan, gibbon, and macaque (Mauss, 1910), then lemur and an insectivore (Brodmann, 1914).

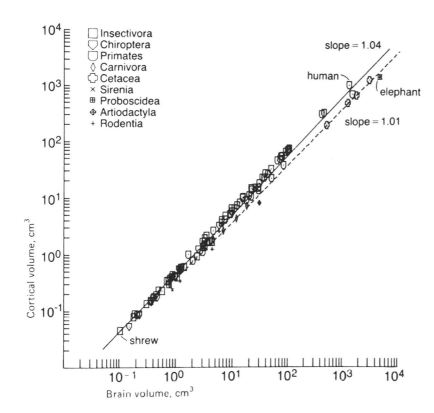

Fig. 2-4 Cortical volume as a function of total brain volume, for a large number of mammals. The slope of the regression line (solid) is 1.04 ± 0.01. The dashed line of slope 1.01 is the result of a best-fit computer simulation of cortical volume. (From Prothero and Sundsten, 1984.)

the volume of that structure to be expected in a basal insectivore of equal body weight. The indices for man are: neocortex, 140–150 (it is 80 for chimpanzee and 40 for monkey); cerebellum, 20; basal ganglia, 14–16. All other brain structures are progressive at lower ratios except the olfactory structures, which are regressive in man.

Cortical Enlargement in Large-Brained Animals Is Produced by an Increase in Cortical Surface Area

The cortical thickness increases modestly over a wide range of animals; from mouse to man the slope of the regression of cortical thickness on brain volume is 0.10–0.20 (Prothero and Sundsten, 1984; Hofman, 1985b). Increase in the size of the cortex in brains without gyri or sulci (lissencephalic) is accounted for by a geometric expansion coupled with the small increase in thickness. Fig. 2-5 shows that

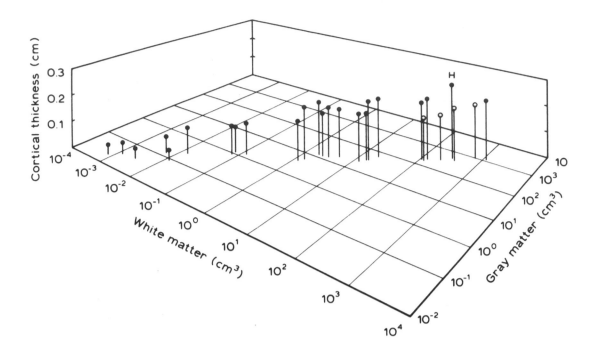

Fig. 2-5 The multivariate distribution of cortical gray and white matter, and mean cortical thickness. The cortex of whales and dolphins (O) is thin relative to the cortical volume. H = *H. sapiens.* The thickness of the cortex changes virtually not at all for volumes above about 3 cm³, and is then asymptotic at about 0.25 cm. (From Hofman, 1989.)

for brain volumes greater than about 3 cm³, thickness reaches an average value of 0.25–0.28 cm. Further increases in cortical volume are accomplished by a nongeometric increase in surface area, absent a radical change in shape. Over the range of animals from mouse to man there is no significant change in the number of neurons beneath any surface unit of the cortex (Rockel et al., 1980; Hendry et al., 1987; Jones, 1990a); what changes is the cellular packing density, which decreases as thickness increases, with an elaboration of the neuropil. The almost linear increase in cortical surface as a function of brain volume is shown by the graph of Fig. 2-6 (Prothero and Sundsten, 1984). The result is folding and gyrification, which I consider in a following section. With further increases in brain size, particularly in the hominids, the rate of increase in the volume of the white matter of the cerebral hemisphere exceeds that of the gray matter (Frahm et al., 1982). This is presumably due to an increase in cortical connectivity and/or an increase in the proportion of myelinated to unmyelinated fibers, for the diameter of myelinated fibers in the corpus callosum does not change from mouse to monkey (Jerison, 1991).

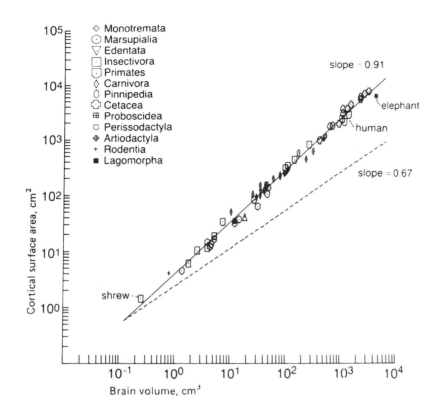

Fig. 2-6 Total cortical surface area shown as a function of total brain volume; logarithmic plot, for 13 orders of mammals. The slope of the fitted regression line is 0.91, which contrasts with the slope of the dashed line, 0.67, predicted by the two-thirds relation. Larger brains are also more convoluted than are smaller brains. The inference is that folding allows an increase in surface area beyond that predicted by the symmetrical expansion of a sphere. (From Prothero and Sundsten, 1984.)

The Cortical Surface Has Increased by the Addition of Ontogenetic Units: The Elaboration of New Cortical Areas

The cerebral cortex is constructed in mammalian ontogeny by the formation of elementary ontogenetic units. These are generated by small sets of progenitor cells of the neural epithelium, the proliferative units of Rakic. Each ontogenetic unit, or *minicolumn,* is produced by the iterative generative action in a proliferative unit (a polyclone) in the neuroepithelium (Chapter 8). The ontogenetic unit is a chain of about 80–100 neurons that extends across layers II–VI of the neocortex. All the major neural cell phenotypes of the mature cortex are present in each minicolumn.

The *cortical column* is the common operating unit in the mature cerebral cortex. It is formed by the union of many adjacent ontogenetic units, bound together by common extrinsic connections and by intense vertical and horizontal intrinsic connections. Its neurons have in common a set of static and dynamic functional properties upon which others are superimposed. The binding of minicolumns into the larger functional columns results from both cell-autonomous and secondary factors controlling the sequence of gene expression. Column size varies only from 300 to 500 μm in diameter between species whose brains differ in volume by nearly three factors of 10. Chapter 7 contains detailed descriptions of and supporting evidence for columnar organization.

The importance of the mechanism of cortical histogenesis pertains to the question, upon what source of variability did evolution operate selectively to yield the enlargement of the cortex observed in mammalian phylogeny? Such a variation could be produced by uniform accumulation of ontogenetic units (Hofman, 1985a; Rakic, 1990b), the result of a uniform increase in the number of symmetric divisions of cells in the germinal epithelium during the proliferative phase that precedes migration. An accumulation of units would produce a uniform and undifferentiated increase in the volume and surface area of the cortex. It appears likely that beyond such a general effect, mutation in one or another local zone of the neuroepithelium could lead to a larger number of ontogenetic units in the topographically related zone of the postmigratory cortex. Simultaneously with the increase in the number of ontogenetic units and the cortical surface in speciation, new cortical areas appeared in new species. These almost certainly resulted from the interaction between increasing numbers of ontogenetic units as well as other factors operating in the temporal sequencing of cortical histogenesis in the postmigratory period; e.g., the elaboration and differentiation of afferent corticipetal systems, the influence of background neural activity, a differential control of cell death, etc. (these subjects are considered in Chapter 9). Whether these changes could have accumulated on the classic idea of phyletic trend and led to speciation, or whether they occurred as more rapid events interspersed in a state of evolutionary equilibrium, is discussed in a following section.

Enlargement of the Cortical Surface Led to the Formation of Fissures and Gyri

The nearly linear relation between total cortical surface and brain volume predicated fissurization of the cortical surface of large brains. A radical change in shape did not occur. It is obvious that in its enlargement in primates, and especially in hominids, the brain was constrained to fit a cranial cavity of a size and form that could be balanced upon and carried lightly on the upper end of the spinal column, in the erect, bipedal position. The flexion of the neuraxis in hominids influenced the relative position of major brain parts— e.g., the brain stem, thalamus, and cerebellum—but appears to have had little effect upon the details of the gyral/sulcal patterns of the cerebral cortex. Cortical folding in large-brained mammals is the result of factors intrinsic to the developing cortex and is not due to extrinsic mechanical constraints. Fissurization begins shortly after neuronal migration is complete, in humans at the start of the third trimester of intrauterine life, and reaches its final pattern several months after birth. Fissurization occurs before the cranial sutures are closed.

The gross form of the brain, independently of gyral formation, is influenced by the nearly simultaneous development of other cranial structures, such as the orbits. However, those structures do not in their development produce or influence significantly the patterns of gyral and sulcal formation. Highly convoluted brains display more and more novel cortical areas, and more complex patterns of connectivity, than do less convoluted ones. It is a long-standing dogma in neurobiology that animals with large, highly convoluted brains are more complex than are those with smaller, less convoluted brains. Particularly, the former are regarded as more intelligent and behaviorally and perceptually more sophisticated than the latter. Thus, it is important to know how gyrification comes about and whether the degree of convolutedness per se is of functional significance beyond its importance in allowing for more cortex; whether convoluted or not, it is the volume/area of cortex that counts! Welker has provided a scholarly review of this complex subject (Welker, 1990).

Models of Fissurization

Several models of the folding process have been described. Hofman (1985b, 1989) proposed a multivariate scaling model, taking into account cortical volume, surface area, and thickness. The model, for total surface S_t and outer surface S_o, is as follows:

$$S_t = 1/d \, V_g$$
$$S_o = a(1/d \, V_g^3)^{1/4}$$

where d = cortical thickness and V_g is the volume of the cortical gray matter and a is a constant. Analyses using this model showed that increased cortical thickness led to a reduction in fissure formation, whereas decreased thickness yielded an increase. The latter is the case for the thin cortex of cetaceans. The ratio S_t/S_o is the fissurization index, FI, which is obviously 1 for lissencephalic brains and which ranges over terrestrial mammals up to 2.83 for man. Zilles et al. (1989) proposed a similar index (2.56 for man) and showed that in anthropoids it co-varies with neocortical volume. A geometric model described by Todd (1982) indicated that sulci form along lines parallel to the minimal cortical curvature, on the assumption of uniform cortical growth.

Prothero and Sundsten (1984) present a scaling model, illustrated in Fig. 2-7. They varied values for cortical thickness and the height, length, and width of gyri over a wide range of values in iterative simulations, and obtained reasonable fits to empirical data. Explorations of the extremes of variant values led to the conclusion that the enlargement of the convoluted brains of terrestrial mammals is self-limiting, for as size increases so does fissure formation, along with small increases in cortical thickness and gyral width. In the limit, when gyral width equals twice cortical thickness, gyri are completely closed to axonal access, for the gyral windows disappear. The limiting value on brain size in their simulations was about 10 kg, but the optimal range of brain sizes with open gyral windows was in the range of 1.5–4 kg. The brain of the elephant (4–6 kg) is a bit beyond that optimal range.

The major gyri, like the postcentral, the precentral, and other primary gyri, appear in characteristic patterns in orders, families, and species; they may compose heritable patterns (Welker, 1990). The lesser gyri and sulci are far less constant and may even defy identification in highly convoluted brains. There are many examples of brains in which sulci mark the borders between cortical areas defined by both cytoarchitectural and functional criteria; for example, the central sulcus, that in every convoluted primate brain examined, marks the transition from the somatic sensory cortical areas behind it to the motor areas in front. Such precise correlations have been established only for the heterotypical sensory and motor areas (Rademacher et al., 1993), and many cases are known in which gyri and sulci do not uniquely identify functional areas in the homotypical cortex. The latter occupies about 95 percent of the neocortex of man. A

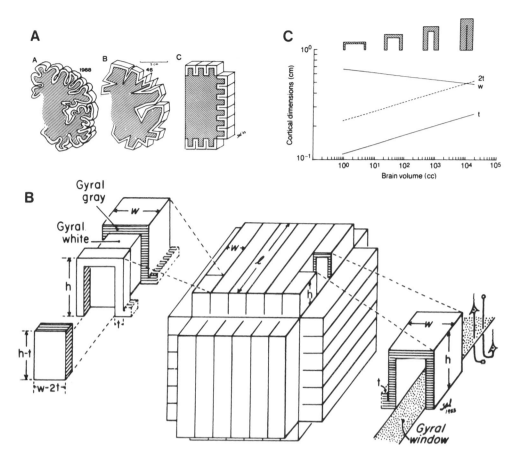

Fig. 2-7 The model of cortical folding suggested by Prothero and Sundsten. (A) Diagrams showing the resolution A–B–C of the cortical surface of a slab of brain to an idealized model. (B) The full model. A gyrus is defined by length *(l)*, width *(w)*, height *(h)*, and cortical thickness *(t)*. A gyral window is shown in dots; it is the area through which fibers leaving and entering the cortex must pass. (C) The maximum brain size permitted by this model: since gyral width decreases and cortical thickness does not decrease with increases in brain size, there is a hypothetical brain size at which the gyral windows close, as shown by the crossing points of the lines for width *(w)* and twice thickness *(2t)*, in (C). The brain of the elephant approaches this limiting size. (From Prothero and Sundsten, 1984.)

The Phylogenetic Development of the Cerebral Cortex

31

major question remains to be answered: are gyri functional entities in highly convoluted brains? My own conjecture is that this is true only in certain special circumstances.

Evolution of the Cortex in Hominids

Enlargement of the brain, the adoption of the bipedal posture and mode of locomotion, the development of manual skills, the invention of a useful technology, the acquisition of spoken language, and the development and generational transmission of culture are all features that appeared in the evolution of hominids. Paleoneurology has as a major aim to discover what correlations exist between the appearance and development of these features and changes in the volume and systematic organization of the brain, including, especially in the present context, the neocortex. The data base upon which to construct these correlations and, if possible, causal relations is thin at best and questionable in some respects. The primary data are endocranial volumes obtained from fossil crania that have been dated and identified by species. Intact fossil crania are rare, the number available for any given species is small, variability between crania within a species is high, and species identification is always difficult and sometimes uncertain. External brain geometry can be observed in naturally formed endocasts or in those prepared from empty crania. Patterns of sulci and gyri can sometimes be seen on the surfaces of endocasts; they are copies of the impressions made in life upon the inner surface of the skull. However, these markings are most clear in immature forms, much less certain in adults, and frequently faint or absent altogether. A persisting problem in paleoanthropology has been greatly eased by the development of accurate "molecular clocks." A half-dozen such clocks are in use; they vary in the times over which they are most accurate—from the radiocarbon method, for times up to 30–40,000 years, to the uranium series and K/Ar isotope methods, appropriate on the scale of millions of years. The best of these methods appear to have coefficients of variation of no more than 1–2 percent, but for some it exceeds 10; thus for the latter the confidence intervals are broad, and the range of error in determining the age of any given fossil may be considerable. Given these uncertainties, it is a tribute to the tenacity and insight of the relatively small group of paleoanthropologists that they have been

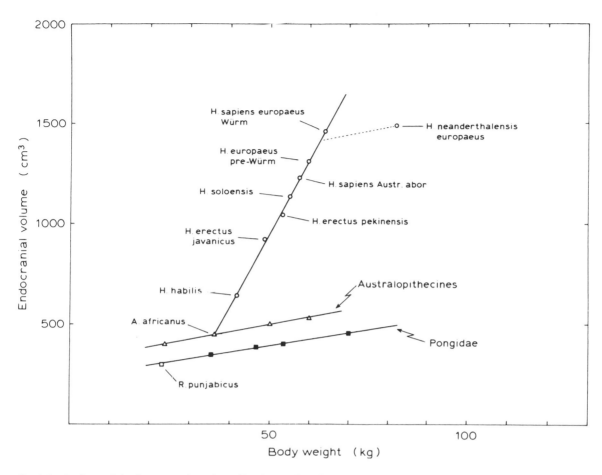

Fig. 2-8 Endocranial volume as a function of body weight, plotted on a linear scale to emphasize the remarkable expansion of brain size in the genus *Homo*. (From Hofman, 1983.)

able to establish a train of events in hominid brain evolution that can be accepted with some degree of confidence.

The double-logarithmic plot of Fig. 2-1 tends to obscure by compression the enlargement of the brain in hominid evolution in the last 3–4 M.Y., which is illustrated by the linear plot of Fig. 2-8 and pictorially in Fig. 2-9. This change is thought to have begun 5–7 million years ago (M.Y.A.), with the separation of the hominid and pongid lines from a common hominoid ancestor. This event occurred toward the end of the period from 22 M.Y.A. onward in which primates prolif-

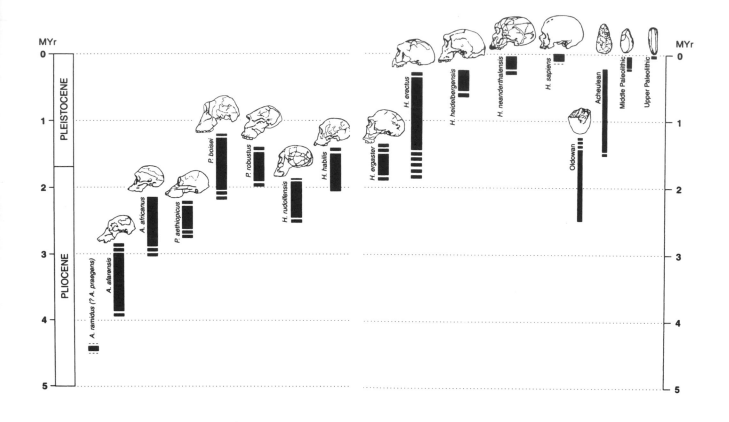

Fig. 2-9 A pictorial display of the skulls of human ancestors, from *Australopithecus ramidus* at 4.5 M.Y.A. to modern *Homo sapiens.* Solid black lines indicate time of existence; the breaks, uncertainty over dates. To the right the names and times of the various associated tool cultures are indicated. (From Tattersall, 1995.)

erated, including those of the genus *Dryopithecus,* who spread over much of Africa and Eurasia. The dryopithecines are the leading candidates for the common ancestor of the hominids and pongids, but much uncertainty surrounds this designation (Simons, 1981; Tobias, 1982).

Recent studies of marine sediments indicate that the climate of Africa varied greatly from 2.8 M.Y.A. onward, concurrently with the onset of glacial cycles in the northern hemisphere (deMenocal et al., 1995). The east African climate trended toward aridity and coolness, and away from that of humid tropical forests. These major changes during the Pliocene-Pleistocene period, combined with geographic

The Phylogenetic Development of the Cerebral Cortex

conditions, were conducive to the success of arid-adapted species and, it is surmised, to the evolution of the hominid line.

Raymond Dart discovered in South Africa (Dart, 1925) a fossil of what is now recognized as one of the earliest hominids, *Australopithecus africanus*. Fossils of related species, *A. afarensis*, were later discovered in Tanzania and Ethiopia and dated in the range of 3.9–3.0 M.Y.A. (Johansen and White, 1979; Kimbel et al., 1994). Two gracile and two robust species of the genus *Australopithecus* have been identified and more than 500 fossils of individuals discovered, providing one of the richest fossil records of any ancient genus. The brain of the *A. afarensis*, at approximately 425 grams, and that of *A. africanus*, at approximately 475 g, are of the same order of size as the brains of extant pongids, but these ancient australopithecines possessed several distinctly hominid characteristics. A recent version of the australopithecine-hominid ancestral tree is shown in Fig. 2-9 (Tattersall, 1995). Some uncertainty still remains concerning which australopithecine stands at the root of the ancestral tree (White et al., 1981). Fossil evidence of two morphologically more primitive and more ancient bipedal hominids has recently been discovered in Africa: *A. ramidus* (4.3–4.5 M.Y.A.) in Ethiopia (White et al., 1994), and *A. anamensis* in Kenya (3.9–4.2 M.Y.A.) by M. G. Leakey et al. (1995). How these four are related to each other is still uncertain; hominid evolutionary trees remain provisional, subject to change as the fossil record accumulates.

A prominent hominid characteristic was the further development of the bipedal posture and mode of locomotion, illustrated dramatically in the sets of australopithecine footprints petrified in volcanic ash at Laetoli in northern Tanzania, discovered by M. Leakey. These were dated to about 3.5 M.Y.A., and thus presumably of *A. afarensis* (Leakey and Hay, 1979; Leakey, 1981) (Fig. 2-10). This primary hominid characteristic met the need for food by foraging over a wide range required by the thinning of the forests to a quasi-open savanna that began in east Africa after 10 M.Y.A. Bipedal locomotion required a major change in body function, and its necessary motor control was achieved without a parallel change in the gross form or size of the brain. Such a radical adaptation must have been enabled by changes in the dynamic operating characteristics of the brain systems controlling movement, the massively interconnected systems of cerebellum, brain stem, basal ganglia, and neocortex, changes of course now beyond study. The change to the form of bipedal progression charac-

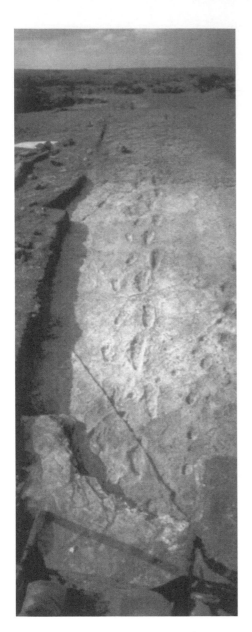

teristic of *Homo* must have occurred gradually. For example, high-resolution computed tomographic studies of the labyrinths of fossil crania reveal that it is *H. erectus* who first possessed a labyrinthine morphology resembling that of modern humans. The labyrinth of the australopithecines resembles that of the extant great apes (Spoor et al., 1994). This suggests that the bipedal mode of the australopithecines was a primitive one, perhaps combined with a form of arboreal climbing.

The second distinctly hominid characteristic is that the australopithecine brain, as revealed by endocasts, shows an enlargement in the inferior frontal lobe, prominent developments of the dorsal frontal and the parietal lobes, and some suggestion of hemispheric asymmetry, all more characteristic of hominid than of pongid brains. A major result of bipedalism was a freeing of the hand for manipulation. Increasing manipulative skills and accuracy in throwing were undoubtedly accompanied or enabled by development of the sensory and motor systems innervating the arm and hand, especially the somatic sensory and motor areas of the neocortex. The postcranial skeleton shows some hominid characteristics, particularly in the adaptation of the iliac and the innominate bones for weight transmission in the erect posture, though these changes differ from both the *H. sapiens* and the pongid patterns (Ashton, 1981). There is only limited evidence that the australopithecines used tools, for no stone tool culture has been found in their places and dated to their time. In sum, one can conjecture that, even without a major increment in brain size, significant organizational changes occurred in the brain and particularly the cerebral cortices of the australopithecines, concomitantly with their increased use of the bipedal posture and mode of progression and the use of the hand (Holloway, 1983).

An equally dramatic step was the cladistic split in the australopithecines that occurred about 2.0–2.5 M.Y.A. (Tobias, 1983). One evolving branch led to species with larger bodies and thus slightly

Fig. 2-10 The trails of hominid footprints discovered by Mary Leakey at Laetoli, Tanzania, in 1978. The trails, which were preserved in volcanic ash, have been uncovered for a distance of 80 feet, and 70 footprints cleared. They are dated to about 3.5 M.Y.A., and thus were most probably made by *A. afarensis*. The footprints in the main trail were made by two individuals, the second treading in the prints made by the first. The smaller footprints in the trail just to the left were made by a much smaller individual, perhaps a child. The trail curving off to the right was made by an ancient horse. (From Leakey, M.G., 1981.)

Table 2-1. A timetable of human ancestors, with brain sizes and some other characteristics (modified from Stebbins, 1982).

Species or genus	Time of appearance (years ago)	Time of disappearance (years ago)	Cranial capacity (cm^3)	Other characteristics
Homo sapiens				
Modern	100,000–30,000	Still living	Male: 1434 Female: 1325	Magdalenian, Aurignacian cultures
Neanderthal	200,000–100,000	30,000	1470	Mousterian culture; early rites and ceremonies
Archaic	300,000	200,000	1300	Late Acheulian culture
H. erectus (? *ergaster*)	1.3 million	400,000 (?–30,000)	900–1200	Acheulian culture; first use of fire
H. habilis	2.0–2.5 million	1.6 million	650–700	Oldovan culture; first use of chipped stone tools
Australopithecus robustus	1.8–1.7 million	?	?	walked erect; no known tools; ? vegetarian; probably not ancestral
A. africanus	3.5–2.5 million	2 million	475	walked erect; probably ancestral
A. afarensis	3.9–3.4 million	2.5 million	425	walked erect; probably ancestral
A. anamensis	4.2–3.9 million	?	?	
A. ramidus	4.5–4.3 million	?	?	
Ramapithecus	14 million	10 million	?	
Dryopithecus	22 million	12 million	?	

larger brains, *A. boisei* and *A. robustus.* These are sometimes given generic status as *Paranthropus boisei* and *P. robustus;* they are thought to have existed simultaneously with the australopithecines and overlapped the appearance of *H. habilis* and *H. erectus,* but they trended to extinction 1.6–1.2 M.Y.A., for reasons still uncertain (Klein, 1988). The line of development shown in Fig. 2-9 led to genus *Homo,* and through the successive stages of *H. habilis* and *H. erectus* to early *H. sapiens* (see Table 2-1). It remains uncertain whether these three evolved in succession by phyletic trend or whether they represent the successful branches of cladistic events. It was *H. habilis* who displayed most certainly the behavioral and morphological features characteristic of hominids. He made habitual the bipedal posture and mode of locomotion in standing, walking, and running, with the associated adaptive modification of the postcranial skeleton for weight bearing in the upright position. *H. habilis* shows structural modifications of the upper limb and hand to accomplish the manipulative skills revealed in his manufacture and use of chipped stone tools. Susman (1994) showed that *H. habilis* is the most ancient hominid to have developed the expanded first metacarpal head characteristic of hands capable of the precision grip. The *habilis* brain at about 650 g was enlarged 45 percent over that of the australopithecines and possessed several hominid characteristics: prominent enlargement of the dorsal frontal and parietal lobes of the neocortex, with increased transverse dimensions; signs of hemispheric asymmetry; enlargement of the inferior frontal lobe, an area presumed to be homologous to Broca's area in the human brain; and a prominence in the inferior parietal lobule, an area presumed to be homologous to Wernicke's area in the human brain. The brain of *H. habilis* shows what are interpreted by some as the external signs of the cerebral machinery for language, and Tobias (1987, 1991) has concluded he was the first obligate speaker in the hominid line. However, recent evidence indicates that Broca's area—in hominids that possess it—is concerned with a high level of motor programming and control, particularly the temporal sequence of movements of the hand and arm, as well as—in man—control of the motor apparatus for speech. Thus, the presence of a "Broca's cap" cannot, by itself, be taken as direct evidence of the possession of language. If *H. habilis* did possess a rudimentary language, his verbal capacity must have been very limited, for he lacked the low larynx and shape of the oral cavity characteristic of hominids with verbal skills. Others have argued that the acquisition of language was a much later event in hominid evolution, even so recently as about 40,000 years ago, with the appearance of modern *H. sapiens* (Noble and Davidson, 1991). No measurements of volume and form of the brain reveal anything about possible internal rearrangements of connectivity, or changes in dynamic operating characteristics within the cerebral cortex that would be required for the increasingly sophisticated motor capacities of tool making and speaking.

H. habilis is the least well documented of the fossil hominids. Apparently he persisted in his African homeland for half a million years. Then there appears in the fossil record a new species with an enlarged brain, *H. erectus,* dated in Africa from 1.5–1.8 M.Y.A.; he thus may have overlapped *H. habilis* as the latter trended to extinction. Knowledge of *H. erectus* has been greatly expanded since the discovery in 1984 of what is most unusual among all fossils, a nearly complete skeleton of a juvenile, male *H. erectus* (now placed by some in a separate species as *H. ergaster*), near Lake Turkana, Kenya (Brown et al., 1985). This fossil was studied intensively for nearly a decade by its discoverers, A. Walker and R. Leakey, who then summarized their results in a general monograph (1993). The brain weighed about 900 grams and showed clear surface protuberances in the putative Broca and Wernicke areas only in the left hemisphere. Together with other signs of hemispheric asymmetry, these features suggest that this *Homo* was right-handed. The calculated height at maturity is over 6 feet, and body weight 68 kg. The postcranial skeleton of long, thin limbs is a characteristic adaptation to hot, dry climates by the modern men who live in them. An encephalization quotient calculated by Jerison's equation is 4.48 (for modern *H. sapiens* it is 7). Somewhat later, *H. erectus* developed a sophisticated stone tool culture, the Acheulian tools, greatly advanced over those of *H. habilis*. We may conjecture that this was accompanied by a further elaboration of the sensory and motor systems of the brain controlling a hand of increased dexterity, including aimed throwing.

Fossils now classified as *H. erectus* have been identified widely over the Eurasian continent, from Europe to India, China, and Java. These fossils show a wide variation in cranial volume, with brain weights ranging up to the 1040–1200 g of the brain of Peking man, but all are classified in the single species of *H. erectus*. The fossils of *H. erectus* found outside of Africa were originally dated to less than 1 M.Y.A. Thus, it was long accepted among paleoanthropologists that *H. erectus* evolved in and then migrated from Africa to colonize the Eurasian continent. A mystery remained: no sign of the Acheulian stone tool culture developed by *H. erectus* in Africa has ever been found with *H. erectus* fossils in Eurasia. This generally accepted "out of Africa" migration hypothesis has now been questioned by new dating studies of the *H. erectus* fossils discovered in Java decades ago. Swisher et al. (1994) have used an accurate isotope dating method (^{40}Ar–^{39}Ar) to show that the Java fossils are about 1.8 M.Y. old. The question is now open whether *H. erectus* migrated out of Africa long before hitherto supposed, and before he developed the Acheulian tools, or indeed whether he evolved separately in Africa and Asia, perhaps from a

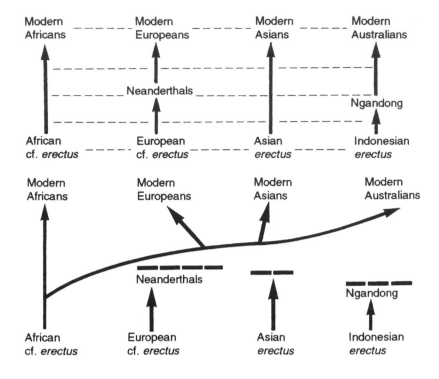

Fig. 2-11 Outlines of two ideas concerning the origin of modern humans, the multiregional hypothesis *(top)* and the "out of Africa" hypothesis *(below).* The dashed lines in the multiregional model indicate an assumed gene flow between regions, thus preventing speciation. (From Stringer and Gamble, 1993.)

common precursor (Fig. 2-11). Some evidence supporting this last conjecture has come from recent discoveries in Longgopo cave, Sichuan province, China. Wanpo et al. (1995) show from newly discovered fossils that the first hominid to arrive in Asia was a species other than *H. erectus,* and that this more primitive *Homo* possessed a stone tool technology. This pre-*erectus* hominid in China is dated to 1.9 M.Y.A. He provides an antecedent for the evolution of *H. erectus* within Asia.

There followed the transition from *H. erectus* to *H. sapiens* through the stages indicated in Table 2-1 (Stebbins, 1982), leading through archaic to modern man—who appeared as recently as 100–30,000 years ago. A recent redating of the *H. erectus* skulls found in Java indicate that he may have persisted until so recently as 27–53 thousand years ago, and thus lived contemporaneously with *H. sapiens* in southeast Asia (Swisher et al., 1996). *H. sapiens neanderthalensis* is now usually regarded as a subspecies who appeared in Europe and the Middle East about 100,000 years ago, and persisted until about 30,000 years ago. Modern man and the Neanderthals must have co-

The Phylogenetic Development of the Cerebral Cortex

existed for several thousands of years; neither is regarded as the predecessor or descendant of the other. The cultural and social advances of *H. sapiens* (see Marshack, 1985) have been achieved without changes in brain size, for the volume and external morphology of the brain of *H. sapiens* have remained almost unchanged through the transition from archaic to modern man.

There is considerable variation in brain sizes in normal adult humans, as shown in Table 2-2, taken from the recent studies of Filipek et al. (1994), made with a 3D magnetic resonance imaging scanning technique. It is not known whether these differences are due to differences in neuron or glial cell numbers, cell sizes, elaborations of the neuropil, etc. What is clear is that there is no well-established causal or even correlative relation between individual brain sizes in mod-

Table 2-2. Volume (in cm^3) of the principal structures of the human brain, determined by magnetic resonance imaging of 10 male and 10 female young adults (from Filapek et al., 1994). SD = standard deviation; CV = coefficient of variation.

Structure	Mean±SD	CV (%)	Min	Max	% Total
Whole brain	1380.1±113.9	8.3	1173.3	1625.6	100.0
Total cerebrum	1192.1±102.5	8.6	1007.5	1403.5	86.4[a]
Neocortex	688.8±65.0	9.4	573.7	828.5	57.8
White matter	443.8±42.4	9.6	376.2	515.8	37.2
Caudate	9.5±1.3	13.8	7.3	11.7	0.8
Lenticulate	14.1±1.1	8.6	11.9	16.6	1.2
Putamen	10.1±0.9	8.4	8.7	1.4	0.9
Pallidum	3.9±0.5	12.6	3.1	5.2	0.3
Hippocampus	9.9±1.2	12.4	7.2	11.5	0.8
Amygdala	5.5±0.8	13.9	4.0	7.0	0.5
Central gray nuclei	20.5±1.7	8.3	18.1	24.1	1.7
Total Cerebellum	143.4±12.5	8.7	123.8	175.1	10.4[a]
Cortex	119.7±10.6	8.8	102.9	146.3	83.5
Central mass	23.7±2.9	12.5	19.1	29.6	16.5
Ventricular system	21.3±7.4	34.7	10.3	36.4	1.5[a]
Lateral	18.1±7.3	39.9	7.3	33.7	85.0
Third	1.3±0.5	36.9	0.3	2.2	6.1
Fourth	1.9±0.6	32.4	1.0	3.6	8.9
Brainstem	23.4±3.1	13.1	19.5	32.3	1.7[a]

a. Percentage of total expressed as proportion of whole brain volume. Other substructures are expressed as proportion of total cerebrum, cerebellum, or ventricular system, respectively.

ern men and their degrees of intellectual or artistic achievement—given at least a size within the normal range. Several widely quoted cases of individuals with very large brains and great achievements are matched by equal numbers of individuals of equally great achievement and modestly sized brains. There is no reliable evidence for differences in brain sizes between the several races of modern man (Tobias, 1981a,b). It would be possible with modern imaging methods to seek for long-term correlations between brain size, determined intermittently throughout life, and life accomplishments.

Whether the *erectus-sapiens* transition occurred in Africa and was followed by a (second) worldwide outward migration displacing all regionally evolving hominids (the replacement hypothesis) or whether *H. sapiens* evolved separately in different parts of the world (the regional hypothesis) is a subject of intense study and debate (cf. Wilson and Cann, 1992; Thorne and Wolpoff, 1992; Wolpoff et al., 1984; see Fig. 2-11). The results of the first mitochondrial studies were interpreted to support the replacement hypothesis (Cann et al., 1987). The idea has been strengthened by the recent mtDNA sequencing results of Horai et al. (1995), which indicate that the last common ancestors of African and non-African humans lived about 150,000 years ago. The results of a new method of genetic absolute dating, based upon the stepwise mutation model, also indicate that the deepest split in human phylogeny occurred between African and non-African populations, also about 150,000 years ago (Goldstein et al., 1995). Matrix correlation tests (Waddle, 1994) are interpreted to support a single origin of modern man from either Africa or the Levant, and recent studies of the genetic variations in modern humans yielded similar results (Bowcock et al., 1994). Ayala (1995) has recently reviewed new molecular evidence obtained in analyses of DNA polymorphisms in a number of worldwide populations. The evidence invalidates the "mitochondrial Eve" hypothesis, but does favor a recent African origin of modern humans. Studies of nuclear DNA variability strongly support the "second out of Africa" hypothesis: that anatomically modern man evolved in and then migrated out of East Africa about 100–300,000 thousand years ago (Tishkoff et al., 1996). There remains, however, an incompatibility between these new observations and the fossil record (see Smith and Spencer, 1984; Mellers and Stringer, 1989; and the review by Spuhler, 1988). Many of these latter authorities read the evidence to indicate that *H. sapiens* originated by regional transitions from regional populations of *H.*

erectus, and not by a worldwide migration from any single place. Those who support the multiregional model cite as evidence a fossil continuity in different global regions in the transition from *H. erectus* to archaic humans to modern man. The replacement hypothesis requires that a population of *H. sapiens* immigrated from Africa to flood the world and replaced all then-evolving hominids without mixing; i.e., he was a separate species and did not breed with any hominids encountered. While this is certainly possible and is strongly supported by the nuclear DNA evidence (Stringer et al., 1984), it appears to others to be unlikely (Wolpolf, 1989).

The incompatibility between many of the dating findings and the fossil record remains unresolved. For example, an early *H. sapiens* skull unearthed in China a decade ago has been reliably dated to more than 200,000 years ago, as early as any discovered in Africa. This finding lends some support to the regional continuity model of the evolution of *H. sapiens* (Tiemei et al., 1994).

It is important to emphasize that the several races of man share the large majority of both their nuclear and mitochondrial gene pools. It is clear that in these evolutionary transitions there appeared the powerful and mutually positive interactions between cultural and social evolution, behavior, and brain structure. One aspect of human behavior in all cultures is the capacity to interpret the behavior of self and others in terms of mental states, such as desires and beliefs. This "theory of mind" is regarded by some as a recent event in the evolution of *Homo,* to have occurred within the last 2–3 million years (Povinelli and Preuss, 1995). The ability to regulate behavior through the use of representations of the mental states of others and oneself is attributed by some to the differential enlargement of the homotypical cortex in *Homo,* particularly of the frontal lobe, but little is known beyond this familiar generalization.

Phyletic Trend or Punctuated Equilibrium?

The generally accepted theory of evolution is based upon a model of gradual evolutionary change caused by changes in gene frequency in a population. When these changes lead to behavior that achieves excessive reproductive success, they are favored by natural selection, are incorporated in the gene pool, and lead to new species formation even in an actively breeding population with free gene flow. A second model, called "punctuated equilibrium," was proposed by Eldredge and Gould in 1972 (see also Eldredge and Tattersall, 1975; Stanley, 1979). It is surmised on this model that long periods of evolutionary stasis or equilibrium are from time to time interrupted by rapid genetic changes (rapid, i.e., on the geologic time scale; e.g., a few thousand years) leading to speciation. These changes are thought to occur when a cohort of the population is isolated geographically from its parent population, in a new environment, thus breaking gene flow with that parent and rewarding genetic change of adaptive value. The changes are thought to be in gene regulation and rearrangement and are overall neutral as regards "progression"; many are maladaptive and do not survive.

Punctuated equilibrium suggests that some long-term trends are due to the success of some particular species and not others, and not or not only to the slow progress of adaptation within a continually evolving population. Stanley (1975) designated this process as "species selection," an operation of Darwinian natural selection at the level of species. This model has been vigorously defended by its authors, Gould and Eldredge (1977, 1993). They say: "The record of human evolution seems to provide a particularly good example (i.e., of punctuated equilibrium): no gradualism has been detected within any hominid taxon, and many are long-ranging; the trend to larger brains arises from differential success of essentially static taxa." The model has been just as vigorously criticized (Cronin et al., 1981), and certainly some gradualism can be seen in the increases in brain size in *H. erectus*. In the opinion of Wilson (1992, pp. 88–89), however, the swift evolution subsumed under the punctuation hypothesis differs only semantically from macroevolution, which is simply the most rapid rate of evolution on the continuum from micro- to macroevolution, and is fully accommodated in neo-Darwinian theory.

The two models make different predictions for the fossil record. Phyletic gradualism predicts that with a perfect fossil record intermediary forms in the evolutionary trend will eventually be found. Only a few have been discovered to the present time (Simons, 1981), but the australopithecine line is becoming more crowded. Punctuated equilibrium, contrarily, predicts that fossil gaps are real, represent prolonged periods of evolutionary stasis, and should be treated as data.

The meteoric increase in brain volume and of the cerebral cortex in hominid evolution, described above, occurred in what are assumed to be speciations from: the australopithecines to *H. habilis* (+45 percent increment in brain volume); from *H. habilis* to *H. erectus* (+46 percent); and from *H. erectus* to archaic *H. sapiens* (+51 percent) (Tobias, 1987; Hofman, 1983), with the caveat that this may not have been a direct progression. Holloway (1995) has emphasized that the doubling in size of the brain from *H. habilis* to *H. sapiens* occurred after three major reorganizations had occurred in the brains of earlier hominids. These were: (1) a change from the pongid pattern of minimal cerebral asymmetries to the human pattern of increasingly greater left-right asymmetries; (2) a reorganization of the third inferior frontal convolution, leading to a "Broca's cap"; (3) a relative reduction in the size of the primary visual cortex (area 17), and an increase in the relative size of the posterior parietal cortical areas.

The subsequent evolution of archaic *H. sapiens* to modern man has apparently occurred without further increase in brain volume, although nothing can be said regarding whether changes in connectivity patterns and/or changes in modes of dynamic operation might have occurred and been of adaptive value. During this period in the late evolution of man, culture was certainly a major driving force in evolving human behavior, and cultural changes have proceeded without change in brain size. The major transitions from the australopithecines through to *H. sapiens* suggest to some the punctuated mode. However, other scholars in the field take the view that hominid evolution fits neither the model of punctuation nor that of phyletic trend perfectly; they say it is best regarded as consisting of gradual change interspersed with varying rates of more rapid evolution (Holloway, 1983; McHenry, 1982, 1994; Tobias, 1990). Indeed, the marked variation in brain size in fossils now classified as *H. erectus,* as well as evidence that ranges from the postcranial skeleton to the fossil signs of culture and behavior, have led some to suggest that the species boundary between *H. erectus* and *H. sapiens* should be abandoned in favor of a slow phyletic trend without further speciation within the genus *Homo.*

What predictions do these different hypotheses make about the evolutionary development of the brain? Neither makes any prediction whatsoever about the neocortex; indeed it appears clear that the transitions from archaic to modern *H. sapiens,* with its attendant revolutions in behavior, technology, and culture, took place *without significant change in brain size or, it is assumed, in relative volume or area of neocortex.* It is difficult to imagine, however, that these evolutionary developments could have occurred without accompanying changes in *brain function*. The inference is that these necessary changes were in dynamic operating characteristics, or even in system organization and connectivity, changes that took place without changes in overall brain size, external geometry, gyral patterns, or relative size of the neocortex. Holloway has summarized the evidence that a very strong natural selection existed in the evolution of the genus *Homo* for successful communicative behavior (Holloway, 1993, 1995). This is thought to have led to a reorganization of the distributed connectivity of both the parietal and frontal lobes, with a tripling in brain size from the late australopithecines to modern man. The changes are inferred to be an increase in the connectivity in the homotypical cortex for sensorimotor integration, particularly in the inferior parietal lobule, and for the simultaneous processing of inputs from several sensory systems, which laid the foundation for neural circuits involved in language perception, a late acquisition in hominid evolution. These changes are thought to have been accomplished by a strong evolutionary advantage for visuospatial skills such as tool using and throwing with accuracy and force.

I wish to emphasize two points. First, allometric studies such as those described are of great value in tracking the phylogenetic development of the brain and the cerebral cortex. Jerison (1991), for example, has shown by a multivariate factor analysis the efficiency of brain size as a statistic for estimating the size of brain parts, olfactory bulbs excepted. Second, the results obtained in such studies are of limited scope, for they deal with volumes, weights, surface areas, and in some cases external morphology. Such studies do not reveal other major changes that have taken place in brain evolution; e.g., the development of hemispheric asymmetry, reorganization of and the appearance of new intracerebral connectivity patterns, the appearance of specialized cortical areas, such as those inferred from the theory of Holloway, described above. While there is some evidence, reviewed in a following chapter, that the major neuronal phenotypes have not changed remarkably in size and form over the range of mammals, no similar statement can be made as regards dynamic synaptic and neuronal circuit operations. Little is known about the similarities or differences between different cortices for the dynamic network processing of neural activity.

Confidence in volume as a measure of progression in cortical development is based upon the rule of columnar similarity. There is evidence that this rule holds over many mammalian species for cell types and numbers, but less certainly for intracolumnar connectivity. There is no evidence one way or the other concerning dynamic intracolumnar operations. Volume increases alone may seriously underestimate increasing complexity in brains and particularly in intracortical operations, where it is likely that the emergent properties of ensembles of neurons contribute heavily to increases in brain complexity (Bullock, 1993). The possibility that these operating modes may differ between different locations in the same neocortex, and between the cortices of different mammalian species, cannot be dismissed out of hand. It is unknown whether changes in these cortical attributes occurred and were of selective advantage in the evolution from archaic to modern *H. sapiens*. Deacon (1990) has proposed that a competitive displacement of some neural connections by others during ontogenesis and postnatal secondary histogenesis may explain the differential enlargement of the neocortex in the evolution of the human brain. It is important to emphasize, as Holloway has done (Holloway, 1983), that brain size per se is not an item acted upon by natural selection, which rather operates upon the behavioral capacities associated with large brains. It is my own conclusion that the brain mechanisms enabling those behavioral capacities are not revealed by brain size alone. How all these factors may have interacted in evolution is suggested by Holloway's 1983 model, shown in Fig. 2-12.

Summary

A salient feature of vertebrate and especially mammalian evolution is the increase in the size of the brain. The relation between brain weight and body weight is adequately described by the allometric equation, a power function with an exponent of about 0.75. Encephalization is measured as that portion of brain not required for direct somatic functions. It is described by the index c in the allometric equation, where $E = cP^a$: E = brain weight, P = body weight, a is the power exponent and thus the slope of the major axis fitted to the log-transformed data, and c is the intercept of that axis at 1 on the y axis. When fitted for different taxa, the encephalization index varies from less than 1 for rodents to more than 7 for man.

The enlargement of the brain in mammalian evolution is largely due to enlargement of the cerebral cortex, produced by the addition of numbers of ontogenetic units. Increments in cortical size are pro-

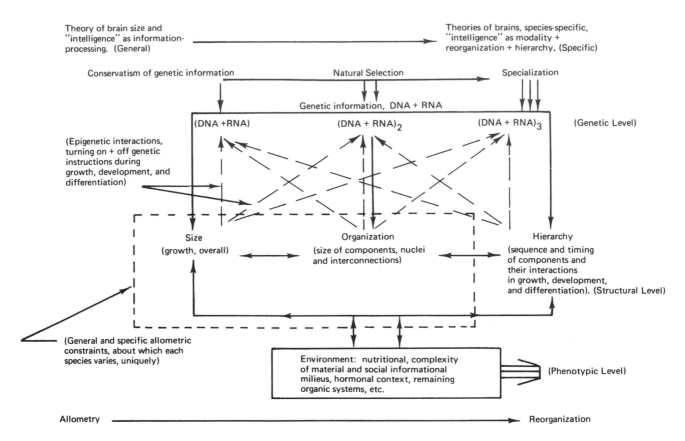

Fig. 2-12 Outline of a general model proposed by Holloway to illustrate that brain size alone cannot account for species-specific modes of behavior, nor for unique evolutionary histories like that which led to *H. sapiens*. The model explicitly states that the final phenotype is the complexed result of the interaction between structural and regulatory genes, so that natural selection may operate upon at least three levels of genetic information. (From Holloway, 1983.)

duced by increases in its surface area, with only minimal increases in thickness. Absent any radical changes in brain shape, the increase in surface area led inevitably to the formation of gyri and sulci, a process produced by mechanisms intrinsic to the cortex itself and not to surrounding structures.

Large, highly convoluted brains possess more new and novel brain areas, and have more complex patterns of connectivity, than do smaller brains. Larger brains generate and govern more complex patterns of behavior, and mammals possessing them are more intelligent and behaviorally and perceptually more sophisticated than are mammals with smaller brains. It is cortical area per se and not the degree or pattern of gyrification that varies with this increased capacity for complex behavior.

The genus *Homo* arose from its australopithecine ancestors about 3.5 M.Y.A., after an earlier split between the latter and the line that led to modern pongids from a common ancestor. The evolutionary trail—so far as it can be established in the midst of much uncertainty—led thereafter through *H. habilis* (650 g brain weight) and *H. erectus* (950+ g brain weight). A major uncertainty surrounds the subsequent evolution from ancient to modern *H. sapiens* (1370 g brain weight). One hypothesis supposes that those steps occurred first and only in Africa, and that modern *H. sapiens* migrated out of Africa less than 200,000 years ago and replaced all the evolving lines over the entire world, without gene flow to the populations encountered but with acquisition of their cultures, leaving no trace of his own African origin. The alternative idea is that there occurred regional evolutions of *H. erectus* to *H. sapiens,* with sufficient gene flow to prevent regional speciations, and that these regional evolutions led to the modern races of man. Although these matters remain unsettled, what is certain is that there are no significant differences in brain size or structure between the ancient and modern *H. sapiens,* or between the modern races of man.

The distinctive features of the brain of *Homo* evolved after he appeared on the African scene about 3 M.Y.A.—a blink in evolutionary time, during which his brain has tripled in size. This phase of *Homo* brain evolution is thought to have occurred in a feedback relation with the development of hand skills and the appearance of social structures like family and group. The brain of modern *H. sapiens* has not changed size during the last 50–100,000 years. Yet in that time he has progressed from a cave-dwelling scavenger to the font of modern cultural and technological achievement—to civilization. When man's evolution is viewed in the context of brain size only, the suggestion is that this has occurred through the mutually reenforcing feedback loops between social and civilizing factors and human behavior. It is possible, however, that in that time important changes occurred within a constant brain size and unchanging external morphology—changes in the dynamic operating characteristics that had major adaptive advantages. Unfortunately this attractive hypothesis is, I believe, untestable.

Cells and Local Networks of the Neocortex

An understanding of the cortical mechanisms in sensation and perception requires knowledge of the morphology of the cortical neurons, of the intrinsic microcircuits that link them together, and of the ways these circuits are arranged on a larger metric in columnar and cytoarchitectural organizations. Cortical neurons differ in shape, in the pattern of their extended neurites, and in their internal biochemical mechanisms, transmitter agents, axonal targets, etc. I provide here a description of the several generally recognized classes of cortical neurons and a brief review of intrinsic neocortical connectivity. This general subject is further elaborated in Chapter 7, on columnar organization, and in Chapter 11, on dynamic operations. A description of cortical architecture is given in Chapter 4.

A major theme of this and the following chapter is that a degree of uniformity obtains in the midst of diversity. *Uniformity* is imposed by the ontogenetic development of the cortex (Chapters 8 and 9) and is shown in the mature cortex by several characteristics. Neurons within major cell classes are generally similar, and there is a uniform distribution of cell numbers and major cell types in all neocortical areas in all mammals studied. The striate cortex of primates has more than twice the number of neurons beneath any unit surface than do other cortical areas, but that number is constant for the striate cortices of all primates studied. The intrinsic cortical circuits—so far as they are known—are generally similar from one area to another, though some areal specializations occur. Cortical *diversity* is shown by equally cogent facts. Cortical areas differ in their patterns of extrinsic connections. There are clearly defined cytoarchitectural differences between cortical areas. Variations in cell form and the distribution of dendrites and axons occur between subpopulations within each major class. Biochemical mechanisms differ between those populations. Different cortical areas are specialized for different processing operations, which are thought to be determined largely by differences in the sources and targets of the extrinsic afferent and efferent connections of cortical areas. The uniformity of cell types and numbers suggests some degree of uniformity of intrinsic operation in different areas of the neocortex. The nature of that operation is unknown, but recent discoveries indicate that synaptic transmission is similar in different neocortical areas (Chapter 5). It is likely that local neural network operations, when they are discovered, will display a basic similarity, upon which areal and dynamic specializations will be superimposed. Some cortical areas have unique properties, which may depend upon the interaction between columnar structure and the horizontal connections that link columns together (Gilbert, 1992). It is likely that modulatory systems afferent to the cortex can change the operations of the intrinsic circuits rapidly, in an unchanging anatomical connectivity, and that those changes could differ from one area to another and from time to time in any one area in a fraction of a second. This critical problem remains unsolved.

Every major advance in knowledge of cortical neuronal cytology has depended upon new experimental methods. The history of the field and summaries of many aspects of cortical structure and function are described in a series of multiauthored volumes edited by Peters and Jones (1984–1994). A major contribution was made by Camillo Golgi in the 1880s, who showed that single neurons could be impregnated with a silver stain that (mysteriously) selects only a few of the many neurons in thick sections of the cortex. The stain penetrates the cell completely in optimal preparations, revealing the form of the cell body and dendrites, the ramifications of the dendritic tree, and the direction but rarely the target or mode of axonal termination. Santiago Ramón y Cajal, who exploited the Golgi method over several decades after Golgi, described the varieties of neurons in the cerebral cortices of several mammals and established the cytological basis for one of the major dogmata of neuroscience, the neuron theory. (DeFelipe and Jones, 1988a, have translated Cajal's writings on the cerebral cortex from Spanish to English.)

The era of Golgi cytology reached an apogee in the work of Lorente de No, who summarized his discoveries in 1938. It was he who first described the synaptic linkage into vertical chains of neurons extending across the cellular layers, or laminae, of the cortex in a direction normal to the pial surface. Lorente's anatomical studies could not reveal to him that these chains are not continuously overlapping in the horizontal dimension, as he supposed, but are arranged in disjunctive groups that we now know are the operating units of the neocortex, the cortical columns (Mountcastle, 1978; see Chapter 7).

Cortical Neurons Can Be Classified by Several Defining Characteristics

Cajal classified cortical neurons by the form of the cell body; by the length of the axon; and by the extent and spatial distribution of the dendritic trees. The morphology of cortical neurons is best revealed by intracellular injection of markers that are transported throughout the cell and visualized in histological preparations. (See Fig. 3-1.) Cell form is frequently used for classification together with other criteria: the laminar position of the cell body; the axonal target; the type of synaptic terminals and thus the direction of trans-synaptic action; the presence or absence of dendritic spines; differences in transmitter molecules, synaptically active polypeptides, calcium-binding pro-

Fig. 3-1 The principal types of nonpyramidal cells in the sensory and motor areas of monkeys, drawn from Golgi stains. (A) arcade cells; (B) double bouquet cells; (C) small basket cell; (D) chandelier cells; (E) "peptide cells"; (F) spiny nonpyramidal cell, an excitatory interneuron of layer IV; (G) neurogliaform; (H) large basket cells. The dark rectangles to the right locate the zones of termination of specific thalamocortical afferents. (From Jones, 1975.)

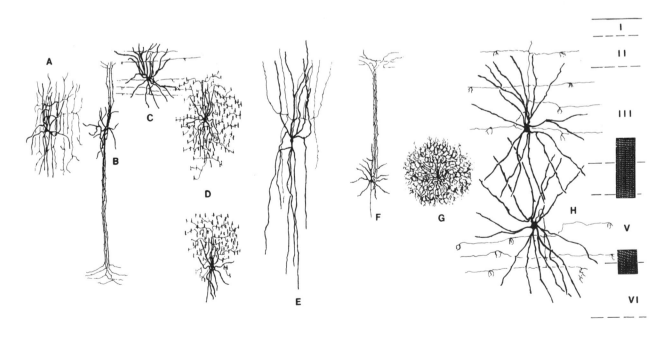

Cells and Local Networks of the Neocortex

Table 3-1. Properties of some classes of neocortical neurons.

Cell Type	Transmitter	Terminal Type	Peptides	Targets
Spiny pyramidal	Glutamate	Asymmetric Excitatory	None	Extracortical structures Intrinsic, recurrent to all cell types
Spiny nonpyramidal	Glutamate	Asymmetric Excitatory	None	Intrinsic Pyramidal and nonpyramidal
Large and small basket cells	Gamma-aminobutyric acid	Symmetric Inhibitory	None	Intrinsic Pyramidal cell somata
Double bouquet cells	Gamma-aminobutyric acid	Symmetric Inhibitory	Substance P Somatostatin	Intrinsic Pyramidal cell spines Nonpyramidal cells
Chandelier cells	Gamma-aminobutyric acid	Symmetric Inhibitory	Corticotrophin releasing factor	Intrinsic Pyramidal cells (initial segments)
Large peptide cells ("bipolar")	Gamma-aminobutyric acid	Symmetric Inhibitory	Cholecystokinin Vasoactive intestinal peptide Neuropeptide Y Somatostatin Tackykinins	Intrinsic all cell types
Neurogliaform	Gamma-aminobutyric acid	Symmetric Inhibitory	Cholecystokinin Vasoactive intestinal peptide Neuropeptide Y Somatostatin Tackykinins	Intrinsic Spiny nonpyramidal cells

teins, and membrane-bound receptor molecules; and differences in biophysical properties (Amitai and Connors, 1995). The classes of cortical cells most commonly recognized are described in Table 3-1, but the reader should note that authorities in this field use several different classification schemes.

Two main types of synapses occur, differentiated mainly on the basis of postsynaptic densities. Asymmetrical, excitatory synapses make up about 75–80 percent of intracortical synapses. They are derived from spiny pyramidal cells and from the axon terminals of corticipetal fiber systems. The remaining cortical synapses are symmetrical in ultrastructure and are the axon terminals of smooth, nonpyramidal interneurons of the cortex. These are inhibitory. Excitatory terminals contain small, round synaptic vesicles, whereas the vesicles in inhibitory terminals are pleomorphic.

Spiny Pyramidal Cells of the Neocortex

Pyramidal cells make up 70–80 percent of neurons in the mammalian neocortex (Feldman, 1984). Long-axoned pyramidal cells are the output channels of the networks in which they lie; the major targets of

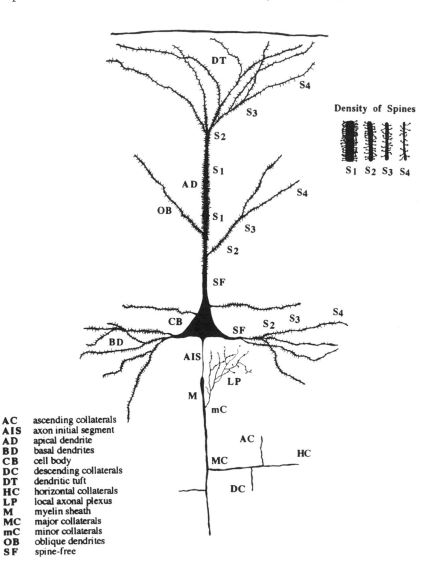

Fig. 3-2 Schematic diagram of a typical pyramidal cell of the neocortex, drawn from Golgi preparations. Minor axon collaterals *(mC)*, thin and unmyelinated, generate a terminal plexus near the cell body. Major axon collaterals *(MC)* are thick and myelinated; for many pyramidal cells of layers V and VI the axons emit exuberant recurrent collaterals that project to the upper layers, and some horizontal ones that project to relatively distant patches of cortex in the same cortical area. (From DeFelipe and Farinas, 1992.)

AC	ascending collaterals
AIS	axon initial segment
AD	apical dendrite
BD	basal dendrites
CB	cell body
DC	descending collaterals
DT	dendritic tuft
HC	horizontal collaterals
LP	local axonal plexus
M	myelin sheath
MC	major collaterals
mC	minor collaterals
OB	oblique dendrites
SF	spine-free

Cells and Local Networks of the Neocortex

their axons are elsewhere. Pyramidal cells are located, in different densities, in all cortical layers except layer I. A composite drawing of a "typical" pyramidal cell is shown in Fig. 3-2 (DeFelipe and Farinas, 1992). The myelinated axon leaves the cortex after emitting sets of recurrent collaterals. An apical dendrite ascends through the overlying layers of the cortex and many dendrites, but not all, end in a tuft of diverging terminal branches in layer I; oblique dendritic branches leave the apical dendrite during its ascent. A branching system of basilar dendrites is emitted and distributed within and near the layer of the cell body. Although the dendritic shafts and branches appear to be covered with spines, on average spines occupy only 2–3 percent of the dendritic surface. The classical image of the pyramidal cell seen in Fig. 3-2 does not reveal that pyramidal cells are heterogeneous, with variations in morphology and in their physiological and biochemical characteristics.

The Extrinsic Targets of Pyramidal Cell Axons

Pyramidal neurons in different cortical layers have different external targets, as listed in Table 3-2 (Jones, 1984b; Jones and Wise, 1975; Gilbert and Kelly, 1975; Lund et al., 1975). Pyramidal cells in the same layer in different cortical areas are uniform in size, except for the corticospinal neurons of area 4, which differ in size as a function of the length of their projecting axons. The density of pyramidal cells in a given layer is disjunctive in the horizontal direction, waxing and waning with spatial periods of a few hundred microns. All cortical areas do not emit all the efferent systems listed in Table 3-2. Some areas and some parts of areas do not emit corticospinal axons, others do not emit callosal axons, etc. The projecting axons of different layers of a cortical column carry the outputs of intracortical operations in different, but overlapping, transcortical channels. The nature of the intracortical operations expressed in those different outputs is unknown. The targets listed in Table 3-2 are central tendencies, and the probability is low that a supragranular pyramidal cell projects to an infragranular target, and vice versa, though exceptions occur.

The Intrinsic Targets of Pyramidal Cell Axon Collaterals

Pyramidal axons emit collaterals before the stem axons enter the white matter (Fig. 3-2). The local distribution of this branching system is confined within 100–200 μm of the cell of origin, projecting

Table 3-2. External targets of neocortical pyramidal cells with projecting axons (from Jones, 1984b).

Source	Targets
Layer II	Ipsilateral cortical areas
Layer III	Contralateral cortical areas
Layer IV	Generally none*
Layer V	Spinal cord, pons, medulla, midbrain, generalized thalamic nuclei, basal ganglia
Layer VI	Principal thalamic, nuclei Claustrum

*Area 17 contains some neurons in Layer IV whose axons project to other cortical areas.

upward through the cortex, frequently for two or more laminae. The concentration of these ascending collaterals increases in the supragranular layers, though few reach layer I. The asymmetric axon terminals end on dendritic spines and shafts, but not upon those of the cell of origin. A major projection is to the dendritic spines of closely adjacent pyramidal cells, providing for a powerful positive feedback for the local population of pyramidal cells. Many of these asymmetric terminals end upon the dendritic shafts of one of the classes of GABAergic, inhibitory, nonspiny cells described below. Antidromic excitation of pyramidal cell axons, and thus dromic activation of their intrinsic collaterals, evokes monosynaptic excitatory potentials, followed by disynaptic inhibitory postsynaptic potentials, in adjacent pyramidal cells. More powerful inhibition occurs in cells of the spatial surround, which contains the lateral spread of activity about an active cortical column. This feedback loop provides a mechanism tending to synchronize the activity of pyramidal neurons in a local cortical area.

Biochemical Characteristics of Cortical Pyramidal Cells

It was first inferred from indirect evidence that amino acids such as glutamate or aspartate are excitatory synaptic transmitters in the nervous system (Curtis et al., 1960; Krnjevic and Phillis, 1963; Streit, 1984; Fonnum, 1984). Use of a specific immunocytochemical method (Hepler et al., 1988; Storm-Mathiesen and Ottersen, 1990) has led to the conclusion that all cortical pyramidal cells use glutamate (or aspartate) as an excitatory transmitter agent in the classic mode of synthesis or uptake, vesicular storage, and quantal release (Maycox et al., 1990). The majority of cortical neurons having glutamate or aspartate as transmitters are pyramidal cells (Conti et al., 1989; Valtshanoff et al., 1993). Glutamate concentration in the asymmetric synaptic terminals of cortical pyramidal cells is several times that in the cytosol or in nonpyramidal neurons; it drops rapidly when the terminals are degenerated by removal of the pyramidal cell bodies. Glutamate (or aspartate) is released in a Ca^{2+}-dependent manner by electrical depolarization of brain slices or synaptosomal preparations, and directly from the terminals of active pyramidal cell projection systems. It excites postsynaptic cells in modes determined by its binding to one or more of the several glutamate receptor molecules in the postsynaptic membranes (see Chapter 5). The target neurons are directly activated by local iontophoresis of glutamate, a synaptic action blocked by glutamate antagonists. The membrane of pyramidal cell terminals contains a specific, high-affinity, Na^+-dependent uptake system for glutamate (aspartate), which rapidly terminates trans-synaptic action. Blockade of the uptake system prolongs that action.

Some Ca^{2+}-binding proteins, like calmodulin, are present in all eukaryotic cells. Several others, among them parvalbumin, calbindin, and calretinin, are expressed differentially in different classes of nonspiny, nonpyramidal GABAergic neurons of the neocortex. Calmodulin is a "trigger" protein that changes conformation after binding with Ca^{2+} and controls the activity of enzymes and ion channel proteins (Jones et al., 1993). The neuronal Ca^{2+}-binding proteins buffer the concentration of Ca^{2+} (Baimbridge et al., 1992). Immunocytochemical staining for calbindin in some pyramidal cells in the upper layers of the somatic sensory cortex has been described (DeFelipe and Jones, 1992), but it remains uncertain whether this is a general property of pyramidal cells (van Brederode et al., 1990; DeFelipe et al., 1989a,b; Hendry et al., 1989). Until now no firm evidence indicates that cortical spiny pyramidal cells express synaptically active peptides.

Synaptic Inputs to Cortical Spiny Pyramidal Cells

The spiny pyramidal cells of the neocortex receive input from: (1) intrinsic cortical neurons, excitatory from spiny nonpyramidal cells and inhibitory from all other nonpyramidal cells; (2) from the recurrent collaterals of other pyramidal cells, all excitatory; (3) from the axonal terminals of pyramidal cells in other cortical areas, all excitatory; (4) from thalamocortical projections of principal thalamic nuclei, all excitatory; (5) from generalized thalamic nuclei, presumably excitatory; (6) from brainstem monoaminergic systems, some excitatory and others inhibitory; (7) from the claustrum, presumably excitatory; (8) from some less well defined projections, e.g., from the basilar nucleus of Meynert (for review see DeFelipe and Farinas, 1992).

The general characteristics of terminals on spiny pyramidal cells are as follows. Terminals on the initial segments of the axon are symmetric, GABAergic, and thus inhibitory, and derive exclusively from the chandelier cells described below. The number of synaptic terminals per initial segment is low, varying from 2 to 50, with more on supra- than on infragranular pyramids. Terminals on the cell somata are uniformly inhibitory, are of intrinsic origin, and derive almost exclusively from the basket cells. The dendritic shafts and spines are the only cellular zones on pyramids that receive excitatory terminals; they receive some inhibitory terminals as well. The number of terminals on shafts and spines is very large, and counts varying from 4,000 to 20,000 and more have been reported.

Spiny Nonpyramidal Cells of the Neocortex: The Excitatory Interneurons

Glutaminergic excitatory interneurons account for less than 10 percent of nonpyramidal cells, and thus for only 2–3 percent of all cortical neurons (cell F, Fig. 3-1). Their small cell bodies are located in layer IV and lower layer III in almost all areas of the cortex, but their densities vary between areas. The dendrites project in all directions from the cell body but are limited in extent to the immediate spatial surround. The axon branches form narrow vertical bundles that project upward through all the overlying cellular layers, except layer I, to end in asymmetric terminals on the spines and the shafts of spiny pyramidal dendritic branches, on other spiny nonpyramidal cells, and on the dendrites of nonspiny, nonpyramidal cells. The spiny nonpyramidal cell is a major target of excitatory thalamocortical fibers, and it therefore plays a central role in the excitation of spiny pyramidal cells and of the superimposed inhibitory loops described below.

Cells and Local Networks of the Neocortex

Nonspiny, Nonpyramidal Cells of the Neocortex: The Inhibitory Interneurons

Several classes of nonspiny, nonpyramidal cortical neurons are defined by their cellular morphology, by their dendritic distribution, and especially by their axonal targets. Their axons remain intrinsic to the cortex and innervate other cortical neurons. These cells make up about 20 percent of all neurons in the primate neocortex. All known classes of nonspiny, nonpyramidal cells are inhibitory, use gamma-aminobutyric acid (GABA) as the classical transmitter, and generate symmetric synapses. GABAergic neurons vary between 10 and 30 μm diameter of the cell body.

Synaptically Active Peptides

Neuropeptides are co-localized with GABA in some classes of inhibitory interneurons in the neocortex (Hendry et al., 1984a,b; Jones and Hendry, 1986; Hendry, Jones, and Beinfeld, 1983; DeFelipe, 1993). However, all classes of GABAergic cells are not also peptidergic. Classic transmitters are synthesized in nerve terminals and stored in vesicles before release. Peptides are generated ribosomally in the cell body as large protein precursors and are moved by axonal transport to the nerve terminals, where enzymatic degradation to the release form is completed and vesicular storage effected (Chapter 5).

More than forty such synaptically active peptides have been identified in neurons; they are grouped into several families by similarities in amino acid sequence. Peptides may elicit either postsynaptic excitation or inhibition, depending upon the appropriate postsynaptic receptor. Those identified in neocortical neurons exert a slow postsynaptic excitation, although they are stored in and released from GABAergic "inhibitory" neurons (Nicoll et al., 1990). The following are among the many synaptically active peptides identified in neocortical neurons: somatostatin (SRIF)—14 amino acids; neuropeptide Y (NPY)—36 amino acids; vasoactive intestinal peptide (VIP)—28 amino acids; cholecystokinin (CCK)—8 amino acids; the tachykinins (TKY), which include substance P(SP)—11 amino acids, and substance K and neuromedin K, with 10 amino acids each; and corticotrophin releasing factor (CRF), with 40 amino acids. The identifications and localizations of peptides in cortical neurons have been made with the immunocytochemical method. Some cells express peptides transiently during development, not thereafter (Parnavelas et al., 1988).

Classes of Neocortical Inhibitory Interneurons

Chemical diversity is a salient feature of nonspiny, nonpyramidal cortical neurons, and many co-localizations of classic transmitters, Ca^{2+}-binding proteins, and peptides have been described. Typical cell types are shown in Fig. 3-1 (Jones, 1975; for reviews, see DeFelipe, 1993; Jones, 1993; Jones et al., 1994; Fairen et al., 1984). (See also Table 3-2 and Fig. 3-4.)

The *large basket cells* are the largest nonpyramidal cells in the neocortex, with cell diameters of 20–33 μm. They occur in all cortical layers, but in highest density in layers III and V/VI of the motor, somatic sensory, and visual areas. The dendrites diverge widely, as shown by cell H of Fig. 3-1 and by Fig. 3-3. Basket cells emit myeli-

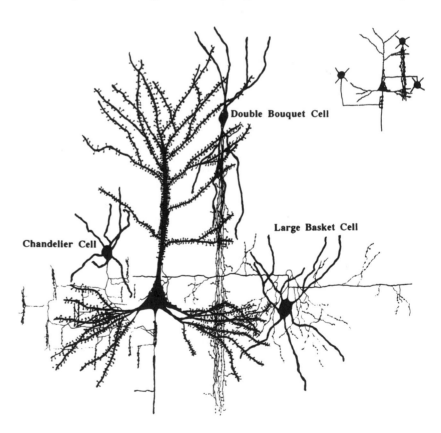

Fig. 3-3 Drawings from Golgi preparations to illustrate the synaptic relations between double bouquet, chandelier, large basket cells, and pyramidal cells in the cortex. The inset schema shows that each of the three nonpyramidal inhibitory interneurons projects to a different target zone on pyramidal cells. (From DeFelipe and Farinas, 1992.)

Cells and Local Networks of the Neocortex

nated axons that project horizontally for distances of 1 mm or more, in or close to the layer of origin, and generate nest-like arrays of symmetric terminals that ensheathe the somata and proximal dendrites of pyramidal cells; this arrangement results in a markedly divergent but minimally convergent system (Jones and Hendry, 1984; Marin-Padilla, 1974). Basket cells are GABAergic and thus inhibitory (Hendry, Houser, et al., 1983; DeFelipe, Hendry, and Jones, 1986). They express the Ca^{2+}-binding protein parvalbumin (Hendry et al., 1989; Akil and Lewis, 1992; Williams et al., 1992), but they are not known to express neuronal peptides (Jones and Hendry, 1984). Basket cells, by virtue of their disjunctive axonal distributions, appear suited to contribute to the pericolumnar inhibition described in Chapter 7.

The *double bouquet cells* are small, intrinsic cortical neurons (somal diameters 10–18 μm) that occur in different densities in all areas in all species studied. They are concentrated in layers II and III of the primate cortex, especially in the sensory and temporal areas. The double bouquet axon divides close to its origin into short ascending and longer descending branches that reach all the cellular layers of the cortex (cell B of Fig. 3-1). The vertically directed axons of local groups of several double bouquet cells are grouped into tight bundles that contribute to the vertical striations of the cortex seen in sections stained for fibers. The axonal bundles occur in a regular pattern with a center-to-center spacing of about 30 μm. Double bouquet cells are GABAergic and inhibitory (Somoygi et al., 1985). They generate symmetric synaptic terminals ending upon both dendritic shafts and branches of other inhibitory interneurons and the spines and small dendritic branches of pyramidal cells (Fig. 3-3) (del Rio and DeFelipe, 1995; Somoygi and Cowey, 1981). Double bouquet cells are biochemically heterogeneous, for many express the Ca^{2+}-binding protein calbindin, while others express tachykinins or somatostatin, rarely co-localized (DeFelipe et al., 1989b).

The vertical distribution of the double bouquet axons, their inhibitory synaptic actions, and their impingements both upon other inhibitory interneurons and upon pyramidal cells in all layers indicate that they contribute to the vertical channelling of neuronal activity in cortical columns, and thus contribute to a dynamic, microcolumnar distribution of neural activity (DeFelipe et al., 1990).

Chandelier cells are small neurons (somal diameters 10–15 μm) most densely concentrated in layers II/III; they occur in lower densities in the infragranular layers (cell D, Fig. 3-1). Axonal targets are uniform and specific: chandelier cells synapse upon the initial segments of pyramidal cell axons (Somoygi, 1977). These neurons are GABAergic and their terminals are symmetric and contain pleomorphic vesicles: they are inhibitory. Each pyramidal cell receives input from only 1–3 chandelier cells, but each chandelier cell innervates many pyramidal cells. The divergent numbers vary from 100 to 400 between different cortical areas (Marin-Padilla, 1987). The initial segments of supragranular pyramids are more densely innervated than are those of infragranular pyramids (DeFelipe et al., 1985). Chandelier cells express the Ca^{2+}-binding protein parvalbumin (DeFelipe et al., 1989a; Williams et al., 1992) and the neuronal peptide CRF.

The large basket, double bouquet, and chandelier cells are the best known of cortical inhibitory interneurons. Their relations to pyramidal cells are shown in Fig. 3-3, and their connections in intrinsic cortical circuits in Fig. 3-4. One can only infer their functions in in-

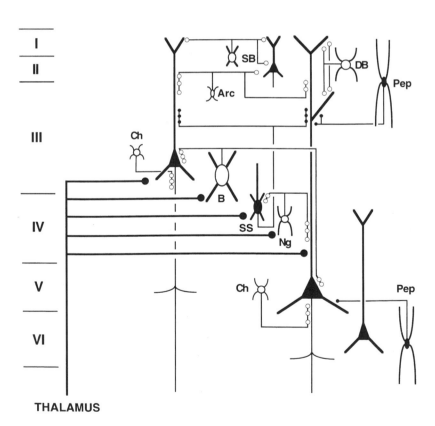

Fig. 3-4 Schematic outline of cortical neurons and their interconnections, including terminations of specific thalamocortical afferents. Solid dots are excitatory terminals; open circles, inhibitory terminals; solid cells, excitatory; shaded cells, inhibitory. Cell designations are: *Arc,* arcade; *B,* large basket; *Ch,* chandelier; *DB,* double bouquet; *Ng,* neurogliaform; *Pep,* "peptide"; *SS,* spiny stellate, or spiny nonpyramidal; *SB,* small basket. (From Jones, 1991; modified by Yoshioka, 1997.)

　　　　Cells and Local Networks of the Neocortex

trinsic cortical operations from their patterns of connectivity. What is missing is precise information about the afferent inputs to these cells and knowledge of their dynamic action in a working cortex. They all receive both asymmetric and symmetric axon terminals, and thus one cannot eliminate any of the known afferent or intrinsic cortical systems as sources of input to these cells.

Several other classes of nonspiny, nonpyramidal neurons are recognized, although the class parameters for them are blurred and investigators differ on categories. It appears reasonably certain that all are GABAergic and thus inhibitory (Hendry and Jones, 1981; Houser et al., 1983).

The *peptide cell* is so named because, although several classes of cortical interneurons express neuronal peptides, it is the quintessential producer of peptides. (See cell E in Fig. 3-1; it is sometimes called "bipolar" or "bitufted," as in Jones et al., 1987.) These small-bodied neurons are most common in layers II/III and VI, but are present in all the cellular layers except IV (Kuljis and Rakic, 1989), and have been identified in all areas of the neocortex examined. This cell generates a massive axonal and dendritic arborization oriented vertically in both directions to reach, for some cells, all the cellular layers of the cortex. Dendritic (and perhaps axonal) processes project to form dense plexuses in both the supra- and infragranular layers (Hendry et al., 1984b). Some neurites are in close but nonsynaptic relation with cortical blood vessels (Hendry, Jones, and Beinfeld, 1983); their axonal targets and terminals have not been clearly defined. Different sets of cells co-localize SRF, NPY, and GABA, while others co-localize CCK, VIP, and GABA (Jones et al., 1987, 1988).

The *neurogliaform cells* (also clewed or spiderweb cells) are the smallest nonspiny interneurons in the cortex, with somal diameters of 10–12 μm (cell G, Fig. 3-1) (Jones, 1975, 1984a). They are present in all layers in many species, including man, but in primates they are most densely concentrated in layers III and IV, particularly in the motor, somatic sensory, and visual areas. The cell emits short, repeatedly branching dendrites that form a dense local arborization 300–400 μm in diameter. The thin axon branches repeatedly and with rare exceptions is confined within the radius of the dendritic field. It is surmised that the axons synapse upon locally adjacent neurons, among them the excitatory spiny nonpyramidal cells.

The *small basket cells* have been identified in many cortical areas, including the somatic sensory cortex of the monkey (Fairen et al.,

1984). They are small replicas of the large basket cells, with somal diameters of about 12 μm, and are preferentially but not exclusively located in layers II and III. Their basket-like endings ensheathe the cell bodies and proximal dendrites of the small pyramids of layers II/III (cell C, Fig. 3-1).

The *Martinotti cells* are multipolar, sparsely spiny, nonpyramidal neurons located largely in layers V and VI and present ubiquitously in mammalian neocortices. Their axons, myelinated in adult life, frequently join in bundles to run vertically toward the pia. These axons may generate local plexuses in layers V and II/III, but their principal target is layer I, where their axons turn to run horizontally for 400–500 μm, forming part of the horizontal fiber plexus of layer I (Wahle, 1993). They terminate upon the apical dendrites of pyramidal cells, but the nature of those endings is unknown; the GABAergic nature of Martinotti cells suggests they are inhibitory (Hedlich et al., 1990). The afferent input to Martinotti cells is uncertain, and thus likewise their role in cortical operations.

Interstitial cells are pleomorphic neurons scattered in the white matter below layer VI, some spiny and quasipyramidal in form, others nonspiny and clearly nonpyramidal. They are the survivors of cell death in the subplate during the neonatal period (see Chapter 10), and of the transverse migration of cells of the third and innermost component of the primordial plexiform layer (DiDiego et al., 1994). A higher proportion of subplate neurons survive in the human than in other mammalian brains, and differentially so in different areas; e.g., many more are found beneath the sensory and motor than the visual area (Meyer et al., 1992). Many of these neurons are GABAergic, and different sets express NPY, SRIF, or CCK. They are assumed to be inhibitory, but direct evidence is lacking.

The Intrinsic Circuitry of the Neocortex

The cell-to-cell connectivity patterns described in the previous sections have a basic similarity throughout the cortex, a pattern upon which area-specific variations are superimposed. The variations are clear in the striate cortex of cats and monkeys, and specializations have now been described in areas of the homotypical cortex of the frontal lobe in the monkey (Kritzer and Goldman-Rakic, 1995; Lund and Yoshioka, 1991; Lund et al., 1993). Descriptions of the intracortical circuitry based on use of the Golgi method established the classical translaminar patterns of the flow of activity through the cortex. These methods have established some of the cellular linkages in the neocortex described in earlier sections of this chapter; see as examples of many papers those by Lund and Yoshioka (1991) and Lund, Yoshioka, and Levitt (1993). There has followed a period of intense research using cell-marker methods. In one class of these experiments, small quantities of cell markers are injected into the extracellular space. After inward membrane transport into adjacent neurons, the markers are moved throughout the cells, outlining the morphology of the cell completely and allowing three-dimensional construction from serial sections. The combination of this method with electron-microscopic analysis reveals the type of synaptic ending and the postsynaptic targets of the cell reconstructed. More recently, markers have been injected via intracellular micropipettes, followed by cell recovery from serial sections and reconstruction. The functional properties of the cell can be determined by recording through the intracellular micropipette before injection. This laborious method has been used by a number of research groups, notably by Gilbert and Wiesel (1979, 1983, 1989; Gilbert, 1993) and by Martin and Whitteridge (1984; Martin, 1988). A large catalogue of cortical neurons studied in this way has accumulated, with descriptions of their laminar locations, three-dimensional forms, types of synaptic endings, and postsynaptic targets. While this information is still not adequate for a full flow diagram, the promise for a full description in the near-term future is great.

Specific Thalamocortical Afferents

In the somatic afferent system, thalamocortical (TC) afferents derive from the cytochrome oxidase–rich, parvalbumin-positive, rod-like lemniscal relay zones in the ventral posterior nuclei of the thalamus and project to areas 3b, 1, and 2 of the postcentral gyrus (Rausell and Jones, 1991a,b). Groups of fibers with similar properties of place and mode terminate in patches of 400–500 μm dimensions, separated by zones of about equal width in which TC innervation is much less dense. This arrangement raises a difficult question, for body parts are represented in tight contiguity in the postcentral gyrus—there are no blank spots in the representation pattern. Each TC afferent divides to form a burst of terminal axon segments and synaptic boutons that distribute throughout its particular patch (Jones, 1995). Double labeling of thalamic neurons by retrograde transport of different tracers is seen only if the two injections are less than 500 μm apart on the cortical surface (Rausell and Jones, 1995).

Neurons in layers III–VI of S1 cortex in the monkey receive direct TC synaptic input; these include the pyramidal cells of III, V, and VI and the spiny nonpyramidal interneurons of IV (Fig. 3-4). The latter also receive a strong excitatory input via the re-entrant ascending axon collaterals of the pyramidal cells of VI. The excitatory terminals of the TC afferents all end on dendritic spines. They occupy only a small proportion of the postsynaptic spines of the spiny, nonpyramidal cells, yet their excitatory input to those cells is very strong. These synapses sustain high-frequency transmission, and synaptic transfer across them survives even deep levels of general anesthesia. The large basket and the neurogliaform cells also receive direct TC synaptic inputs. This is confirmed by observations made in cortical slice experiments, that electrical stimulation of corticipetal axons just below the cortex evokes strong disynaptic inhibitory postsynaptic potentials (IPSPs) in pyramidal cells in layers II and III.

The TC afferents are less dense in homotypical areas, and in them the zone of termination is confined to layer III, even though a granular layer IV exists in those areas. However, the apical dendrites of the spiny nonpyramidal cells project from IV into the zone of terminations in IIIb, indicating that the portal of entry of TC afferents may be quite similar in all cortical areas. The vertically directed axonal projections of the excitatory interneurons probably engage neurons in all cellular layers. The local laminar zone of excitation in IV and IIIb is quickly converted to a vertical zone extending across all layers. The specific TC afferents also terminate in layer VI, though less densely than in II/IIIb. They provide through that linkage a pathway for a tightly focused re-entrant loop via the corticothalamic cells of VI back to local zones in the ventral posterior thalamic nuclei. Given the strong vertical internal organization (described in Chapter 7), it appears likely that within two or three synaptic transmissions every cortical cell will receive synaptic impingements generated initially by impulses in TC afferents.

The lemniscal relay rods of the ventral posterior nuclei are embedded within, and partially surrounded by, a matrix in which neurons are smaller and less densely packed. They stain only weakly for cytochrome oxidase and contain the Ca^{2+}-binding protein, calbindin. The matrix regions of the ventral posterior medial (VPM) and ventral posterior lateral (VPL) thalamic nuclei receive ascending inflow from the nucleus caudalis of the trigeminal system and from the spinothalamic system. Elements of these systems are activated by nociceptive stimulation of peripheral tissues. The matrix cells project upon layer I of the somatic sensory cortex, where they have access to the apical dendritic expansions of almost all the pyramidal cells in the cortex. What role this system plays in intrinsic cortical operations is unknown.

Intrinsic Circuits

The pattern of the translaminar progression of activity evoked in the cortex by a TC afferent volley has been known for a long time: from the entry points in IV and lower III upward to II/III, and from thence downward to V and then to VI, and then upward to all superior laminae again, especially to layer IV. In recent years efforts have been made to specify this flow pathway in terms of neuron types and their synaptic connections with other neurons (Fig. 3-4; Jones, 1991). How this pattern of cellular connectivity contributes to the columnar organization of the neocortex is described in Chapter 7; see the section, "Anatomical Basis of Columnar Organization." Briefly, the cellular network is as follows. The TC afferent terminals articulate directly with the pyramidal cells of III, V, and VI and with three classes of interneurons: the inhibitory basket cells, the neurogliaform cells, and the excitatory, nonspiny, nonpyramidal cells. Activity is relayed over the axons of the excitatory interneurons vertically to the pyramidal cells of II/III, and probably to the many classes of inhibitory interneurons shown in Fig. 3-1. The pyramidal cells of V/VI are strongly activated by the collaterals of the emerging axons of the pyramidal cells of II/III. The recurrent collaterals of the pyramidal cells of V/VI then activate all classes of cells in superior laminae. Some pyramidal cells of both the supra- and infragranular layers emit collaterals that run for some distances within the cortex, to terminate in patchy, intermittent axon terminal distributions. I describe that system in the following section.

It is important to emphasize the pervasive role of inhibition in the intrinsic operation. The cortex is replete with short inhibitory circuits: the basket cells to the somata of pyramidal cells; the chandelier cells to the initial segments of pyramidal cells; neurogliaform cells to the excitatory interneurons; and the vertically directed double bouquet cells to the dendrites of pyramidal and nonpyramidal cells in all layers. Moreover, many terminals of inhibitory interneurons are applied to the smooth dendritic shafts of other inhibitory interneurons.

The dynamic intrinsic operations of the neocortical microcircuits are described in Chapter 11.

Horizontal Intracortical Connections

Powell and his colleagues made narrow vertical lesions in the monkey visual cortex by passing a microelectrode normal to the pial surface down through all the cellular layers. They used an axonal degeneration method to show that 90 percent of the horizontally projecting axon terminals ended within 1 mm of the lesion edge; the remainder projected horizontally for long distances through the cortex—in some cases for several millimeters (Fisken et al., 1973, 1975). The introduction of axon-tracing methods based upon axoplasmic flow revealed in full detail these horizontally projecting collaterals of pyramidal cells. The collaterals terminate intermittently in local patches about 400 μm in diameter in the cat visual cortex, spaced by intervening terminal-free regions of about the same size. These projections elaborate columnar distributions of axonal terminal branches through all the cellular layers of the target modules (Gilbert and Wiesel, 1979, 1983; for reviews see Gilbert, 1992, 1993). Similar observations were made by Martin and Whitteridge in their studies of intracortical connectivity (Martin and Whitteridge, 1984; Martin, 1988; Kisvarday et al., 1986, 1989). Ninety percent of the terminal boutons in the target patches are asymmetric and thus excitatory; 80 percent end upon dendritic spines, the remainder on the smooth dendritic shafts of nonspiny interneurons, probably those of small basket cells. The system thus impinges upon both the excitatory and inhibitory mechanisms in the target modules. The terminals on spines are glutaminergic and are linked to postsynaptic N-methyl-D-aspartic ion (NMDA) and non-NMDA receptors (Keller, 1993). These synaptic linkages can be strengthened or weakened under appropriate conditions in the mode of long-term facilitation or depression (Chapter 6).

There are two such systems. One arises from the pyramidal cells of layers II/III, the second from pyramids of layers IVb/V. The layer IVb/V system is fully mature by the seventh week of postnatal life, while that of layers II/III is completed only after the sixteenth week

(Burkhalter et al., 1993). The former is shaped by axonal pruning in the interdigitated areas, while the latter is patchy in distribution, de novo.

A number of studies have shown that neurons of the source and target modules of the visual cortex have similar properties; for example, in the visual cortex of the ferret they have similar eye preference and orientation specificity (Weilikey, et al., 1995); in the monkey links from the cytochrome+ puffs are restricted to similar puffs, those from the interpuff regions to other interpuff regions (Livingstone and Hubel, 1984). Excitatory correlations exist between neurons in modules linked by horizontal connections in the cat. The spatial pattern of the horizontally distributed systems changes in transit from the primary visual area V1 through V2, V3, V4, and into 7a in the monkey. There is a marked increase in the lateral extent of the distribution, which reaches 7 mm in area 7a. The average interpatch interval increases from 0.61 mm to 1.56 mm between V1 and 7a, but there is no significant change in the patch dimension: it averages 231 μm in V1 and 310 μm in 7a. The clustered order of the projections is preserved in all areas (Amir et al., 1993). Galuske and Singer (1996) have found that in cat area 17 the patch diameters are about 400 μm, with interpatch intervals of 800 μm. Here the horizontal projections appear much longer than in the monkey, reaching 4–8 mm for different cell types. Moreover, in the cat some neurons of the white matter and some intracortical multipolar neurons also contribute to the horizontal system.

This pattern of horizontal projections has been observed in every area of cortex studied: in the monkey somatic sensory (DeFelipe, Conley, and Jones, 1986) and motor areas (Huntley and Jones, 1991a); in the auditory cortex of the cat (Ojima et al., 1991, 1992; Wallace et al., 1991); and in several areas of the dorsolateral frontal cortex of the monkey (Kritzer and Goldman-Rakic, 1995; Lund et al., 1993).

These anatomical discoveries have provoked speculation about what role the horizontal system may play in cortical neuronal processing, particularly in sensory and motor areas. Singer (1995) has proposed that the horizontal connections provide a base for binding together the components of sensory stimuli by the dynamic association of the local modular activities evoked by different stimulus aspects into an assembly in which the population activity is a coherent representation of all. I discuss this subject further in Chapter 12.

The Layer I Circuit

Early in ontogenesis the telencephalic vesicle is invaded by afferent fibers that divide and spread in a branching pattern over its surface, just beneath the pia. This is followed by the appearance of the characteristic neurons of layer I, the Cajal-Retzius cells. These large neurons have widely distributed dendrites and myelinated axons that run horizontally in layer I, sometimes for several millimeters. This primordial plexiform layer (Marin-Padilla and Marin-Padilla, 1982; Marin-Padilla, 1984) is later split into layer I above and the subplate below by the cortical plate, formed by the migrating waves of neurons from the neuroepithelium (see Chapter 9). Cajal-Retzius cells engage synaptically the apical dendritic branches of pyramidal cells whose somata lie in the developing cortical plate (Fig. 3-5). The first set of afferent fibers innervating the Cajal-Retzius cells is the monoaminergic projection that arises from nuclei in the central core of the brain stem.

Cajal-Retzius cells are excitatory, use glutamate as transmitter, and make asymmetric endings upon the apical dendrites in the developing cortex (Rio et al., 1995). Cajal-Retzius cells appear in layer I of the human cortex at about the sixth gestational week, and by the eighteenth week they mature into a polymorphic population consisting of both horizontal and vertical cells (Meyer and Gonzalez-Hernandez, 1993). Three types of calretinin-positive Cajal-Retzius neurons persist into the adult human neocortex: horizontal cells, triangular cells, and multipolar cells (Baloyannis et al., 1993; Belinchenko et al., 1995). The small neurons of layer I differentiate first in the lower half of I, but later appear also in its upper half. These neurons are GABAergic, and express the peptide NPY (Kuljis and Rakic, 1989). Later in development, elements of both intrinsic and extrinsic systems project some of their elements to layer I: the ascending axons of certain intrinsic cortical cells, like the Martinotti cells; afferents from the basal forebrain (cholinergic), from the raphe nuclei of the brain stem (serotonergic), and from the locus ceruleus (noradrenergic), which arrive early in ontogeny. Projections also reach layer I from the midline, intralaminar, and anterior ventral thalamic nuclei, as well as from some elements of cortico-cortical systems.

The divergent nature of these systems suggests that they exert some generally controlling action upon cortical pyramidal cells, and

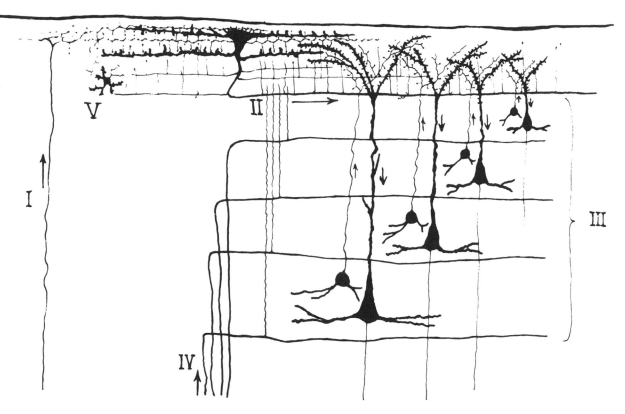

Fig. 3-5 The organization of layer I of the mammalian cerebral cortex. (I) The primitive corticipetal fibers are the first to reach layer I during cortical ontogenesis. (II) The Cajal-Retzius neurons. (III) The outputs of layer I are via the apical dendritic bouquets of pyramidal neurons in different cortical layers. (IV) Projection of specific and nonspecific thalamocortical afferents. (V) The small neurons of layer I that appear late in ontogenesis are probably nonpyramidal inhibitory neurons. (From Marin-Padilla, 1984.)

their early completion hints that they may influence cortical maturation, as well (Vogt, 1991).

The Intralaminar Thalamocortical Afferents

The term *intralaminar* designates cortical afferents from the intralaminar and midline nuclei of the thalamus. This group includes the central medial, paracentral, and central lateral nuclei and, in primates, the center median-parafascicular complex. The several small midline nuclei include the rhomboid, reuniens, paraventricular, parataenial, and intermediodorsal nuclei. These nuclei are sources of afferent projections to both the cerebral cortex and the basal ganglia.

The intralaminar (IL) nuclei were long regarded as diffuse and nonspecific, largely because electrical stimulation at any one point within them elicited widespread changes in the electrical activity of the cortex, accompanied by global changes in behavioral state: sleep, arousal, attentiveness, depending upon locus and frequency of stimulation. The term *diffuse* is inappropriate, for recent studies show that each nucleus consists of many cellular groups, each of which projects upon a restricted zone of the cerebral cortex or the basal ganglia: these nuclei are multifocal, but not diffuse, in nature (for reviews, see Groenewegen and Berendse, 1994; Macchi and Bentivoglio, 1988; Macchi, 1993). The cortical and basal ganglia target zones are themselves interconnected (e.g., by corticostriate projections). The IL afferents to the cortex are excitatory and terminate densely in layer I, where they have access to the apical dendritic arborizations of almost all the pyramidal cells in the layers below. The IL afferents project less densely to layer VI.

The Corticocortical Afferents

There are two classes of corticocortical afferents: those linking the two hemispheres via the callosum, and those connecting cortical areas within the same hemisphere. Some areas of the cortex, and some modules within any given connected area, are free of callosal connections. The zones of the somatic sensory area of the primate postcentral gyrus in which the apices of the limbs and the face are represented are free of callosal connections, while closely adjacent modules representing other body parts are connected. Callosal connections arise and terminate in column-like areas about 400 μm in diameter, separated by areas in which origins and terminations are less dense—they follow the patch rule that also governs the patterns of termination of the TC afferents. When modules are connected transcallosally, the relation is very precise for connections between homologous areas. The pyramidal cells of origin in III (of the somatic sensory cortex, e.g.) receive directly the callosally mediated input from the contralateral side. The exact relations for heterologously connected areas are uncertain. All callosal efferents are excitatory and glutaminergic, and all terminate upon dendritic spines. What role they play in the dynamic intrinsic processing within the cortex is unknown. The ipsilateral cortico-cortical systems may arise from the middle layers, or from those above or below, and may terminate in intermittent columns in the patch mode; or, convergent projections may engage alternate layers in the target area. The functional meaning of these many patterns is unknown.

Cells and Local Networks of the Neocortex

Afferents from the Central Core and Basal Forebrain

The neocortex is engaged by a dense three-dimensional network of afferent fibers projected monosynaptically from a number of discrete nuclei distributed along the anteroposterior axis of the brain from the basal nucleus of Meynert to the raphe nuclei of the central core of the brain stem. These modulatory systems engage the cortex in a noncolumnar manner; they enter the cortex and both as systems and as single axons project tangentially, in some cases for long distances, emitting axon collaterals and terminal branches as they project. In the primate much more so than in the rodent, the patterns of the terminations of these systems display some areal and laminar specificities that differ between systems and between lobes of the cortex. Nevertheless, the neocortex viewed through the aperture of the central core systems is scarcely recognizable to an observer conditioned by views from the specific thalamocortical systems. Viewed through the former, the cortex appears as a large, thin sheet of closely packed neurons organized by laminar and columnar parameters, but otherwise heavily innervated by several systems that engage it tangentially and divide it imprecisely on the large scale of lobes and zones, only occasionally innervating classical cytoarchitectonic areas differentially.

Each of these systems operates with a specific transmitter: the basal nucleus of Meynert with acetylcholine, the peri-hypothalamic regions with histamine, the substantia nigra and ventral tegmental area with dopamine, the locus ceruleus–subceruleus system with norepinephrine, and the raphe nuclei with serotonin (Table 3-3). Some of these afferents co-localize neuroactive peptides. Moreover, cortical neurons contain several varieties of postsynaptic receptors for each of these transmitters, which may account for the varied effects of these afferents upon cortical neurons.

It is generally held that these systems exert modulating effects upon their postsynaptic targets. Their trans-synaptic actions are slow, may differ from time to time depending upon the activity state of the postsynaptic cell and the dynamic pattern of its other synaptic inputs, and may even include action at a distance by volume conduction, in addition to synaptic input. They may influence glial cells and blood vessels as well as neurons. A large body of evidence indicates that these systems are involved in the regulation of forebrain excitability, the sleep-waking cycles, appetitive and other drives, and

Table 3-3. Biochemical features of modulatory afferent systems.

Transmitter (type)	Co-localized peptides	Source	Receptors
Acetylcholine (excitatory)	Vasoactive intestinal peptide Luteinizing hormone releasing hormone Tachykinins Somatostatin Neurotensin Galanin	Basal nucleus Medial septal nucleus Diagonal band	Muscarinic (M-1 and M-2)
Serotonin (inhibition of spontaneous activity)	Cholecystokinin Enkephalin Tachykinins Thyrotropin releasing hormone	Dorsal and medial raphe nucleus	Serotonin-la–d Serotonin-2 Serotonin-3 Serotonin-4
Dopamine (excitatory, inhibitory)	Cholecystokinin Enkephalin Neurotensin	Substantia nigra Ventral tegmental area	D1–D5
Norepinephrine (inhibition or diminishing of spontaneous activity)	Neuropeptide Y Enkephalin Neurotensin Somatostatin Vasopressin Corticotrophin releasing factor	Locus ceruleus	Alpha-1 Alpha-2 Beta-1 Beta-2

more generally the affective tone of thought and action. Disorders of these systems are thought to be important in the pathogenesis of psychotic states, although the mechanisms of these brain disorders remain elusive. Many hundreds of papers appear annually describing various aspects of the regulatory systems and their role in controlling behavior, but the exact mechanism of those controls is still unknown. Important reviews are those in the handbook volume edited by Floyd Bloom, particularly chapters 1–4 and 14 (Bloom, 1986), and those by Steriade and Buzsaki (1989), Saper (1987), and Morrison and Hot (1992).

I describe as an example one of these systems, that which originates in the raphe nuclei of the brainstem and operates with the transmitter serotonin.

Two overlapping serotonin projections arise from the median and dorsal raphe nuclei. Dorsal raphe axons are very fine, those from the median nucleus are somewhat larger and contain large, beaded varicosities thought to be transmitter release points. The cortical projections of these two sets considered together include in the monkey all layers in all neocortical areas. The fine axons predominate in layers II–VI, particularly in IV, the larger axons with beaded varicosities in layer I (Molliver, 1987; Wilson and Molliver, 1991a,b). There are, however, selective variations in the densities of the serotonin projections; e.g., the postcentral sensory cortex is heavily innervated, the motor cortex only lightly (Fig. 3-6). Raphe neurons discharge slowly during the waking state, increase their rates during phasic arousal, decrease during slow-wave sleep, and may be silent during periods of paradoxical sleep. Iontophoretic application of serotonin near cortical neurons produces either excitation via the serotonin-2 (5-HT-2) receptors or inhibition via the serotonin-1 (5-HT-1) receptors, or complex sequences of the two, but most commonly a profound inhibition (Davies et al., 1987). The postsynaptic potentials are slow in onset and long in duration, compared with direct synaptic responses. Many of the terminals and axonal varicosities are located upon the apical dendrites of pyramidal cells; others form terminal baskets about GABAergic inhibitory neurons. Whether all of these terminal appositions show the ultrastructural signatures of true synapses is still uncertain. Some do not, however, and the possibility of action by volume conduction must be left open.

The Claustrocortical Projection System

The claustrum is a narrow band of neurons located between the extreme and external capsules, which latter separates the claustrum from the putamen. Anatomical studies made with degeneration methods indicate that the claustrum sends efferents to, and receives afferents from, almost every area of the neocortex (for review see Sherk, 1986). Studies with tracer methods have confirmed these reciprocal connections for the visual, somatic sensory, auditory, and motor areas, and for many areas of the homotypical cortex as well. These relations are not random. The claustrum receives a topographically ordered input from the contralateral half of the visual field (Le-Vay and Sherk, 1981; Sherk and LeVay, 1981), a representation of the body surface (Olsen and Graybiel, 1980), and, it is inferred, an

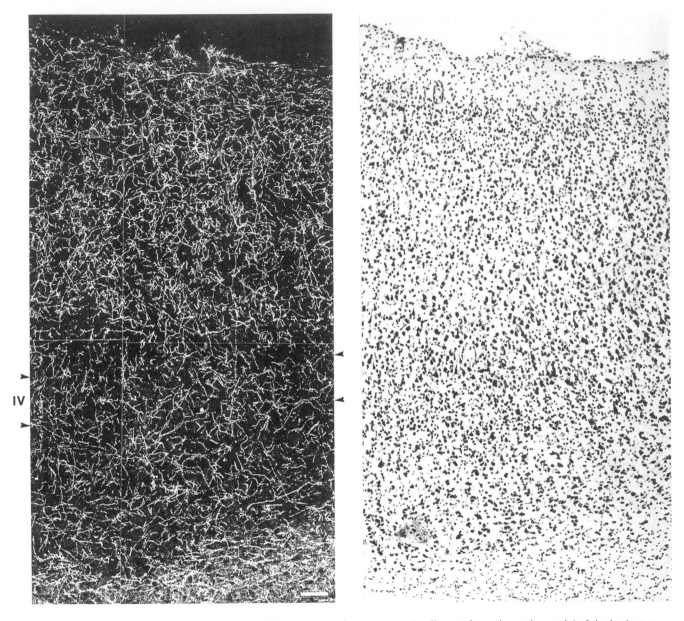

Fig. 3-6 Demonstration of the dense innervation of the neocortex by serotonergic afferents from the raphe nuclei of the brainstem. At left is a section prepared by serotonin histochemistry; area 3b of the somatic sensory cortex of the postcentral gyrus of a macaque monkey. The innervation is more dense in the supra- than in the infragranular layers. There is a narrow zone of thinner innerva tion in the deepest part of layer IV (arrows). The micrograph to the right is of an adjacent section stained with Cresyl Violet. Scale bar = 100 μm. (From Wilson and Molliver, 1991a.)

ordered input from the auditory system. The subcortical sources of these projections to the claustrum have not been defined completely. The reciprocal connections between the claustrum and the three primary sensory areas of the cortex fit with this topographic pattern, with a considerable overlap between the systems.

The claustrum contains a class of large, spiny, pyramidal-like cells thought to be excitatory neurons with cortical projections. It also contains a numerically larger class of small, nonspiny, nonpyramidal neurons presumed to be interneurons, but still of unknown synaptic action. If inhibitory, they are virtually unique among telencephalic inhibitory neurons in being non-GABAergic. Little is known of the function of the claustro-cortical projections in any area other than the striate cortex of cats (V1). Here they make their densest terminations in layer IVB, where they make up a small percentage of the excitatory terminals on the spines of the spiny nonpyramidal cells (Ahmed et al., 1994). They make less dense projections to layer VI. All the cortico-claustral projection neurons are located in layer VI. They are a class separate from the much more numerous corticothalamic cells of that layer. Claustral axons terminate upon both complex and simple visual cortical neurons (Bopyapati and Henry, 1985). Sherk and LeVay (1983) discovered that after a lesion of the visual portion of the claustrum the percentage of visual cortical neurons with end-stopped inhibition and directional selectivity was greatly reduced, a finding described also by Bopyapati and Henry (1985). This observation indicates that the claustral afferents play a role in composing the distinctive properties of visual cortical neurons. What more general role the system may play in the wide areas of both hetero- and homotypical cortex it innervates is unknown.

The Organization of the Neocortex

Any biologist confronted with a system as complex as the human brain, especially its cerebral cortex, is consumed with a desire to divide it into smaller parts—if he does not turn away in dismay. He portions it out in the hope that by a persistent analysis of the structure and function of parts he may someday be able to reconstruct the whole. This reductionist effort has been pursued with vigor and ingenuity for nearly two hundred years, and as a result there are now a variety of ways of dividing and classifying different areas of the cerebral cortex. Architectural methods are cast at a level of analysis midway between the unaided visual inspection of brain sections and observations at high magnification of the structure and ultrastructure of nerve cells. They range from the classical methods of cyto- and myeloarchitecture to present efforts to designate cortical areas by differences in biochemical mechanisms, or by the differential prevalence of transmitter and receptor molecules. The results obtained with the classical methods have been of immense value for brain science and for clinical neurology. They were generated in an era in which the geographical approach dominated thinking about the brain, however, and they tell us little about the *function* of the cerebral cortex. They do provide the base for studies of the dynamic aspects of cortical function that will surely dominate the future of neuroscience.

I review some of these geographic and numerical facts in the present chapter.

The Cytoarchitecture of the Neocortex

Brief study with low-power magnification of Nissl (thionin)-stained serial sections of the neocortex, cut normal to the pial surface, is sufficient to convince even the skeptic that he views a laminated structure. The layers are produced by differences in depth below the pia in cell types and packing density; they are aligned horizontally parallel to the pial surface. Further study shows that these properties differ between different cortical locations. This is the factual base of cytoarchitecture. Myeloarchitecture depends upon variations between cortical areas in the sizes and distribution of myelinated axons, and their differential time of myelination in ontogeny.

The neocortex (also known as the *isocortex*) is defined as cortex that contains six layers in its mature form, or that ever contained six layers during development. It is now customary to define six layers in the neocortex, even though some classical layers are absent in some locations and in others are subdivided to account for obvious intralaminar differences—e.g., layer IV of area 17 in primates. Conversely, layer IV of the motor cortex (area 4), though present early in development, can scarcely be seen in the mature cortex, and in area 3b of the postcentral gyrus layers II and III are inextricably fused. The layers were traditionally defined in terms of the most common cell types within them, but other cell types are now known to occur in each, in lesser numbers. Cytoarchitectural layers are commonly referred to by their roman numerals. The classical layers in sequence from outside to inside are as follows:

I   The plexiform (or molecular) layer contains a feltwork of horizontally running axons and dendrites, the relatively rare Cajal-Retzius cells, and a poorly defined class of small nonspiny, nonpyramidal cells.

II   The layer of small pyramids (or corpuscular layer); it also contains many nonpyramidal cells, such as the small basket cells.

III The layer of medium-sized pyramids (or simply the pyramidal layer), in a gradual transition from layer II; it also contains many nonspiny, nonpyramidal cells—the large basket cells, the chandelier cells, the double bouquet cells.

IV   The granular layer contains many small neurons, cell bodies that are tightly packed in a narrow layer, including the spiny, nonpyramidal cells, neurogliofarm cells, and others.

V   The layer of large pyramidal cells (or ganglionic layer).

VI   The layer of pleomorphic cells, sometimes called the "multiform," or "spindle" layer, contains cells of varying morphology: regular and inverted pyramids, Martinotti cells, etc.

Cytoarchitecture is the study and definition of cortical areas in terms of parameters revealed by stains of the ribonucleic acids of cell bodies. Only the cell soma and the proximal dendritic shafts can be seen; nothing of the full dendritic and axonal arborizations, or of cell-to-cell connectivity, are visible by this type of staining. Nevertheless, a remarkable correlation was obtained, for many areas defined by this simple method correlate well with cortical parcellations determined by other methods.

The field of cytoarchitecture is said to have begun with the work of Meynert in 1867, although earlier discoveries—like that of the white line in the striate cortex by Genari in 1776—hinted at what was coming. The history of the field after Meynert is studded with the names of giants in neuroanatomy: Berlin, Lewis, Campbell, Eliot Smith, Kolliker, Hammarberg, the Vogts, Brodmann, Lorente de No, von Economo, and more recently Sarkisov. The results were detailed parcellations, and hence maps, of the neocortex in many mammals, including man and other primates. The general position was reached that the transition from one cortical field with certain properties to an adjacent field with different ones might be very abrupt at some junctures (1 mm or less), and that the changes occurred almost simultaneously in all the cellular layers. Hence in some cases they could be marked with a line.

Fig. 4-1 shows the most widely reproduced of all cytoarchitectonic maps of the human cortex, that of Brodmann (1905, 1914). Brodmann numbered 52 areas in the human cortex, but with counting gaps only 45 can be made out in Fig. 4-1. He published no photomicrographs, and only brief descriptions of the areas he numbered, yet his general plan has been at least partially confirmed in many recent studies. Brodmann's map for the monkey (thought to have been a cercopithecoid) is shown in Fig. 4-2. This map is known to be incom-

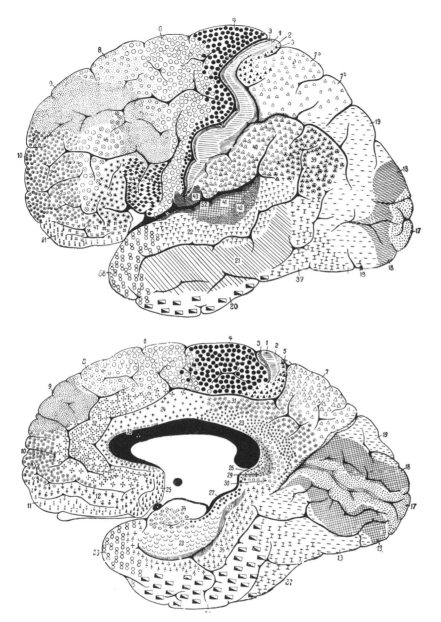

Fig. 4-1 Classical architectural map of the human neocortex; lateral surface above, medial below. (From Brodmann, 1914.)

Fig. 4-2 Brodman's cytoarchitectural map of a monkey, probably a cercopithecoid. (Reproduced from Vogt and Vogt, 1919.)

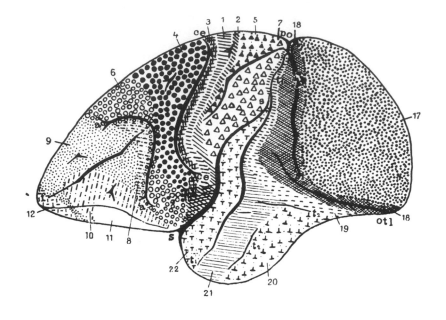

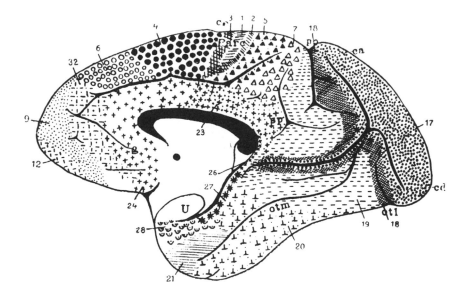

The Organization of the Neocortex

plete and perhaps partially conjectural, but it was until recently the most widely used map of the cortex of Old World monkeys. More exact and detailed maps have since been constructed for different regions of the cortex of the macaque.

The map of Fig. 4-3 summarizes many years of study of the human cortex by Sarkisov and his colleagues at the Moscow Brain Research Institute (Sarkisov et al., 1955). While the general plan of Sarkisov's map is similar to that of Brodmann, many differences are obvious. How these differences will be resolved is uncertain, for cytoarchitectural study is now the experimental occupation of few neuroscientists.

When pursued with diligence by those expert in cytoarchitectural studies, even minute parcellations in the cortex were thought to be valid. An extreme conclusion of some anatomists and neurologists of the first half of the twentieth century was that each of these identified cortical areas should be regarded as a quasi-independent cerebral "organ," each functioning more or less independently of its neighbors—an idea reminiscent of the phrenology of a century before (Spurzheim, 1925). This view evoked a swing to the equally extreme position of Lashley and Clark (1946), who came to regard all but the most obvious differences as subjective impressions (see also Bonin and Bailey, 1947). This uncertainty may have arisen from the variability in the size and exact location of areas now known to occur in individuals of the same species. Haug et al. (1984) measured neuron size and laminar packing densities in a heterotypical area (area 17) and a homotypical area (area 11) in a number of human brains. Neuron size and the laminar packing densities varied in both areas with coefficients of variation of 15–20 percent. Rajkowska and Goldman-Rakic (1995a,b) made a quantitative study of areas 9 and 46 in the frontal lobe of the human brain, using an objective, three-dimensional cell-counting method to lend validity to cytoarchitectural identifications. Fig. 4-4 shows the variability in size and location of these two areas in the left-hemisphere reconstructions of five human brains. Fig. 4-5B shows the overlap of the zones for the two regions in the five brains, to be compared with the delineation of these two areas in the frontal lobe in the three classical cytoarchitectural studies noted above (see Figs. 4-1–4-3).

The conclusion seems certain that the sizes and exact locations of cytoarchitectural areas differ significantly between individual brains, and even between hemispheres of the same brain. This variability

Fig. 4-3 Cytoarchitectural maps of the human cortex, shown in lateral and dorsal views. The areas' sizes and locations in this map differ markedly from those in Brodmann's map (Fig. 4-1). (From Sarkisov et al., 1955.)

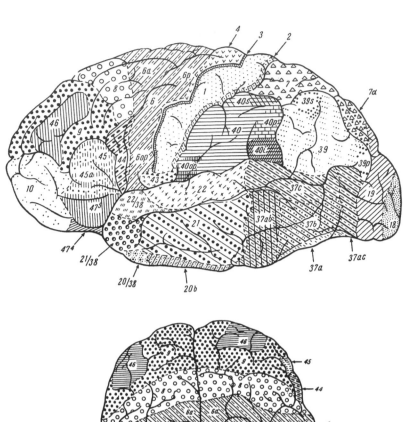

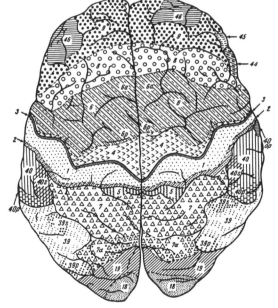

The Organization of the Neocortex

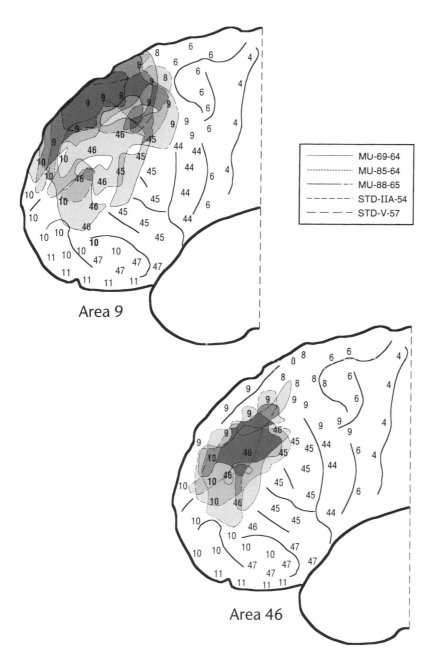

Fig. 4-4 Superimposition of five cytoar-chitectural reconstructions of the frontal lobes of human subjects, illustrating that areas 9 and 46 vary in location and area between subjects. The area of common overlap is shown in black, and variations in gray. Outlines of areas 9 and 46 in individual brains are marked by different line patterns. (From Rajkowska and Goldman-Rakic, 1995b.)

Area 9

	MU-69-64
	MU-85-64
	MU-88-65
	STD-IIA-54
	STD-V-57

Area 46

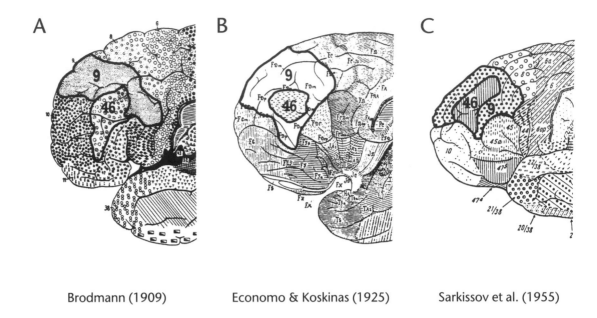

A — Brodmann (1909)

B — Economo & Koskinas (1925)

C — Sarkissov et al. (1955)

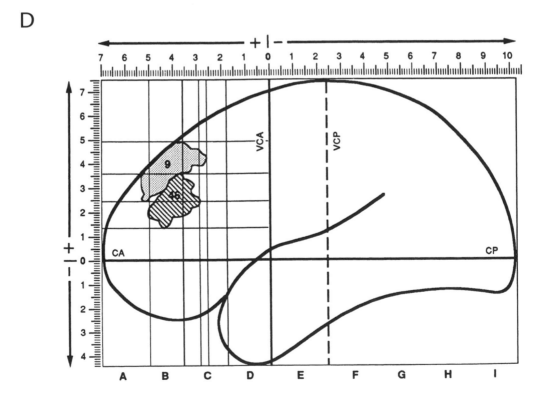

Rajkowska & Goldman-Rakic (1994)

appears to be much greater in the homotypical than in the hetero-typical areas of the cortex. Casual comparison of an identified area in a small number of brains might very well lead one to question the cytoarchitectonic criteria, absent more extensive study. I suspect that almost every neuroscientist, when first confronted with Nissl-stained sections of the neocortex, has been haunted by the doubts expressed by Lashley and Clark and Bonin and Bailey.

Nevertheless, Lashley and Clark were wrong, for discoveries made since their study have confirmed to a remarkable degree many of the parcellations of the cytoarchitectonists. This is especially clear in what von Economo called the heterotypical areas of the cortex, the primary motor and sensory areas. However, exceptions have been discovered in what von Economo called the homotypical (sometimes "association") regions, which appear more uniform when viewed in Nissl-stained sections. Several of these cytoarchitecturally uniform fields have now been shown to contain more than one—sometimes many—clearly separate areas. This was revealed in degeneration and tracing studies of inter-areal connections; by use of the cytochrome oxidase method, in which the enzyme cytochrome oxidase of the neuronal mitochondria is stained, thus differentiating areas by their level of metabolic activity; by immunohistochemical methods that uncovered areal biochemical differences; and by electrophysiological methods that defined the functional properties of the neurons of an area by recording the actions of single neurons. Further parcellations of the classic Brodmann areas have been made in the homotypical cortex of the frontal, temporal, and parietal lobes, but most dramati-cally in the prestriate areas of the occipital lobe. Here as many as thirty areas have been defined in a large region in which Brodmann defined only two, areas 18 and 19. Each has its own—frequently distorted—representation of the visual field; each has a defining set of extrinsic connections; each contains neurons with identifiable sets of functional properties (Felleman and Van Essen, 1991).

Thus a cortical area can now be defined by one of these criteria, and in some cases congruently by all: it may possess a unique architec-

---

Fig. 4-5   The remarkable variation in the locations of areas 9 and 46 is displayed in the classical cytoarchitectonic maps at top, prepared by Brodmann, von Economo and Koskinas, and Sarkisov. At bottom, shading marks the area of com-mon overlap of the five cytoarchitectonic reconstructions shown in Fig. 4-4. (From Rajkowska and Goldman-Rakic, 1995b.)

ture, an identifying set of extrinsic connections, and neurons that have unique sets of functional properties. The cortical projection zones of specific thalamic nuclei converge with cytoarchitecture to define some areas of the heterotypical cortex, but it is now clear that many other cortical areas that receive a major and specific projection from one thalamic nucleus also receive overlapping projections from other nuclei (Jones, 1985, p. 810; Darian-Smith et al., 1997). Fig. 4-6 shows the differences in structure between the precentral motor and the postcentral somatic sensory cortical areas in the macaque monkey. These heterotypical areas have different extrinsic connections; the cells of the motor cortex are active before and during intentional movements, those of the postcentral are activated by mechanical stimulation of body tissues.

The transition from area 1 to area 2 on the exposed surface of the postcentral gyrus, shown in Fig. 4-6, is a more subtle case. Some students of cytoarchitecture have denied that an area 2 exists, although the two regions have different patterns of extrinsic connections and important differences in the functional properties of their cells. Neurons of area 1 subtend receptive fields limited to single fingers; those of area 2 are related to fields that cover the skin of several fingers (Darian-Smith et al., 1984; Iwamura et al., 1980) and are differentially sensitive to the direction of moving stimuli, but insensitive to the frequency of oscillating mechanical stimuli delivered to the glabrous skin of the contralateral hand. The two areas of homotypical cortex that line the banks of the intraparietal sulcus in the monkey resemble one another closely. Experts may discern differences in the pyramidal cells of layers III and V of the two areas, or in the thicknesses of various layers, but these differences are not at all obvious. However, these two areas have quite different patterns of extrinsic connections, receive thalamocortical afferents from different thalamic nuclei, and make different corticocortical connections. Moreover, neurons of area 5 are active in the somesthetic sphere, those in area 7 in the visuo-spatial.

How cytoarchitectural areas are specified and their boundaries established in development is discussed in Chapter 9, particularly whether areas are prespecified in the germinal epithelium before migration and/or after migration and during the development of extrinsic connections. The importance of these two factors in determining neocortical areas appears to differ between species with short and long gestational periods—e.g., between rodents and primates. The

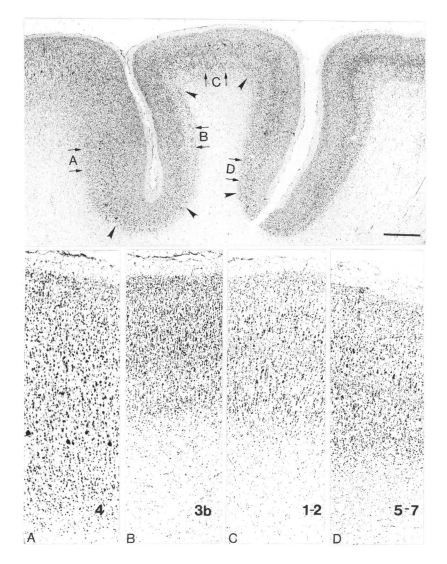

Fig. 4-6 (Above) Photomicrograph of a section of the pre- and postcentral gyri of the cortex of a macaque monkey, made normal to the line of the central sulcus; Nissl stain; calibration bar = 1.5 mm. Large arrows indicate transition points between cytoarchitectural areas. *A, B, C,* and *D* key the locations of the four photomicrographs shown below, respectively from areas 4 (panel A), 3b (B), 1–2 (C), and 5–7 (D). Calibration bar above = 0.4 mm for the lower illustrations. (Photomicrographs by Professor Stewart Hendry.)

second proposition is that both cytoarchitectural and functional differences between cortical areas are the result of differences in the sources, targets, and densities of the afferent and efferent extrinsic connections of different cortical areas. This generalization converges with the notion that the neuronal processing mechanisms within neocortical areas are more alike than different: a basic uniformity prevails, upon which local differences may be superimposed. Alternatively, it might be that the nature of intracortical processing differs in different regions because the local synaptic and circuit operations differ. I believe this problem can be solved by a further development and application to many different areas—and especially in primate brains—of the methods of electrophysiological study in brain-slice preparations described in Chapter 5.

The facts of cytoarchitecture provide a language in which to speak of different cortical areas. They served for decades as guides to experimental procedures such as lesion making or electrophysiological recording. The classic Nissl method has now been combined with new methods by which cortical areas can be specified more exactly and their extrinsic connections defined. The result is an explosion in our knowledge of the number of cortical areas and their connectivity, which has led to the new qualitative understanding of neocortical organization described in the following chapters.

The Myeloarchitecture of the Neocortex

Axons within the cerebral cortex are myelinated by the action of oligodendrocytes, each of which myelinates segments of many axons. This process of myelination differs greatly in ontogenetic time between different mammals and between different cortical areas in the same brain. The myelination of axons in the human brain is completed only many months after birth. Flechsig (1920; see also Meyer, 1981) used these differences to classify different regions of the cerebral cortex in terms of their times to maturity of myelination, and on this basis generated the idea of "association" cortical areas, those maturing late and not directly linked to afferent systems (Fig. 4-7).

The majority of axons of intracortical neurons and of the major thalamocortical afferent and the efferent systems are myelinated. The difference in neuron distributions between different layers carries with it the implication of differences in the number and size distributions of myelinated fibers. Cortical areas differ in the pattern of vertical and horizontal myelinated fibers. Some areas, for example, have two clear stripes of Baillarger, others have none. The vertical bundles of fibers may differ in their density and their translaminar extent. Variations such as these are the basis of myeloarchitecture, which has been used to define six layers that are virtually congruent with the six defined cytoarchitecturally. The Vogts (1919) defined

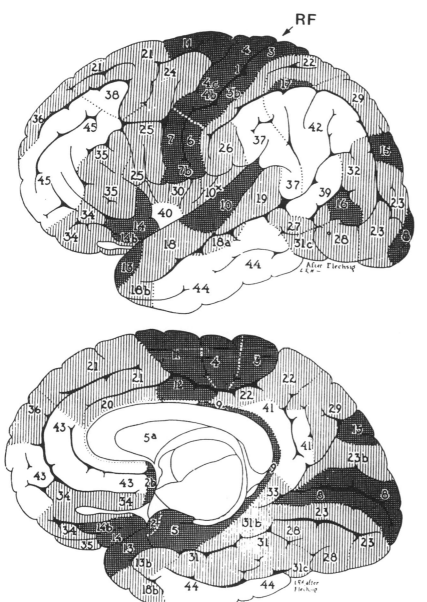

Fig. 4-7 Lateral and medial surfaces of the human hemisphere; diagrams summarize the myelogenetic studies of Flechsig (1920). Cortical fields are numbered in their order of myelination. Shaded zones with low numbers are those whose afferent and efferent fibers are myelinated earliest, unshaded areas with high numbers are myelinated later in ontogenesis and in the neonatal period. For a full explanation, see Meyer (1981).

The Organization of the Neocortex

more than 200 areas in the human cortex with this method and believed that the two sets of areas determined by myelo- and cyto-architecture mapped accurately one upon the other. The myeloarchitectural method has fallen into disuse in recent decades, perhaps because of the capricious nature of the original myelin staining methods. However, recently improved staining methods have been useful in defining areas in the prestriate cortex of the monkey and areas of the primate frontal lobe (Preuss and Goldman-Rakic, 1991). Many cortical areas contain local, repetitive variations in cyto- and myeloarchitectural structure. The most intensively studied of these is the barrel area in the somatic sensory cortex of rodents, described in Chapter 7.

Chemoarchitecture

Chemoarchitecture is the selective definition of cortical areas by the expression of different molecules within neurons in those areas. Specification in terms of different synaptic transmitters used by systems afferent to different areas falls under another rubric, one that includes the cholinergic, dopaminergic, adrenergic, and serotonergic systems arising from the brainstem and the basal forebrain. These systems impose their own special architecture upon the neocortex.

The oldest of the true chemoarchitectural methods is pigmentoarchitecture, which depends upon the fact that some neurons store in the cytoplasm of the cell body a neurally specific and selectively stainable pigment, lipofuscin. The amount of pigment stored varies between neuronal phenotypes: pyramidal cells are frequently heavily pigmented, nonpyramidal cells seldom so. The degree of pigmentation also varies between the neurons in different cortical layers, and pigment stains reveal the classical six laminae with particular clarity. (See the histological preparation of the human pre- and postcentral gyri in Fig. 4-8.) The pattern of organization also varies between different cortical areas, and Braak has used this areal variation in extensive architectonic studies of the cortices of many mammals, including humans (Braak 1980, 1984). His (still incomplete) pigmentoarchitectonic map of the human cortex is shown in Fig. 4-9. Braak found the combination of Nissl and Golgi stains to be especially useful. The method has not been widely applied in studies of the cerebral cortex, however, perhaps because the degree of pigment deposit in cortical neurons varies greatly and increases with age. It has thus

The Organization of the Neocortex

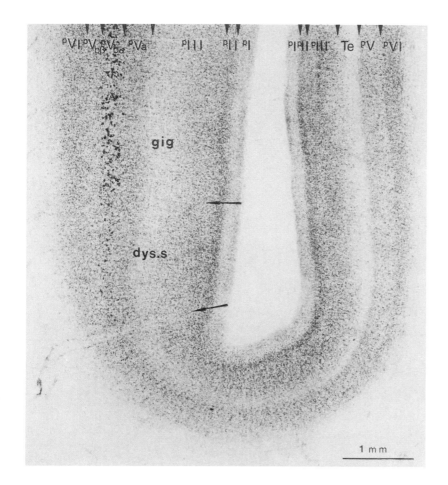

Fig. 4-8 A microscopic section of the human neocortex cut at a right angle to the central sulcus close to the paracentral lobule to display the motor and somatic sensory areas, left and right. The pigment-stained section reveals the large Betz cells in the motor cortex and the fusion of layers II, III, and IV in area 3b of the postcentral somatic sensory cortex. Compare with the Nissl-stained section of Fig. 4-6. The one labeled *gig* is the "gigantoganglionic core field." The transition to the dysgranular cortex *(dys)* may mark a transitional zone to area 3a. The postcentral cortex to the right, called the parietal granulomatous core, is more or less equivalent to area 3b. (From Braak, 1980.)

been useful in studies of aging of the brain and of certain neuro-pathological conditions.

The advent of the new methods of molecular biology, as well as fluorescent- and immunocytochemistry, in the last decades stimulated a large and still continuing research program in many laboratories. Its aim is to explore whether a cortical architecture could be defined in terms of the differential expression of molecules in neurons in different cortical areas, and/or upon a differential distribution of transmitters and their receptor molecules. This effort is now in full flower, and what the final outcome will be is uncertain, but until now no set or sets of cell markers have been identified that label cortical areas with the precision of the older methods of cyto- and myeloar-

Fig. 4-9 A map of the major regions of the human neocortex, prepared with the method of pigment staining. Compare with the maps of Brodmann, Fig. 4-1, and of Sarkisov, Fig. 4-3. *ag,* anterogenual core; *cm,* cingulate magnoganglionic core; *e,* entorhinal region; *fb,* frontal paraglionic belt; *fgc,* frontal ganglionic core; *ifm,* inferofrontal magnopyramidal region; *ob,* occipital paragranulous belt; *pg,* paragenual belt; *pgc,* parietal granulous core; *pl,* paralimbic areas; *pm,* parietal magnopyramidal region; *ps,* parasplenial belt; *rs,* retrosplenial core; *s,* subcentral region; *sfm,* superofrontal magnopyramidal region; *tb,* temporal paragranulous belt; *tgc,* temporal granulous core. The regions indicated by fine stippling have not been specified in detail. (From Braak, 1980.)

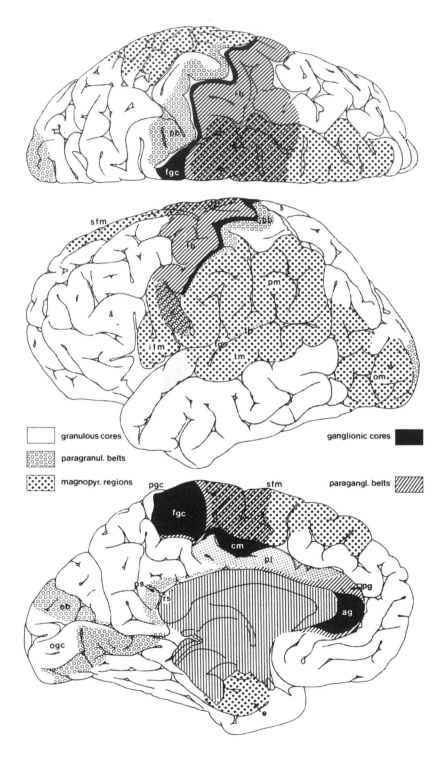

granulous cores	ganglionic cores
paragranul. belts	
magnopyr. regions	paragangl. belts

The Organization of the Neocortex

chitecture. The general result appears to be that a chemoarchitecture does exist that is mapped on a larger and less precise scale than that of previously defined cortical areas, for some clear differences and more often gradual trends have been observed between such large entities as cortical lobes.

A clear example is the discovery by Levitt and his colleagues that a particular cell-surface glycoprotein is expressed only by neurons of the limbic lobe, and nowhere else (Levitt, 1984; Zacco et al., 1990). This limbic-associated membrane protein (LAMP) is expressed on the surfaces of both axons and neuron somata of the developing limbic structures, but in the mature cortex only on the somata of limbic lobe neurons (Horton and Levitt, 1988). There is some evidence that LAMP is a nondiffusible attractant molecule for thalamocortical axons growing into the developing limbic cortex, and that it is important for this specific pattern of thalamocortical connectivity (Barbe and Levitt, 1992). A second example is the discovery that a large extracellular proteoglycan, CAT 301, is specifically expressed by the motion-sensitive components of the visual system in cats and monkeys from the level of the lateral geniculate to the prestriate visual cortex (DeYoe et al., 1990). This discovery suggests that there may develop a system-specific chemical architecture not limited to a single cortical area.

Spatial Distribution of Cell Numbers and Cell Types

The Size and Surface Area of the Human Brain

A persistent problem in human neuroanatomy has been to determine precisely the weight and volume of the human brain and the surface area of the human cerebral cortex; witness the wide variations in measurements tabulated in the monograph by Blinkov and Glezer (1968). Filapek et al. (1994) used the method of magnetic resonance imaging to obtain precise measures of brain volumes in 20 young adults. When converted from volume to weight, the mean value is 1,370 g (SD = 81 g) (Table 4-1). The brain nears adult size by the age of 6 years and grows somewhat more rapidly in females than in males during the first four years of life (Kretschmann et al., 1979). The measurements of Filapek et al. support the general conclusions of many earlier studies that the overall volume of the female brain of young adult humans is about 10 percent less than that of males. This difference was observed by them in a population of 10 males and 10

Table 4-1. Numerical measures of the human brain.

Measure	Value	Range
1. Brain weight	1,370 g	1,130–1610 (3 SDs)
2. Cortical surface	2,600 cm^2	1,830–3,560 cm^2
3. Cortical thickness	1.4–4.0 mm	
4. Number of neurons	27.4 × 10^9	CV = 12 percent
5. Number ontogenetic units of diameter 30 μm	368 × 10^6	258–505 × 10^6
6. Number of columns of diameter 300 μm	3.7 × 10^6	2.6–5.0 × 10^6
7. Ontogenetic units per column	c. 100	
8. Neurons per ontogenetic column	c. 75–80	
9. Neurons per column	c. 7,500–8,000	
10. Neurons beneath 1 mm^2 surface	c. 113,000	

Notes:
1. From Filapek et al., 1994; weight = volume/1.05.
2. General average of many studies; values vary from 2,000 to 3,000 cm^2.
3. Thinnest in area 17, thickest in area 4.
4. From Braengaard et al., 1990.
5–8. Calculated using the counts of Powell and Hendrikson in frozen sections (79.4 per counting unit with surface of 25 × 30 μm, through the depths of area 18 in monkeys).
4–6. Ranges are calculated from brain surface area, on the assumption of linear change in neuron number with surface area.
5. Calculated as total surface area/surface area of a minicolumn of 30 μm.
6. The ontogenetic unit is thought to be the equivalent of the minicolumn.
7. Neutrons beneath 1 mm^2 surface area of the striate cortex are about 2.5 × this figure.

females, but was barely significant. The difference was mainly due to larger volumes of the cerebellum and cerebral white matter in males, partially offset by a larger volume of the caudate nucleus and the hippocampus in females. Sexual dimorphisms of the brain have been described in many species and studied intensively, but the causes of these differences and their meaning for brain function remain uncertain (see Gorski, 1985; Goy and McEwen, 1980; Kimura, 1992; Kertesz et al., 1990).

An unsettled question is whether there is any correlation between brain size in humans and intellectual or artistic achievement. I believe it fair to say that no general correlation has been established. However, some extraordinary cases have been studied. For example, a study of the brain of Albert Einstein has just been made. Witelson et al. (1997) compared Einstein's brain with those of 35 men who had undergone intelligence testing and were free of neurologic or psychiatric disease. Einstein's brain was in the normal range in overall size (fresh brain weight 1,230 grams) but was unique in the morphology of the sylvian fissure, in both hemispheres. This resulted in a remarkable expansion of the parietal lobes. The brain width at the parietal level was 15 percent above the average value. These two features resulted in an enlargement of the retrosylvian expanse of the parietal lobe in both dimensions. The authors suggest that the parietal enlargement may have provided a substrate for an extraordinary ability to generate and manipulate mental images. What is needed now is an extended study of brain volumes in living gifted individuals, using methods of imaging such as that used by Filapek et al.

The true value for the surface area of the human brain is uncertain, but 2,600 cm^2 is modal for many measurements, which vary between 2,000 and 3,000 cm^2 (see, e.g., Elias and Schwartz, 1971; Haug, 1987; Hofman, 1982). Surface area varies directly with brain size, as shown in Figs. 2-6 and 2-7. It is not known whether differences in brain size are due to differences in number of neurons or in number of glial cells, to variations in the volume of extracellular space, or to some combination of these. Several values of Table 4-1 are based on the assumption of a linear relation between neuron number and surface area, for which there is no direct evidence. The thickness of the human cortex varies from 2.5 mm in striate area 17 to 4.0 mm in motor area 4, with an average of 2.87 mm (Schlenska, 1969). Thickness varies by less than a factor of 3 over a wide range of mammalian cortices.

Values for the brain of the macaque monkey, the primate most commonly used in brain research, are: weight, 90–100 g; surface area, from 100 to 200 cm^2 (widely varying values reported); total neuron number, 1.8–2.3 billion.

Numerical Parameters of the Neocortex

Simple inspection of a microscopic section of the cerebral cortex reveals that cell density and cortical thickness vary between different layers and areas in the same brain, as well as between different species. Neurons are more closely packed in layer IV, for example, than in other layers, and in general the cortex is thicker in large brains than in smaller ones. How cortical thickness differs between different areas is shown for areas 4 and 7a in Fig. 4-10. The greatest differences in thickness occur in the pyramidal cell layers III and V. It was therefore totally unexpected that careful counts of the number of cells beneath any unit area of the cortical surface in any one of a number of mammals yielded virtually identical values. Powell and his colleagues (Rockel et al., 1974, 1980; Powell, 1981) counted the number of neurons and the proportions of the major neuron types in a vertical cylinder extending from the pial surface to the white matter in a number of areas and species, including man. The numbers are virtually identical for all areas in all species, except for area 17 in primates, where the counts are more than doubled (7 primate species examined). The original counts were made in fixed brains without compensation for shrinkage; they ranged around 100–110 cells per counting unit, i.e., the column of cortex beneath a pial patch 25×30 μm in size. Later counts by Powell and Hendrikson (1981) made in frozen sections with presumably minimal shrinkage yielded counts of about 75–80 cells in the same counting unit, except for the commensurably higher count in area 17. Table 4-2 shows these extraordinary results, here transformed to take account of tissue shrinkage.

These findings were confirmed and extended by Hendry et al. (1987) in studies of the distribution of GABAergic nonpyramidal neurons in the monkey neocortex. These latter authors observed a uniformity of counts in 7 different areas of neocortex and in 5 different monkeys (Table 4-3). In this study the ratio of cell numbers in area 17 to that in other areas was about 2.0. The data of Hendry et al. provide evidence for a similarity in the proportions of neuron numbers, and of the different cell types, in different areas of the neocortex in the primate. The identity of the numbers of neurons in vertical arrays extending across the cortical layers normal to the pial surface is wholly consonant with—in fact is predicted by—the radial unit hypothesis of Rakic described in Chapter 8.

The Number of Neurons and Glial Cells in the Cerebral Cortex

Gunderson, West, and their colleagues at the Aarhus University in Denmark have solved the problem of the total neuron counts in the cerebral cortex by applying new stereological and optical dissector methods that allowed them to make unbiased estimates of the total number of neurons in the human neocortex (Braengaard et al. (1990); Gunderson (1986); for description of the methods, see West,

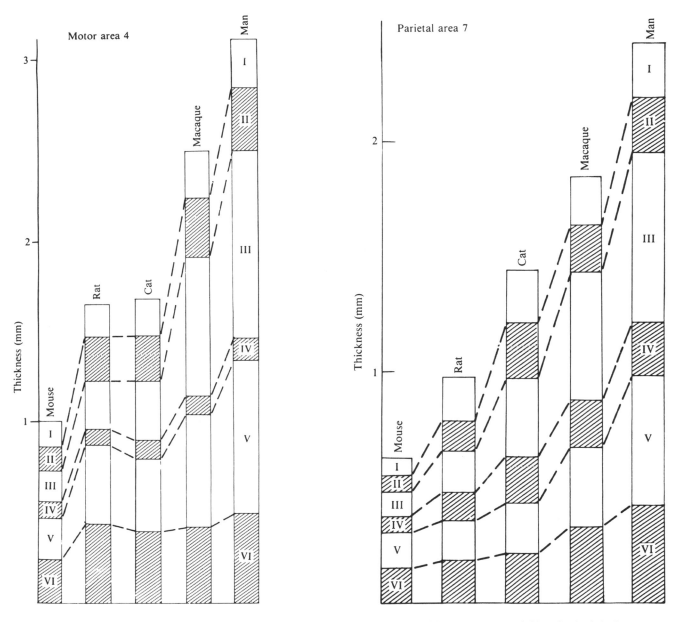

Fig. 4-10 Comparison of total cortical thickness and thickness of each of the cortical layers in areas 4 *(left)* and 7 *(right)* of mouse, rat, cat, macaque monkey, and man. The total number of cells is virtually the same in the vertical dimension of the cortex, except for primate area 17; see Tables 4-2 and 4-3. (From Rockel et al., 1980.)

Table 4-2. Number of neurons beneath pial patches (25 × 30 μm) in several areas of the cerebral cortex in five mammals.

Mammal	Translaminar cell count (± SD)						
	Motor	Sensory	Frontal	Temporal	Parietal	Visual	Means
Mouse	73.4±4.5	75.2±4.6	74.5±6.8	74.3±4.4	70.4±6.8	75.4±4.30	73.8±4.6
Rat	72.7±3.9	71.9±6.8	70.1±6.8	72.4±6.2	70.7±4.6	72.4±5.3	71.6±4.9
Cat	69.8±5.1	71.6±6.8	72.6±4.2	76.5±4.9	74.3±6.7	73.8±6.7	73.6±4.9
Monkey	74.1±6.3	73.5±6.3	75.3±7.5	73.8±6.9	77.0±6.7	180.0±9.2	—
Man	68.7±6.5	69.7±3.9	69.4±5.8	72.4±5.0	70.0±8.4	174.0±10.6	—

Note: Numbers transformed from original counts of Rockel et al. (1974) to account for section shrinkage. Patches of area 25 × 30 μm = 750 μm² were noted to display linear shrinkage of 18 percent. Original size of the patches was therefore 25/.82 × 30/.82 = 1,116 μm². A conversion factor of 750/1,116 = 0.672 was therefore multiplied by the original counts.

Table 4-3. Number of neurons in a 50 × 30 μm patch running from the pial surface into the white matter, for 5 cynemolgus monkeys.

Area	Count (±SD)					Mean
	CM 181	CM 187	CM 183	CM 189	CM 184	
4	158.9±16.1	159.4±16.3	161.7±15.3	161.6±17.0	157.1±15.5	159.7
3b	152.7±4.9	154.9±11.7	157.9±12.2	156.5±12.7	160.4±11.0	156.5
1–2	154.8±14.2	157.9±16.1	154.3±11.6	158.8±11.9	154.9±9.7	156.1
5	163.1±10.6	160.6±14.1	155.3±9.4	155.5±12.0	158.1±13.0	158.4
7	158.2±9.4	158.8±14.8	157.6±11.8	160.1±16.5	159.9±11.7	158.9
18	157.3±10.1	157.9±15.0	152.0±9.1	157.5±17.5	158.4±16.2	156.6
17	315.7±19.4	309.9±22.7	309.8±17.1	321.3±23.6	319.6±21.4	315.3
21	161.4±10.4			156.4±11.2		158.9
Infero-frontal	157.6±9.0			158.9±12.2		158.3
Lateral frontal	163.1±12.1			160.4±14.1		161.8

Note: Except for some difference in the counts for area 17, these numbers are comparable to those in Table 4-2 (i.e., for unshrunk tissue). Reprinted from S. H. C. Hendrey et al., "Numbers and proportions of GABA-immunoreactive neurons in different areas of the monkey cerebral cortex," *Journal of Neuroscience* 7(5): 1505 (1987).

1993). They found the total number of neurons in the cortices of five 80-year-old men to average 27.4 billion, with a coefficient of variation of 12 percent. It is virtually a miraculous coincidence that if one multiplies the count of 75–80 neurons in Powell's unshrunk cylinders and the average surface area of the human neocortex of 2,600 cm^2, the total number of neurons in the human neocortex is between 26.0 and 29.3 billion! O'Kusky and Colonnier (1982) found the number of glial cells in the visual cortex to be one-half that of neurons. However, they conjectured that the glia-to-neuron ratio might be 2–3 times that value in other areas of the neocortex. This was confirmed by Haug (1987), who found that overall the densities of glial and neuronal cells were about the same, even though he also noted a much wider variation in glial cell than in neuron numbers.

Powell et al. used ultrastructural criteria to identify and count pyramidal, large nonpyramidal, and small nonpyramidal cells in the neocortex (Winfield et al., 1980; Sloper, 1973; Sloper et al., 1979). They found a nearly constant ratio between these cell types in all areas studied in rat, cat, and monkey. About two-thirds were pyramidal cells, less than a third small nonpyramidal cells, and less than 10 percent large nonpyramidal cells. The proportions were the same in different areas, even though the total numbers of neurons differed by a factor of 2.6 between striate and other areas of the monkey cortex. This implies that an identical number of efferent axons (of pyramidal cells) is emitted from each unit area of the neocortex, save for area 17. Differential distributions of the major neuron types were observed in different layers of the neocortex in different areas, a factor that contributes to the architectural differences described above.

The Number and Types of Synapses in the Cerebral Cortex

There are about 440×10^6 synaptic terminals per cubic millimeter in the visual cortex, where each neuron on average receives 3,900 synaptic terminals (Beaulieu and Colonnier, 1985). Of these, 17 percent are GABA-positive and thus inhibitory, as are 20 percent of visual cortical neurons. It is clear from these findings, and from earlier studies of Hendry et al. (1987), that the proportions of excitatory and inhibitory neurons are similar in the visual and other areas of the monkey cortex. In the latter, excitatory terminals (i.e., GABA-negative) were found almost exclusively upon the dendritic spines and shafts of target neurons, and only rarely on cell bodies. The surprising finding was that 88 percent of the inhibitory synapses were also located on dendritic spines and shafts, and only 12 percent on cell bodies. It is not yet possible to give exact divergent-convergent numbers for any synaptic transfer in any transcortical channel, but cortical neurons are with few exceptions heavily invested with presynaptic terminals. Estimates vary from the 3,900 per visual cortical neuron in the monkey (Beaulieu et al., 1992) to 6,000–18,000 for cells in the rat visual cortex (DeFelipe and Farinas, 1992). The numbers of synapses per neuron and the distribution between initial segments, somata, dendrites, and spines vary greatly from one cell type to another, and from one area to another, but the numbers are uniformly large. This contrasts with the fact that any single presynaptic stem axon in the cortex seldom delivers more than 10 terminals to any single target cell, and frequently only 1 or 2. Intracortical synaptic systems are thus highly divergent and convergent, with ratios that vary between 100 and 1,000, except for the irreciprocal relations between basket and chandelier cells and pyramids, where divergence is great, convergence small. The arrangement so described raises the general question of how to account for the elegantly precise cortical operations if they are carried out in such a sloppy system. The answer is by population coding, described in Chapter 11.

The Relation of Numerical Parameters to Cytoarchitecture: Resolution of a Paradox

An apparent contradiction exists between the two sets of facts described above: cytoarchitectural differences exist in a neocortex with uniform numbers of neurons beneath any unit surface area. These differences could be created in two ways, and perhaps both play a role. The differences in phenotype numbers and packing densities in different layers and in different areas could be produced by a nonlinear distribution of stop-points in the transcortical dimension of neurons migrating from the neuroepithelium into the cortical plate, given differences in those nonlinearities between different areas. They could also be produced by differences in afferent innervation patterns. Heterotypical areas receive a heavy thalamocortical input and a much lighter one from other cortical areas, while homotypical areas receive a more balanced innervation. These differences in efferent and afferent innervation patterns commonly occur at the transition points between cortical areas defined by cytoarchitectural criteria.

Synaptic Transmission in the Neocortex

Three sets of discoveries form the basis for present knowledge of synaptic transmission between cerebral cortical neurons. The first is the ionic hypothesis of Hodgkin and Huxley, a major principle of neuroscience that provides explanations for excitation and conduction in nerve axons. All neural action depends upon the slight temporal stagger between the changes in Na^+ and K^+ membrane conductance Hodgkin and Huxley discovered to be the critical events of the nerve impulse (Fig. 5-1; Hodgkin, 1964). The ionic hypothesis is now incorporated in all schemes of synaptic transmission, and its principles apply to ligand- as well as voltage-gated channel action. A molecular explanation of the voltage-gated signaling in nerve axons has been provided by the cloning, subunit sequencing, and determination of the physical structure of the relevant Na^+, K^+, and Cl^- channels.

The second major step in understanding synaptic transmission is the series of discoveries made by Bernard Katz and J. C. Eccles, whose work revealed the nature of the transfer of excitation from one cell to another: from nerve axon to muscle cell at the neuromuscular junction (Katz, 1969), and from primary afferents to motoneurons in the mammalian spinal cord (Eccles, 1964). They established the chemical nature of peripheral and central synaptic transmission. Eccles's discovery of the local excitatory and inhibitory postsynaptic responses of neurons led to an understanding of integrative action at the cellular level. This model of synaptic transmission was established by Eccles (1964) in experiments carried out on spinal motoneurons more than forty years ago.

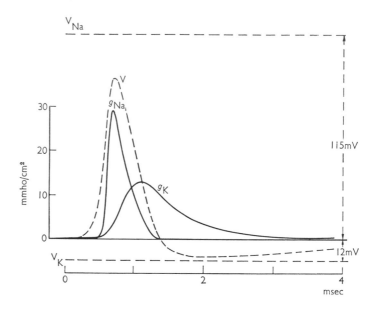

Fig. 5-1 Theoretical solutions for the propagated action potential and Na$^+$ and K$^+$ in the giant axon of *Loligo;* temperature 10.5 °C. The opening and closing of the voltage-gated Na$^+$ and K$^+$ channels follow different time courses. Na$^+$ conductance rises rapidly, and the inward flow of Na$^+$ions (4/33 pmole/cm^2) accounts for the rising phase of the action potential. K$^+$ conductance (4.26 pmole/cm^2) rises more slowly, and the outward flow of K$^+$ ions accounts for the falling phase. The slowing in the rise in Na$^+$ conductance is due to an inactivation process, that of K$^+$ to repolarization. Membrane potential is graphed in millivolts (scale at right) and conductance in mmho/cm^2 (scale at left). (From Hodgkin and Huxley, 1952.)

The third foundation of our knowledge of synaptic transmission rests on the use of new methods to outline the morphology of cortical neurons, the introduction of the cortical slice preparation for studying the biophysical properties of cortical neurons and their synaptic responses, the perfection of the method of intracellular recording in the intact and recently in the waking mammal, and the use of the methods of molecular biology to identify transmitters, receptors, and second-messenger systems. A major discovery is that plasticity is an almost universal property of central synapses.

The Biophysical Properties of Cortical Neurons Vary with Neuron Type

The integration of its biophysical properties with its responses to synaptic inputs determines a cortical neuron's pattern of impulse discharge. The biophysical properties of neurons observed by recording intracellularly in explanted slices form the basis for a functional taxonomy of cortical neurons. Identifications are made by the shape and the time course of the action potential, the response of the cell to brief threshold currents, and the pattern of discharge evoked by sustained suprathreshold current stimuli. The differences observed between cells are attributed to differences in the density and spatial distribution of voltage-gated ion channels in cell membranes.

The responses of three major classes of cortical neurons to trans-membrane current pulses are shown in Fig. 5-2, and the properties of the several classes are summarized in Table 5-1 (Amitai and Connors, 1995; Connors and Gutnick, 1990).

Regular-Spiking Neurons

Regular-spiking neurons (RS-1, RS-2) respond to brief transmembrane depolarizing pulses with single impulse discharges. After sustained depolarizations, they respond with repetitive discharges that slow from an initial peak at 200–300 spikes/sec to a steady rate of 50–100 spikes/sec after 500 msec (for class RS-1 cells) or to zero (for RS-2

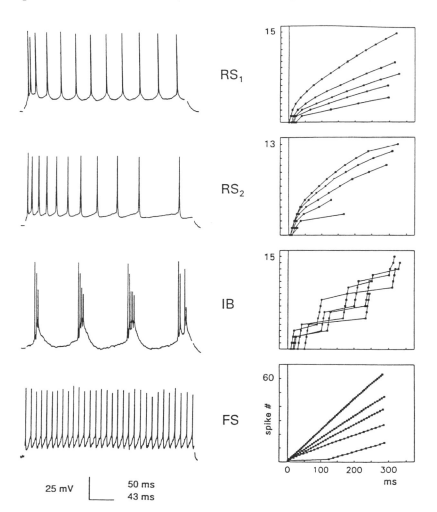

Fig. 5-2   Patterns of impulse discharge of different classes of cortical neurons. The intracellular records of the left column were made in slice preparations of the mouse somatic sensory cortex; the neurons were activated by step current pulses delivered intracellularly between the two artifacts (blanks). Regular-spiking neurons (RS-1 and RS-2) and intrinsically bursting (IB) cells are spiny pyramidal cells; fast-spiking cells (FS) are nonpyramidal inhibitory interneurons. RS-1 and RS-2 cells differ only in rate of spike adaptation; RS-2 are found only in the infragranular layers, and the IB cells only in layer V. The varying amplitude of the FS spikes is a digitalization artifact. In the right column are graphs with each spike plotted serially in time after stimulus onset—they are instantaneous frequency plots. The time scales differ for the RS and FS records. A. Agmon and B. W. Connors, "Correlation between intrinsic firing patterns and thalamocortical synaptic responses of neurons in mouse barrel cortex," *Journal of Neuroscience* 12(1): 319–329 (1992).

Table 5-1. Biophysical properties of cortical neuron classes.

	Cell class			
	Regular spiking (RS-1)	Regular spiking (RS-2)	Intrinsically bursting (IB)	Fast spiking (FS)
Spike duration[a]	0.5–1.0 msec	0.5–1.0 msec	0.5–1.0 msec	0.2–0.3 msec
After potentials[b]	Fast, medium, and slow AHP; medium ADP	Monophasic AHP	Strong AHP	Brief, strong AHP
Response to brief stimuli	Single spike at threshold	Single spike at threshold	Threshold response 3–5 spikes at 150–200/sec	Train of high-frequency spikes
Response to maintained depolarization	Adaptation to 50–100 spikes/sec	Rapid adaptation to zero	Bursts recur at 5–15/sec	Nonadapting high-frequency response to 300–500 spikes/sec
Cell morphology	Spiny pyramidal or spiny nonpyramidal	Spiny pyramidal or spiny nonpyramidal	Spiny pyramidal or spiny nonpyramidal	Nonspiny, nonpyramidal inhibitory interneuron
Axonal target	Corticocortical	Corticocortical	Brainstem and spinal cord	Local intracortical
Layers	II–VI	V–VI	IV–V (concentrated in lower V)	II–VI
Response to thalamocortical afferent	Disynaptic EPSPs; late IPSPs[c]	Monosynaptic EPSPs; disynaptic IPSPs	Disynaptic EPSPs; weak, late IPSPs	Strong monosynaptic EPSPs; ?IPSPs

a. Durations are at one-half spike amplitude; values from McCormick et al. (1985). Values for RS and IB cells vary with species and preparation, but are always much longer than are those for FS cells.

b. AHP = after-hyperpolarization; ADP = after-depolarization.

c. RS-1 cells of the infragranular layers may respond with monosynaptic EPSPs to thalamocortical volleys.

cells). Spike frequency adapts to the sustained depolarization because the activation of two K^+ currents (I_M and I_{AHP}) tends to hyperpolarize the cell membrane. Spiny pyramidal cells and spiny nonpyramidal cells are both RS-1 cells. RS-1 cells of the supragranular layers respond to thalamocortical volleys with disynaptically relayed excitatory postsynaptic potentials (EPSPs). RS-1 cells of the infragranular layers, all RS-2 cells, and spiny nonpyramidal cells respond with monosynaptically evoked EPSP's. Both classes of RS cells produce disynaptically evoked IPSPs that are more powerful in supragranular than infragranular cells. RS spiny pyramidal cells project their axons to other cortical areas; the axons of the spiny nonpyramidal cells project locally to other cortical neurons.

Intrinsically Bursting Neurons

Intrinsically bursting (IB) neurons respond to brief depolarizing current pulses at, or slightly above, threshold with a high-frequency burst of 3–5 impulses riding on an intense depolarization. Sustained depolarization evokes a train of bursts at 5–15/sec that, over a few hundred milliseconds, may change to the single-spiking mode. That mode may be evoked directly by depolarizing pulses delivered on a background depolarization of e.g., −60 mV membrane potential. IB neurons are spiny pyramidal cells concentrated in layer Vb. Their axons project out of the cortex to brainstem and spinal cord.

Although the RS and IB cells of layer Vb are both spiny pyramidal cells, they differ in morphology (Chagnac-Amitai et al., 1990; Kasper et al., 1994). IB cells have larger somata and more extensive basilar dendritic trees, and their apical dendrites reach and arborize widely in layer I. IB axonal collaterals are limited to layers V and VI. RS neurons have smaller somata, their apical dendritic tufts are more limited and many do not reach layer I, and their ascending axonal collaterals branch widely in the supragranular layers. Gray and McCormick (1996) have recently identified a subclass of bursting neurons in the supragranular layers of the cat striate cortex that contribute to the gamma-band oscillations evoked by visual stimuli (see Chapter 12).

Fast-Spiking Neurons

Fast-spiking (FS) neurons discharge action potentials that repolarize rapidly (Fig. 5-3) (McCormick et al., 1985). They are nonspiny, non-

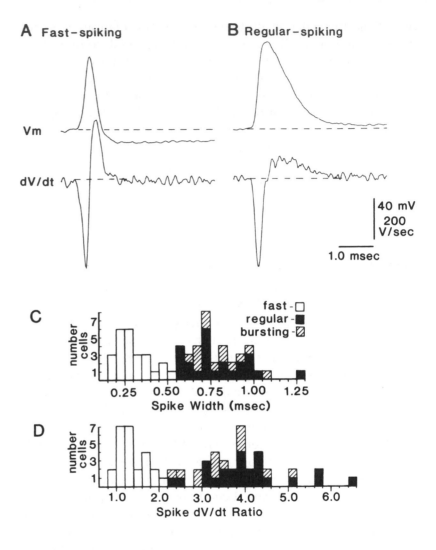

Fig. 5-3 Comparison of the properties of fast-spiking, regular-spiking, and initially bursting cortical neurons. Intracellular records were made in cortical slice preparations of guinea pig cortex. (A) Action potential of a fast-spiking neuron, the first spike evoked by a suprathreshold depolarizing current step. V_m = voltage trace; *dV/dt* = differentiated voltage record, positive downward. (B) Similar records for a regular-spiking neuron. (C) Distribution of the spike widths for RS, FS, and IB neurons, measured at half height. (D) Distribution of ratio of *dV/dt* for the rising phase of the spikes to *dV/dt* for the falling phases, for the three classes of cells. (From McCormick et al., 1985.)

pyramidal cells, the inhibitory interneurons of the cortex. FS neurons respond to brief transmembrane current pulses with high-frequency discharges (Fig. 5-2). Thalamocortical volleys evoke monosynaptically relayed EPSPs and disynaptic IPSPs in FS cells. These observations, made in cortical slice preparations, have been confirmed and extended by Baranyi et al. (1993a), who succeeded in obtaining stable intracellular recordings from a large number of neurons in the motor cortex of the waking cat. The researchers observed two subclasses of the initially bursting neurons, one inactivating and one

Synaptic Transmission in the Neocortex

not, but otherwise the findings of these several groups are similar. Baranyi et al. (1993b) also described the biophysical properties of the several classes of neocortical neurons.

The Single-Trigger-Zone Model of Central Synaptic Transmission

Eccles developed and used the methods of intracellular recording and the current clamp experiment in his studies of mammalian spinal motoneurons (Eccles, 1964). Some of his discoveries are illustrated in Fig. 5-4. An afferent volley excitatory for a motoneuron evokes a local depolarizing change in membrane potential, the excitatory postsynaptic response. The EPSP equilibrium potential is close to zero membrane potential, which indicates an increase in conductance for both Na^+ and K^+ (Fig. 5-4A). The excitatory transmitter at this synapse has since been identified as glutamate. Impulses in afferents inhibitory for the motoneuron under study evoke, via a linking inhibitory interneuron, a hyperpolarizing, inhibitory postsynaptic response. The IPSP equilibrium potential is several mV more negative than the resting membrane potential (Fig. 5-4B), indicating increases in either Cl^- or K^+ conductance. The transmitter of this inhibitory interneuron has since been identified as glycine, although GABA also induces inhibitory responses in spinal motoneurons.

The initial segment of the motoneuron's axon (the axon hillock) has a lower threshold for electrogenic action than do the soma or dendrites of the cell, which means that this part of the cell discharges an action potential before any other part (Fig. 5-4D), whether the cell is activated synaptically or antidromically (by stimulation of its own axon). The core proposition of the single-trigger-zone model is that the local postsynaptic currents are summed algebraically at the initial segment. The resultant determines the rate of discharge of action potentials by the cell (Fig. 5-4C). This summation may occur in either a linear or a nonlinear manner (Rall et al., 1967; Fig. 5-5). Nonlinearities result when active regions of postsynaptic membrane are close together, indicating that electrotonic extensions of local responses in one position can affect the driving potentials for local responses in adjacent regions of membrane.

Transmission at neocortical synapses is complicated by the biophysical properties of the various classes of neurons, by the electrogenic capacity of dendrites and the chemical sequestration function of their spines, by the many transmitters operating at cortical syn-

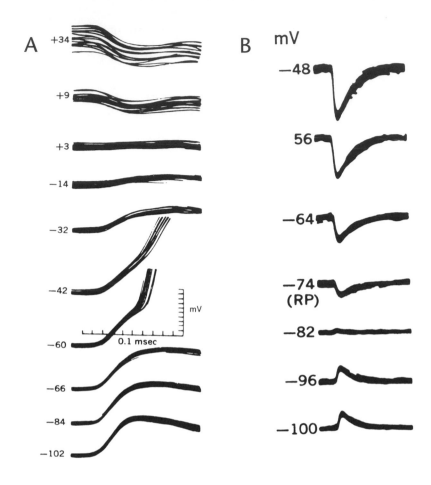

Fig. 5-4 Discoveries of J. C. Eccles and his colleagues in studies of synaptic transmission in the spinal cord.

(A) Records of excitatory postsynaptic potentials (EPSPs) evoked in a cat spinal motoneuron by monosynaptically related excitatory afferent volley. Each record is superimposed traces of about 40 responses. Steady membrane potential is maintained at a series of levels (mV) by passage of current. Depolarization upward; resting membrane potential *(RP)*, −66 mV. The EPSP reversed at about zero membrane potential. (From Coombs et al., 1955b.)

(B) Results of a similar experiment in which the afferent volleys were inhibitory for the spinal motoneuron under study. The inhibitory postsynaptic potential (IPSP) reversed at about −80 mV membrane potential. (From Coombs et al., 1955a.)

Synaptic Transmission in the Neocortex

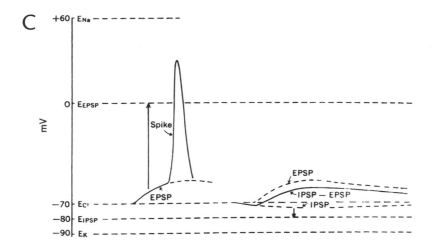

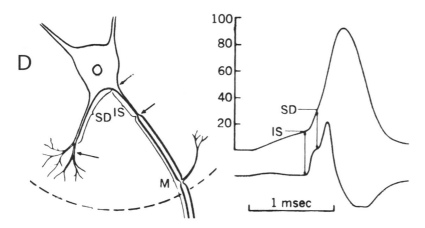

(C) Summary of the action of chemically operated synapses at spinal motoneurons. The equilibrium potentials for Na+, K+, Cl−, EPSP, and IPSP are
marked by dotted lines. At left, the EPSP is shown driving the membrane potential in a depolarizing direction and at threshold eliciting an action potential. At
right, EPSP and IPSP are shown alone (dotted lines) and when they interact (solid
line). (From Eccles, 1949.)

(D) *(Left)* Schematic diagram of motoneuron of cat spinal cord: a recurrent collateral leaves the axon at *M; IS* = initial segment of the axon; *SD* = one of the so-
madendritic parts of the neuron. (From Eccles, 1955.) *(Right)* Intracellular
recording of response of motoneurons to monosynaptically related excitatory afferent volley. The record below is differentiated, and illustrates that the initial segment is the site of spike initiation. (From Coombs et al., 1957.)

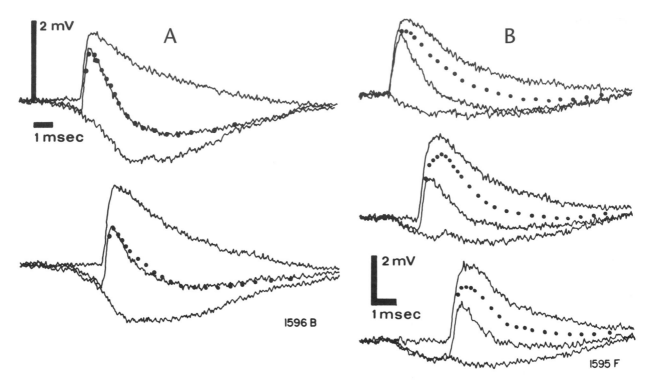

Fig. 5-5 Record of averaged postsynaptic potentials recorded intracellularly in motoneurons of cat spinal cord. Column A illustrates linear summation of EPSPs (upper trace of each set) and IPSPs (lower trace of each set). Middle records in each case were obtained when the two volleys reached the motoneuron simultaneously; they are neatly superimposed by the black dots that represent the algebraic summation of upper and lower records (the summation is linear). Column B illustrates the opposite case, obtained from another spinal motoneuron, where summation is clearly nonlinear. Most motoneurons studied in this way show intermediate degrees of nonlinearity. (From Rall et al., 1967.)

apses and the variety of postsynaptic responses they evoke, and by the number and variety of ion channels in cortical neurons. The general proposition that the axon hillock–initial axonal segment of the neuron is the lowest-threshold trigger zone for the initiation of action potentials has been confirmed in many studies of neocortical neurons.

Two principal modes of synaptic transmission in the neocortex operate through different molecular mechanisms and on different time scales (for reviews, see Jessell and Kandel, 1993; Changeux, 1996). Direct (fast) transmission is initiated by transmitter binding to a transmembrane protein that contains an intrinsic ion channel. The channel protein is composed of several subunits; the combination has allosteric properties. Binding of a ligand to a specific site on the receptor induces a conformational change in the latter and opens its ion channel. The resulting ionic current is determined in sign and amplitude by the ion channel, not the transmitter; the ionic current may be excitatory or inhibitory, but not both. Direct responses have latencies of 1–5 msec and are frequently transient in nature, though some persist for about 100 msec. Indirect (slow) synaptic transmissions are initiated by allosteric binding of a transmitter to a transmembrane protein that does not contain an ion channel but is linked on the intracellular side of the membrane to one of a class of G-proteins that bind guanosine diphosphate (GDP). Activated G-proteins may gate ion channels directly, and/or they may initiate second-messenger cascades by activating specific molecular targets in the cell (Clapham, 1994). The second-messenger cascades lead to phosphorylation and thus regulation of channel proteins, as well as to modulation of transcriptional proteins that control gene expression in the postsynaptic neuron. Indirect transmissions have longer latencies than do direct ones—they may last for seconds to hours.

Storage and Release of Synaptic Transmitters

One of the most important series of discoveries made in neuroscience in the twentieth century is that on neuromuscular transmission by Bernard Katz and a gifted group of collaborators (Fatt, del Castillo, Miledi) during the 1960s; for a summary, see Katz's monograph of 1969. These researchers identified the general sequence of events in chemical synaptic transmission, the basis for understanding how cells in the brain communicate with each other.

A brief outline follows (see Stevens, 1993; Kelly, 1993). Small molecular transmitters are synthesized in nerve cells and packaged in discrete quantities in intracellular organelles called vesicles, discovered by Gray and Whittaker (1960) and independently by De Robertis et al. (1961). Small, clear vesicles (c. 40–50 nm) store rapidly acting transmitters like Glu, ACh, and GABA; larger, dense-cored ones (c. 100–200 nm) store monoamines and polypeptides. Vesicles are formed in the trans-Golgi apparatus and moved by rapid axoplasmic transport to axon terminals, where the small, clear vesicles accumulate transmitter. A subset of the pool of small vesicles within the terminal is docked at special release points on the internal side of the plasma cell membrane (Fig. 5-6).

The arrival of a nerve impulse triggers the essential event: a large, transient, but spatially localized influx of Ca^{2+} into the terminal (Katz and Miledi, 1965). This Ca^{2+} surge evokes a fusion of the vesicle membrane to the plasma cell membrane, the opening of a fusion pore between the two, and bulk flow of the transmitter into the synaptic cleft. Binding of transmitter to postsynaptic receptors leads

Fig. 5-6 Sudhof's division of the synaptic vesicle (SV) cycle into nine successive steps that take place in nerve terminals. (1) SVs filled with neurotransmitter *(NT)* dock at the active zone opposite the synaptic cleft by an unknown targeting process. (2) SVs become competent for fast, Ca^{2+}-triggered membrane fusion. (3) Fusion/exocytosis of SVs is stimulated by a Ca^{2+} spike during an action potential; exocytosis requires less than 0.3 msec. (4) Empty SVs are rapidly internalized and coated during endocytosis. (5) Coated vesicles lose their coats and then are internalized and recycled. (6) Recycled SVs fuse with endosomes. (7) SVs are regenerated by budding from endosomes. (8) SVs accumulate neurotransmitter by active transport driven by an electrochemical gradient created by a proton pump. (9) SVs move back to the active zone either by diffusion or by a cytoskeleton-based transport process. (From Sudhof, 1995.)

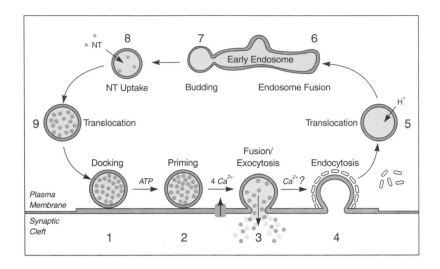

to channel opening and increased conductance of the postsynaptic membrane for Na^+ and K^+ ions, postsynaptic depolarization, and the end-plate potential (EPP) of the muscle cell or the excitatory postsynaptic potential (EPSP) of a central neuron. At inhibitory synapses the transmitter opens Cl^- or K^+ channels, leading to hyperpolarization/stabilization of the postsynaptic membrane potential, the inhibitory postsynaptic response (IPSP) of central neurons. The patch clamp method (Nehrer, 1992; Sakmann, 1992) permits study of the opening and closing of single channels. Ions move through open channels by aqueous diffusion. Transmitters are removed rapidly from the synaptic cleft by enzymatic destruction, re-uptake, and diffusion. Vesicle membrane is incorporated into the membrane of the terminal, then recycled and repackaged with transmitter within the terminal (Fig. 5-6).

The Quantal Nature of Chemical Synaptic Transmission

Fatt and Katz discovered (1952) that the neuromuscular junction is not silent in the absence of nerve impulses. They observed the spontaneous appearance, at a slow rate, of miniature end-plate potentials (MEPPs), which are postsynaptic responses all of a single size or unit multiples of that size. Each of these single-valued events is inferred to be the response to exocytosis of the transmitter contents of a single vesicle. Each site is thought to release one vesicle at a time, and both spontaneous and evoked responses are composed of independent release events. The response evoked by a nerve impulse is produced by a rapid increase in the frequency of quantal releases. Del Castillo and Katz (1954) developed a successful quantitative description of quantal release in terms of the binomial distribution, which with large source populations of vesicles devolves into its limiting form, the Poisson distribution. Quantal analysis has since been used in many studies of central synaptic transmission in attempts to identify whether changes in the efficacy of synaptic transmission are due to pre- or postsynaptic changes, or to both; see, e.g., the studies of long-term potentiation described in Chapter 6.

Neuropeptides are synthesized and stored in the larger, dense-cored vesicles within the trans-Golgi apparatus, and the loaded vesicles are then transported to the terminals. The exocytotic process for the large vesicles is independent of that for the small vesicles (Kelly, 1993). Empty large vesicles are transported to the Golgi apparatus, the site of protein synthesis, for repackaging.

These discoveries have been confirmed in many studies of synaptic transmission ranging from the invertebrate to the mammalian brain (for review, see Redman, 1990). High-impedance whole-cell recording from brain slices provided evidence that both excitatory and inhibitory transmission in the forebrain is quantal in nature. Some features differ from the classic model, however: (1) The probability of transmitter release varies over a time scale of minutes; release may fall to zero and remain there for long periods. (2) The quantal response is small, and there is evidence that only a limited number of receptor channels are located in the subsynaptic membrane, which means that the postsynaptic response may be of constant size even though the number of transmitter molecules released varies. (3) The probability of release may be increased by facilitatory processes, which may introduce significant nonlinearities.

Synaptic Ultrastructure

E. G. Gray discovered that the synaptic endings of cortical neurons are of two classes (Gray, 1959). Class 1 shows an electron-dense thickening of the postsynaptic membrane; an increase in the width of the subsynaptic cleft over the width of the intercellular cleft in nonsynaptic regions, from 20 to 30 nm; prominent presynaptic dense projections; and a line of electron-dense material within the subsynaptic cleft. The presynaptic grid and the dense projections are thought to be involved in vesicle docking and in vesicle release; they are molecular complexes attached to the cytoplasmic side of the presynaptic terminal. Intramembranous particles are aligned at release points, where vesicles are in line. The lateral dimensions of the grid are closely apposed to the sides of the grid of the postsynaptic density. Perforations are seen in some synapses, in both the pre- and postsynaptic specializations, and these are in perfect register on the two sides. The conclusion drawn from ultrastructural studies is that the formation of the specializations on two sides of the synapse is a controlled process, and that the synapse is a structural unit (Lisman and Harris, 1993).

Class-2 synapses show only minimal thickening of the postsynaptic membrane; the subsynaptic space is not widened and contains little or no electron-dense material; the presynaptic dense projections are less obvious and the active zones are smaller (Colonnier, 1981). After hyperosmotic aldehyde fixation, Gray's class-1 terminals contain round synaptic vesicles and class-2 terminals contain pleomorphic and flattened vesicles. Type-1 endings with round vesicles are commonly excitatory in action, type-2 with pleomorphic vesicles inhibitory (Uchizona, 1965, 1967; Colonnier, 1968). The difference in membrane structure at synapses is a reliable indicator of the direction of synaptic action, although rare exceptions to the correlation between vesicle size and shape in aldehyde-fixed material have been observed—e.g., in the cerebellum (Harmori et al., 1990).

A cortical neuron generates either asymmetric or symmetric synaptic terminals, but never both. Excitatory synapses in the cerebral cortex are generated by both spiny pyramidal and spiny nonpyramidal neurons, and by the terminals of afferents entering the cortex from elsewhere. Inhibitory synapses are generated by the nonspiny, nonpyramidal intrinsic cells of the cortex. Long-axoned inhibitory neurons are rare in the central nervous system.

Vesicular Biosynthesis, Transport, and Exocytosis

Specific events in the general outline given above have now been pursued at the molecular level, and explanations sought in terms of the action of specific proteins at each stage of the process. The identification of synaptic vesicles by Gray and Whittaker (1960, 1962) and by De Robertis et al. (1961) opened the field to the methods of biochemistry and molecular biology. It was first shown that the vesicles could be isolated within pinched-off terminals, called synaptosomes, by differential centrifugation of brain homogenates. Vesicles freed from the synaptosomes contain high concentrations of transmitters such as glutamate, acetycholine, and GABA. The granular vesicles with electron-dense cores contain peptides or monamines (Whittaker, 1993; Whittaker et al., 1964; McMahon and Nicholls, 1991). Granules frequently contain more than one transmitter, sometimes both peptides and low-molecular-weight transmitters; vesicles in the central nervous system commonly contain only one of the latter. The common designation of the small molecules as transmitters and the peptides as modulators reflects their rapid and slow release rates and postsynaptic responses, respectively. Many experimental results indicate that as regards fast transmission, the axon terminal is to a degree autonomous over the time scale of seconds and minutes. Driven by action potentials and Ca^{2+} entry, the terminal synthesizes, stores, releases, and takes up again the small molecular transmitters, recycles membrane components of released vesicles, and reconstitutes them for use again. These mechanisms are well suited for the needs of fast synaptic transmission (see Zimmerman, 1993).

Both granules and vesicles are initially synthesized within the trans-Golgi apparatus of the neuron soma. The organelles are moved to the axon terminal by fast, neurotubule-dependent axoplasmic transport. Vesicular traffic in axon and terminal requires interaction of vesicle and cytoskeletal elements. The four proteins of the synapsin family studied by Greengard and his associates (Valtorta et al., 1992) form the link between the cytoskeletal matrix and the vesicle membrane, as these proteins fix the vesicles within a reserve pool within the terminal. Phosphorylation of the synapsins by Ca^{2+}/calmodulin-dependent protein kinase II (CaM-KII) is initiated by the inward surge of Ca^{2+} that accompanies the axon potential. This releases the vesicles from the cytoskeleton and allows their transfer from the reserve pool to an active pool at the release sites.

The Synaptic Vesicle Cycle

The cycle represented in Fig. 5-6 (Sudhof 1995) consists of nine steps. It takes about a minute for any given vesicle to make the rotation. Yet, synaptic transmission requires a fast local release process that can be repeated rapidly and is subject to tight regulation. Exocytosis of transmitter occurs in less than a millisecond, and chemically operated synapses can be activated repetitively at rates of several hundred per second, for short periods of time. This requirement is met by a large pool of vesicles in intermediate stages of the cycle; of these, one portion is continually primed, ready to fuse, and docked at active zones, the release sites, which are studded with Ca^{2+} channels. Almers and Tse (1990) suggested that the presorted vesicles "pre-assemble" fusion pores, presumably in a closed state, so that pore opening and fusion evoked by the Ca^{2+} influx of the action potential may occur within microseconds. The time course of transmitter release and clearance from the synaptic cleft is an important factor controlling synaptic transmission. Detailed theoretical modeling and studies of the alterations in synaptic transmission by low-affinity competitive antagonists suggest that the time course varies greatly between synapses of different sizes, structural conformation, etc. In general, however, transmitter concentration reaches its peak of 1–5 millimoles (mM) almost instantaneously after opening of the fusion pore. Transmitter frequently saturates the postsynaptic receptors and is cleared from the cleft along a biphasic time course with time constants of 100 μsec and 2 msec (Clements, 1996).

Synapses function at long distances from cell bodies, at least as regards the release of small molecule transmitters, for the cycle shown in Fig. 5-6 takes place within the terminal itself. One result of this relative autonomy is that the different synapses of a single neuron may be regulated independently by modulatory mechanisms. A current research program in synaptic neuroscience is aimed at defining the families of proteins that regulate each of the steps in the exocytotic-endocytotic cycle. A large number of proteins—already hundreds—have been characterized and shown to play roles in one or another of the steps in the process (Matthews, 1996). For example, at least 32 protein families have been identified as associated with the synaptic vesicles, and many of these are often expressed in many isoforms (Sudhof, 1995). Jahn and Sudhof (1994) propose a model of these processes that incorporates knowledge of the relevant molecular mechanisms with heuristic speculations. Some important predictions of the model are: (1) that the fusion protein is integral to the vesicle membrane; (2) that the Ca^{2+} receptor molecule is not identical with the fusion protein; and (3) that the molecule acts as an inhibitor not an activator of fusion.

Synaptic Transmission in the Neocortex

Transmitters are driven into vesicles against a strong electrochemical gradient, energized by a proton translocator ATPase. Specific transporters have been identified for glutamate, acetylcholine, GABA, the monoamines, and serotonin. These biochemically distinct transporters are differentially distributed in the brain.

Direct Synaptic Transmission in the Neocortex

The synaptic responses of Fig. 5-7 were recorded intracellularly from neocortical neurons in a cortical slice preparation. They were evoked by electrical stimulation of cortical afferents through an electrode placed just where the afferents enter the cortex from the white matter (McCormick et al., 1993). The record of Fig. 5-7B was obtained from a pyramidal cell of layer III. The afferent volley evoked monosynaptically a short-latency, transient, depolarizing excitatory response, the EPSP. It was followed and overlapped in time by a di- and polysynaptically evoked, double-phased, hyperpolarizing inhibitory response,

Fig. 5-7 Records of an experiment revealing the EPSP of a cortical neuron mediated by NMDA receptors and the two phases of synaptic inhibition mediated by GABA_A and GABA_B receptors. Intracellular records obtained in a slice preparation of guinea-pig neocortex; stimulation of cortical afferents by single electric shocks. (A) A single afferent volley evoked a high-frequency repetitive train of impulses in a fast-spiking inhibitory interneuron. (B) Intracellular responses of a pyramidal cell to a single afferent volley; a monosynaptic EPSP is followed by a prolonged, two-phased IPSP. Application of the GABA blocker bicuculline enhances the EPSP and blocks the GABA_A component of the IPSP, at first partially and then, with higher concentration of the blocker, completely, revealing the prolonged GABA_B-mediated IPSP. (From McCormick et al., 1993.)

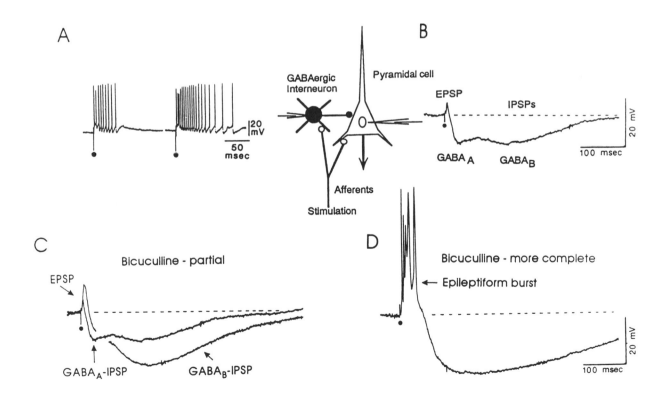

the IPSP (Connors et al., 1988). All afferent fibers entering the cortex at this point are excitatory and glutaminergic. The fast EPSP is produced by the allosteric binding of glutamate to the AMPA receptors (described below) and a resulting inwardly directed depolarizing Na^+ current. The equilibrium potential for the EPSP is about 0 mV membrane potential. Partial pharmacological block of the following fast IPSP causes an increase in the amplitude of the EPSP, reveals the temporal overlap of these two fast responses, and indicates that they interact in synaptic actions in the neocortex (Fig. 5-7C). After more complete block of the IPSP, a single afferent volley produces a powerful depolarization and a burst of action potentials in the pyramidal cell (Fig. 5-7D), a response produced by glutamate binding to NMDA receptors.

The time course and some of the unique properties of the NMDA-mediated excitatory postsynaptic response are shown by the records of Fig. 5-8. The channel is blocked by Mg^{2+} ion bound in its channel at resting membrane potentials. Depolarization to about -60 mV is required to relieve that block and allow glutamate to bind to the receptor. This depolarization is achieved via the AMPA receptors. The open NMDA channel has a high conductance for Ca^{2+}, less so for Na^+. NMDA receptors are both ligand- and voltage-sensitive, and they have the properties of both direct and indirect synaptic actions. The direct increase in Ca^{2+} conductance contributes to the delayed, but nevertheless direct, postsynaptic depolarization; the surge of intracellular Ca^{2+} sets in motion several of the second-messenger cascades described below.

Responses of a fast-spiking inhibitory neocortical interneuron are shown in Fig. 5-7A. GABAergic interneurons of this type produce the di- and polysynaptic early and late IPSPs of pyramidal cells like those of Fig. 5-7B. The transmitter engages simultaneously both $GABA_A$ and $GABA_B$ receptors clustered together in the postsynaptic densities beneath inhibitory presynaptic terminals. GABA binding to $GABA_A$ receptors leads to a fast, inwardly directed, hyperpolarizing Cl^- current through the receptor's intrinsic ion channel. The equilibrium potential of the fast IPSP is close to the resting membrane potential at about -95mV. It is antagonized by bicuculline and the epileptic drug picrotoxin. GABA binding to the $GABA_B$ receptors leads to the indirect, late inhibitory response described below.

The fast postsynaptic events in the neocortex are essential for transcortical actions in rapid tempo, like those of a sensory discrimination for which intracortical times of 200 msec or less are common.

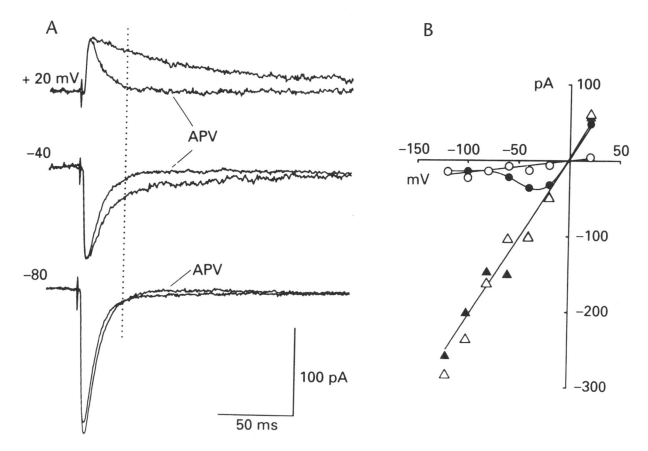

A

+ 20 mV

APV

−40

−80   APV

100 pA

50 ms

B

pA   100

−150   −100   −50   50

mV

−100

−200

−300

Fig. 5-8 Excitatory postsynaptic currents (EPSCs) evoked at glutaminergic synapses on pyramidal cells of slice preparations of adult rat hippocampus. The EPSC has two components, a rapid current evoked via non-NMDA (QA/KA) receptors and a slower, more prolonged current evoked via NMDA receptors. (A) The slow component is not present at hyperpolarized levels of membrane potential (−80 mV), but then it appears and grows with depolarization (−40 mV, +20mV). It is blocked by the selective glutamate antagonist, DL-2-amino-5-phosphonovalerate (APV). (B) Current-voltage plots show that APV has no effect on the early EPSC but blocks the negative-slope conductance measured 25 msec after EPSC onset (vertical dotted line). (From Hestrin et al., 1989.)

The distributed cortical networks (Chapter 10) allow even complex operations within that time. Nevertheless, serial operations are required at local nodes of distributed networks, and input-output times of a cortical column may be limited to a few tens of milliseconds.

Transmitters and Receptors That Mediate Direct Synaptic Transmission in the Neocortex

It is now generally agreed that L-glutamate (Glu) and gamma-aminobutyric acid (GABA) are, respectively, the excitatory and inhibitory transmitters mediating direct (fast) synaptic transmission in the primate neocortex. Several other transmitters also play important roles; among these are a number of polypeptides and glycine (or serine?). Polypeptides are co-localized in a small percentage of the GABAergic inhibitory interneurons. Their trans-synaptic actions are obscure. The afferent modulatory systems projecting to the neocortex from the basal forebrain and the central core of the brainstem operate with system-specific transmitters: acetylcholine, dopamine, serotonin, norepinephrine, or histamine. Many of these terminals also release polypeptides. Monoamines are not transmitters of intracortical neurons in the mature primate cortex.

There are three groups of channels in central neurons: the voltage-sensitive channels, the ligand-sensitive channels, and gap junctions expressed only during cortical ontogenesis. The protein superfamilies are related by some degree of sequence identity, and all have some features in common. Each receptor contains a channel whose selectivity is determined by its diameter and the molecular charges lining it. Ions move through the open channels down electrochemical gradients both by simple diffusion and by rapid loading-unloading at a binding site within the channel. Channels are formed by subunits, 4 for the voltage-gated, 5 for ligand-gated, and 6 for gap-junction channels. Subunits are separate protein molecules except in the voltage-gated channels, where they are tandem repeated homologous domains of a single polypeptide. Each subunit of ligand-gated channels contains 4 transmembrane domains, with the second (M2) of each turned inward to form the pore lining. Binding sites for transmitters are located on the extracellular, N-terminal portion of the molecule, frequently on only one of the subunits.

There are two subfamilies of ligand-gated channels: the glutamate (NMDA and non-NMDA) receptor family (Seeburg, 1993) and the nicotinic ACh and Gly receptor family (ACh, 5-HT, $GABA_A$, and Gly). A large number of subunit proteins are candidate components of the naturally occurring pentameric, ligand-gated, glutaminergic receptors. The particular set of genes expressed varies between different populations of neurons. The glutamate receptors are cation-selective, ionotropic channels named in terms of their pharmacological agonists, as follows.

AMPA	Agonist is alpha-amino-3-hydroxy-5-methyl-4-isoxazole proprionic acid
Kainate	Agonist is the kainate ion (KA)
NMDA	Agonist is the N-Methyl-D-aspartate ion
Quisqualate A	Agonist is the quisqualate ion (QA)

Synaptic Transmission in the Neocortex

The quisqualate and kainate receptors are often referred to together as the non-NMDA receptors because they share a number of similar properties that differ from those of the NMDA receptors. The affinity of these agonists for the different classes of receptors is differential, not absolute.

Twenty-eight GluR subunit proteins have been identified; the addition of splice variants (called "flip" and "flop") brings the total to 45 (for reviews, see Hollmann and Heinemann, 1994; Wheal and Thomson, 1991; Kalb, 1995). Of these, 16 genes coding for subunits of the ionotropic glutamate receptors have been characterized. They generate the subunits of the glutamate receptors that occur naturally. They are:

$GluR_1$–$GluR_4$	Ionotropic AMPA receptors
$GluR_5$–$GluR_7$	Ionotropic, low-affinity kainate receptors
KA_1 and KA_2	Ionotropic, high-affinity kainate receptors
$NMDAR_1$–$NMDAR_{2A-D}$	Ionotropic NMDA receptors
mGluR	The "metabotropic," non-ionotropic receptors generated by a different gene family are discussed below; 7 mGluRs have been identified
Delta-1 and delta-2	Two nonfunctional receptors have also been identified; they do not gate ion flow

The number of possible combinations of subunits forming the naturally occurring receptors is large, and until now it has not been possible to identify the subunit compositions of glutamate receptors.

AMPA Receptors

Subunits of the AMPA receptor show binding affinities in decreasing order for QA > AMPA > Glu > KA. They are present at high densities at the majority if not all the excitatory synapses in the neocortex, more densely in layers I–IV than in V and VI. AMPA receptors mediate fast, excitatory transmission with onset, off-set, and desensitization times in the low msec range. The $GluR_2$ subunit confers on the natural

AMPA receptors their salient features of rapid kinetics, high permeability to monovalent cations and low to divalent ones, and a linear current/voltage *(I/V)* relation.

Kainate Receptors

Kainate receptors, which are about one-fifth as prevalent in the neocortex as are the AMPA receptors, are preferentially distributed in layers I, V, and VI. It is unlikely that any naturally occurring kainate receptors exist that are composed exclusively of only one type of KA subunit. The high-affinity KA_1 and KA_2 receptors do not generate functional channels when expressed alone in oocytes, but they do so when combined with $GluR_6$ or $GluR_7$.

NMDA Receptors

NMDA receptors have strong binding affinities for NMDA, but they have a unique gating requirement for a nearly coincident ligand binding and membrane depolarization, which removes a blocking Mg^{2+} from the channel. The channel has a prolonged open time (100–200 msec) and a high conductance (50 pS) for Ca^{2+}, low for Na^+ and K^+. The transient flow of Ca^{2+} into the cell initiates the Ca^{2+}-dependent second-messenger cascades described below. The properties of coincident voltage/ligand gating and high Ca^{2+} permeability suggest that these receptors are essential for the long-term changes in synaptic efficiency. They are best characterized as coincident detectors; the outcome of that detection is Ca^{2+} entry (Bourne and Nicoll, 1993). The sequence of events in NMDA-mediated synaptic transmission is outlined in Fig. 5-9.

The NMDA receptors have extracellular binding sites for glycine, zinc, the polyamines, and the dissociative anesthetics ketamine and phencyclidine. Glycine (or D-serine?) is an obligatory co-agonist; without it glutamate is virtually ineffective. The polyamines increase the affinity of Gly for its binding site (Ransom and Deschenes, 1990). Zinc is an allosteric inhibitor and selectively blocks the NMDA receptor (Peters et al., 1987). The dissociative anesthetics are channel blockers. NMDA receptors are widely distributed in the nervous system and densely in the neocortex, where they are concentrated in layers I, II, and III. They operate on a slower time scale than do the

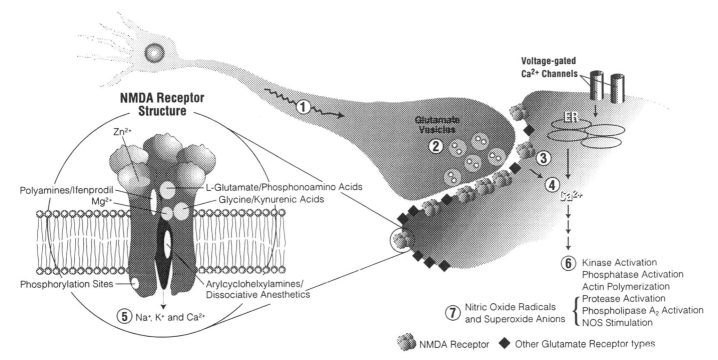

NMDA Receptor Structure

Zn²⁺

Polyamines/Ifenprodil

Mg²⁺

L-Glutamate/Phosphonoamino Acids

Glycine/Kynurenic Acids

Phosphorylation Sites

Arylcyclohelxylamines/
Dissociative Anesthetics

(5) Na⁺, K⁺ and Ca²⁺

Voltage-gated
Ca²⁺ Channels

Glutamate
Vesicles

ER

Ca²⁺

(6) Kinase Activation
Phosphatase Activation
Actin Polymerization
Protease Activation
Phospholipase A₂ Activation
NOS Stimulation

(7) Nitric Oxide Radicals
and Superoxide Anions

NMDA Receptor   Other Glutamate Receptor types

non-NMDA receptors because of slow dissociation of glutamate from the receptor, with synaptic current rise times of about 12–13 msec and decay times of 100+ msec. They contribute to the late phase of the excitatory postsynaptic current illustrated in Fig. 5-8 (Hestrin et al., 1990). The time window for coincidence between NMDA and AMPA receptor activation is about 100 msec; the former contributes to both fast and slow synaptic transmission.

Expression cloning experiments show that the NMDAR₁ subunit possesses all the properties of the naturally occurring receptors, with ligand-binding affinities decreasing in the order Gly > Glu > NMDA > QA; they do not respond to kainate or AMPA. The *I/V* curve (Fig. 5-8) is linear in the absence of Mg²⁺, but in its presence responses are blocked at membrane potentials more negative than about −40 to −20 mV. None of the other subunits identified shows these properties when expressed either homomerically or in combinations with each other. However, co-expression of NMDAR₁ with either NMDAR₂ₐ or NMDAR₂ᵦ increases channel conductance several-fold.

Fig. 5-9 A schematic diagram of the events initiated by binding of glutamate in a postsynaptic mammalian neuron, including the structure of the NMDA receptor. The major events are numbered in sequence. (1) A nerve impulse is conducted along the presynaptic axon and invades the synaptic terminal. (2) Synaptic vesicles fuse with the presynaptic membrane and release glutamate into the synaptic space. (3) Glutamate binds KA/AMPA receptor complexes in the postsynaptic membrane, leading to increased Na⁺ conductance and postsynaptic depolarization. (4) Depolarization displaces Mg²⁺ from the NMDA channels, leading to (5) increased Ca²⁺ influx, which triggers the effects listed at (6). (7) Excessive release of glutamate and activation of glutamate receptors can lead to excessive intracellular Ca²⁺ and production of nitric oxide radicals and superoxide anions, which may be lethal for the cell. The enlargement of the NMDA receptor shows sites at which the function of the receptor is regulated. (From Michaelis, 1996.)

Fig. 5-9 gives a schematic of a glutamate-operated synapse and the chain of postsynaptic events; it also depicts the structure of the NMDA receptor.

Metabotropic Receptors

G-protein-linked, non-ionotropic glutamate receptors (called "metabotropic"—mGluR) are generated by a different gene family; seven or eight subtypes have been identified (Nakanishi, 1994). mGluRs are transmembrane receptor proteins linked intracellularly via G-proteins to second-messenger systems, notably adenylyl cyclase, which it inhibits, and protein kinase C. Through the latter they mediate slow responses to glutamate by modulating through phosphorylation both voltage- and ligand-gated transmembrane ionic channels. L-AP4 (2-amino-4-phosphonobutyric acid) is a potent agonist for three of the mGluRs, one of which, $mGluR_6$, mediates glutamate transmission from photoreceptors to the on-bipolar cells of the retina. Other mGluRs are widely distributed in the nervous system and may serve to modulate changes in synaptic effectiveness, such as long-term potentiation.

GABA Receptors and Synaptic Inhibition in the Neocortex

Inhibitory neurons of the neocortex are intrinsic, nonspiny, nonpyramidal cells, and they use GABA as transmitter (McCormick, 1989) (see Chapter 3, and Figs. 3-3 and 3-4). They make up 17–20 percent of all neocortical neurons. Some still uncertain percentage (10–40 percent) of cortical GABAergic cells also express one or more neuroactive peptides.

$GABA_A$ receptors are Cl^- selective ion channels with five-fold symmetry of subunits surrounding the ion channel, in the mode of other ligand-gated receptors. The open-channel conductance is about 30 pS. The reversal point for the early IPSP is about -95 mV, the Cl^- equilibrium potential. $GABA_A$ receptors incorporate binding sites both for agonists, such as the axiolytics, sedatives, and hypnotics (e.g., the benzodiazepines, barbiturates, alcohol), and antagonists, such as the epileptogenic drug picrotoxin.

Fifteen proteins have been identified as $GABA_A$ subunits by molecular cloning and studied by recombinant expression in cultured cells. They are Alpha$_{1-6}$, Beta$_{1-4}$, Gamma$_{1-4}$, and one Delta (Burt and Kamatchi, 1991; Seeburg et al., 1990). Each subunit has a large N-terminal extracellular domain with GABA and other binding sites, including several glycolysation sites, and a large cytoplasmic domain thought to provide a phosphorylation site. Many possible combinations (about 3,000) of these subunits might form the natural receptors of 5 subunits. The sets present in the naturally occurring receptors are not known exactly, but the combination of 2 Alpha$_1$, 2 Beta$_2$, and 1 Gamma$_2$ possesses many of the characteristics of the natural receptors that occur in the neocortex (McKernan and Whiting, 1996).

Indirect Synaptic Transmission in the Neocortex

Although the separation between fast and slow synaptic responses is blurred by their overlaps in latency and duration, their distinction is clear as regards receptor type and mode of postsynaptic response. Direct transmissions are effected by ligand-gated, membrane-spanning ion channels. Indirect transmissions are effected via G-protein-linked, membrane-spanning proteins that do not contain ion channels but link to second-messenger systems that regulate synaptic transmission by phosphorylation of membrane proteins, including ligand-gated channels. Receptors of the two types exist for each of the common small-molecule transmitters in the neocortex. The records of Fig. 5-8 (Hestrin et al., 1990) illustrate the combined voltage and ligand sensitivity of the NMDA receptor. Its direct contribution to the late synaptic current is significant only at moderate levels of membrane depolarization. What cannot be seen in records like those of Fig. 5-8 is the indirect NMDA action, the second-messenger cascades initiated by Ca^{2+} influx. This produces synaptic modifications essential for the changes in synaptic plasticity characteristic of long-term potentiation, described in the following chapter.

The inhibitory transmitter GABA also has indirect actions, mediated via GABA$_B$ receptors. Although produced indirectly, the late IPSP begins within some tens of msec after the afferent volley, peaks at about 135 msec, and may last for 300–400 msec. It overlaps the direct action of glutamate via the NMDA receptors shown as the late current in Fig. 5-7C. GABA$_B$ receptors are G-protein-linked, and they initiate a second-messenger action—perhaps the phosphotidylinositol biphosphate (PIP$_2$) cascade—that leads to increased K$^+$ conductance. The equilibrium potential for the late IPSP is about -100 mV membrane potential.

The majority of indirect actions persist for much longer than those described and produce their effects by regulating direct synaptic transmissions. They are best understood in terms of the G-protein receptors and second-messenger systems involved.

Mechanisms of Indirect Synaptic Transmission in the Neocortex

The Transmitter–Receptor–G-Protein Linkage

The G-protein-linked receptors consist of seven membrane-spanning domains surrounding a deeply embedded ligand binding site. The cytoplasmic loops linking the intracellular ends of the domains bind to G-proteins of the cytosol; the loop sequence determines the G-protein selectivity of the receptor. G-proteins are heterotrimers; each contains an alpha catalytic unit flanked by beta and gamma regulatory subunits. Receptor activation of the G-protein catalyzes the exchange of its bound GDP for GTP and a transient separation of the catalytic from the regulatory units. This activated state is rapidly reversed by the self-hydrolyzing GTPase action of the G-protein. The active G-protein unit "activates" second-messenger systems that act on time scales from milliseconds to hours, have a wide transmitter receptivity coupled with high sensitivity, and operate with an enormous amplifying power, so that a few transmitter molecules may initiate large-scale postsynaptic responses (Ross, 1989).

The most common postsynaptic responses initiated by G-proteins are activation or suppression of voltage-dependent ion channels by covalent phosphorylation of channel proteins at specific residue sites, frequently serine. On more extended time scales, they modulate the regulatory proteins that control gene transcription and thus the changes in synaptic ultrastructure that accompany long-term changes in synaptic potency. Overlapping ranges of selectivity at each stage of the cascades produce a widely divergent/convergent signal-processing system. Activated G-proteins may gate membrane ion channels directly (Clapham, 1994), forming a pathway to synaptic responses intermediate between the fast, synaptic responses evoked directly by ligand gating and the slower, indirect mode of the second-messenger pathways.

The Second-Messenger Systems

Several second-messenger pathways have been identified in neurons, particularly those whose messengers are cAMP (cyclic adenosine monophosphate); cGMP (cyclic guanosine monophosphate); Ca^{2+}; and the products of the hydrolysis of PIP_2 (phosphotidylinositol biphosphate), IP_3 (inositol triphosphate), and DAG (diacylglycerol). Several other second messenger-cascades have been identified. The cAMP and Ca^{2+} cascades, found in all animal cells, are the most prevalent and the best understood of those in neurons. The sequence for the cAMP cascade, from transmitter to G-protein receptor to activated G-protein to activated adenylyl cyclase, yields the enzymatic synthesis of cAMP from ATP. cAMP activates the cAMP-dependent protein kinases, and the end points of the chain are the phosphorylations of a number of target proteins. These include leak, voltage-gated, and ligand-gated channel proteins, which means that this system can influence both the resting and active membrane potential of the cell. cAMP also phosphorylates the regulatory proteins that control transcription, and thus stimulates protein synthesis.

The Ca^{2+} ion plays roles in neurons as diverse as controlling presynaptic vesicle release, regulating neurite extension during axonal growth, and forming the essential link in the postsynaptic initiation of long-term potentiation. Intracellular Ca^{2+} concentration is held at a low level (0.1–0.2 μmol), compared with its extracellular concentration (1.8 mmol), by a membrane Na^+/Ca^{2+} transporter, by an ATPase-powered, outwardly directed pump, and by sequestration intracellularly in the endoplasmic reticulum. Ca^{2+} moves into neurons down steep concentration and potential gradients through ligand- (NMDA) and voltage-gated ionic channels. The intracellular actions of Ca^{2+} are transient in time and local in space (Kasai and Peterson, 1994; Silver et al., 1994; Sugimori et al., 1994); its effects are imposed within, and limited to, such small cellular regions as the postsynaptic spines, and its actions are repeated rapidly.

The impulsive rise in intracellular Ca^{2+} also has many direct effects. Ca^{2+} activates directly membrane ion channels for K^+, Cl^-, and Ca^{2+} itself; and such membrane-bound proteins as phospholipase-C, whose hydrolysis of phosphotidylinositol biphosphate yields two other second messengers, IP_3 (inositol triphosphate) and DAG (diacylglycerol); and phosphatase K2, which controls still another candidate second-messenger system, the arachidonic acid metabolites. The direct cytosolic targets of Ca^{2+} are protein kinase C, calpain (a protease), and the ubiquitous effector-receptor protein for Ca^{2+}, calmodulin.

The allosteric interaction between Ca^{2+} and calmodulin initiates a second-messenger system, without G-protein intermediation, that influences or controls: (1) activation of CaM-KII, which is heavily concentrated in postsynaptic densities and in presynaptic terminals, where it activates synapsin I, a protein essential for vesicle mobilization and release; (2) activation of isozymes of adenylyl cyclase and diesterase, the two enzymes regulating cAMP levels in neurons; (3) activation of CaM-dependent neuronal NO-synthase, thus controlling the retrograde signal thought to evoke the presynaptic change in long-term potentiation. The second-messenger systems in neurons overlap by having some common extracellular signaling molecules, interactions at intermediate steps in their intracellular biochemical pathways, and overlapping sets of targets.

Neuroactive Peptides

Many neuroactive peptides have been identified in nerve cells (>40, and growing), and about a dozen of these occur in the neocortex, where they are co-localized with GABA in all classes of inhibitory interneurons except the basket and chandelier cells. Only a small proportion of the GABAergic interneurons co-localize a neuropeptide, hence only a small percentage of cortical cells express a neuropeptide (DeFelipe, 1993). Neuropeptides are synthesized in the endoplasmic reticulum of the neuronal cell body, pass through the trans-Golgi network, and are packaged in large, dense-cored, membrane-bound vesicles of 50–200 μm diameter that are moved to the nerve terminals by fast axoplasmic transport. They are released by exocytosis after fusion of the large vesicles with terminal membrane, but the details of this process are unclear. Neuropeptide Y (NPY) is one of the common neuroactive peptides in the neocortex (Colmers and Wahlestedt, 1993). The terminals of NPY neurons are symmetric (inhibitory) and are found on the dendrites and spines of non-GABAergic cells. Many NPY endings do not form classical synapses, however, but make close membrane appositions with the terminals of non-NPY cells (Hendry, 1993). NPY receptors are G-protein-linked, membrane-bound proteins without ionophores, and they affect Ca^{2+}

channel proteins via a second-messenger system, probably that of cAMP (Bleakman et al., 1993).

The inference is made that the trans-synaptic actions of polypeptides on cortical neurons resemble those at peripheral synapses. Slow excitatory or inhibitory postsynaptic responses are evoked there by second-messenger action, including delayed and prolonged trophic responses and differential gene expression, typically but not always enhancing and extending the action of primary transmitters. It is widely believed that neuroactive peptides not only act at receptors in the immediately subsynaptic membrane, but diffuse though the extracellular space to influence other neurons, glial cells, and the smooth muscle cells of small vessels and thus control local blood flow in the cortex. Neuropeptides are not removed by re-uptake into the synaptic terminals, and it is assumed they are inactivated by the enzymatic action of the pervasive peptidases in the extracellular fluid.

Presynaptic Inhibition

A volley of impulses in one set of primary afferent fibers evokes via interneuronal action a depolarization of adjacent terminals upon which the fibers converge. Impulses invading those partially depolarized terminals from their parent axons release less transmitter than otherwise, and thus have decreased potencies for postsynaptic actions. Presynaptic inhibition occurs throughout the nervous system, but is effected by different mechanisms at different levels. Presynaptic inhibition in the spinal cord and brainstem, and at some subcortical structures of the forebrain, is effected in a different way through axo-axonic, terminal-to-terminal synapses, of which the presynaptic member of the pair has the ultrastructural features of inhibitory terminals. The transmitter at these synapses is GABA; in the spinal cord the postsynaptic receptor is the $GABA_A$ type (Stuart and Redman, 1991). The increased membrane conductance produced by opening the $GABA_A$ chloride channel shunts the terminal membrane, which reduces the amplitude of an invading action potential and thus decreases transmitter release.

There is little evidence from studies of ultrastructure that axo-axonic, terminal-to-terminal synapses exist in the forebrain, particularly not in the neocortex. Nevertheless, $GABA_B$ receptors are plentiful in presynaptic membranes of neocortical cells, and local applications of GABA in slice preparations elicit presynaptic inhibition. $GABA_B$ receptors increase K^+ conductance via G-protein-linked, second-messenger pathways, thought to be accompanied by a reduction in Ca^{2+} conductance, thus interfering with transmitter release at the level of vesicle fusion. GABA is thought in these cases to move by simple diffusion from its source in remote synaptic terminals to bind with $GABA_B$ receptors in terminal membranes. If so, this marks an example in which trans-synaptic actions are effected by volume diffusion of transmitter.

Integrative Functions of Dendrites and Spines

The majority of neocortical synapses end on dendrites, almost all of the excitatory terminals on dendritic spines. A major problem is to understand how actions at those spatially distributed synapses are integrated to control the ongoing impulse activity of the nerve cell. One premise of the single-trigger model is that dendrites are electrotonic cables and that the influence of dendritic synapses upon the cell is inversely proportional to their electrotonic distance from the spike-initiating zone (Rall et al., 1967, 1992). Several studies have shown that the dendrites of central neurons contain voltage-gated Na^+ channels that are expressed along the full length of the dendritic trees; dendrites can generate action potentials in the regenerative mode, as well as local synaptic responses (Amitai et al., 1993).

Local transmembrane current pulses or local excitatory input elicit in dendrites local EPSPs and fast Na^+ action potentials, and slower Ca^{2+} action potentials. The local voltage-gated Na^+ channels support the cellulifugal propagation into the dendritic tree of action potentials that originate in the cell body or initial axon segment (Kim and Connors, 1993; Stuart and Sakmann, 1994). Conduction of action potentials in the orthodromic direction seldom occurs. Impulses evoked by local dendritic EPSPs originate in the somatic trigger zone after electrotonic extension. For example, EPSPs restricted to the apical dendrites in layer I of the layer V pyramidal cells elicit action potentials that are initiated in the cell body (Cauller and Connors, 1994). This has also been observed by recording simultaneously with microelectrodes in the dendrite and cell body of the same single pyramidal cell (Stuart and Sakmann, 1994).

Extension of EPSPs toward the spike-initiation site in the soma is facilitated by the fact that EPSPs themselves open Na+ channels in the dendritic membrane. The spike-initiation site can be shifted into the proximal dendrite by strong dendritic depolarization. The antidromic propagation of action potentials from soma to dendrite modulates the integrative properties of the dendrites by activating voltage-gated Ca^{2+} channels and opening NMDA channels. The location of the spike-initiation zone at the border of soma and initial segment is thought to be due to the high density of voltage-gated Na^+ channels in its membrane, a density that decreases gradually from cell body backward through the dendritic tree to its apex. This provides an explanation for the paradox of active back-propagation without the capacity for local initiation of impulses (Mainen et al., 1995). However, the density of Na+ channels in dendrites increases with cortical maturity, so under some circumstances dendrites may conduct action potentials toward the soma (Regehr et al., 1993).

Spencer and Kandel (1961) proposed for hippocampal pyramidal cells that the electrogenic patches in dendritic membranes served to boost the electrotonic extension in the cellulipetal direction of local EPSPs, and this appears to be true also for cortical pyramidal cells. A differential distribution of these electrogenic patches, perhaps concentrated at dendritic branch points, creates local, spatially restricted zones capable of integrative action, for inputs from different presynaptic sources are frequently segregated in different dendritic compartments. Interaction between events at ligand- and voltage-gated channels with passive membrane properties creates a dynamic state of excitability within the dendritic tree that can affect such fundamental properties as the electrotonic length of the cell. (For a recent model of the integrative properties of dendrites, see Jaslove, 1992; for a review, see Yuste and Tank, 1966.)

Dendritic spines were discovered by Cajal more than a century ago, and both Cajal and Tanzi suggested that spines play a role in learning and memory. Spines vary in head and neck diameters and shape and in neck lengths. These differences have led to speculations that changes in these parameters are related to the control of electrical events, such as the electrotonic extension into the dendrite of local EPSPs in the spine head. Indeed, it has now been shown that spine parameters are determined in a dynamic way by levels of presynaptic activity; intense presynaptic input induces the formation of new spines upon the dendritic shaft (for review, see Harris and Kater, 1994). Analyses carried out in modeling experiments suggest a quite different spine function. They "create an isolated biochemical microenvironment around synapses" (Koch and Zador, 1993) and in this way segregate within a local postsynaptic space of one or a few spines the postsynaptic surge of Ca^{2+} produced by NMDA receptor activation. This surge is responsible for the Ca^{2+}-dependent forms of long-term potentiation; it has been observed directly in active dendritic spines by Ca^{2+} imaging methods (Muller and Connor, 1991; Guthrie et al., 1991; Murphy et al., 1994). Llinas and his colleagues have shown that the surge of Ca^{2+} occupies small microdomains of space in such diverse locations as the axon terminal of the giant axon of the squid (Sugimori et al., 1994; Silver et al., 1994) and in the postsynaptic spines of Purkinje cells (Denk et al., 1995).

Volume Transmission Is a Second Mode of Interneuronal Communication in the Neocortex

Interneuronal signaling in the neocortex may take place by the diffusion of transmitter molecules through the intercellular space to act at receptor molecules in neuronal and perhaps glial cell membranes at some distance from the release sites (for review, see Fuxe and Agnati, 1991). Interneuronal actions in this mode may be randomly distributed in the diffusion space, but action may still be target-cell-selective within that space for those cells bearing the relevant receptor molecules. It is unlikely that the small-molecule transmitters like glutamate or GABA operate in this paracrine mode. They are released directly into the synaptic cleft, which will itself slow diffusion, and re-uptake and degradation mechanisms rapidly reduce transmitter concentrations in the cleft to low values.

It is for the cortical terminal distributions of the ascending monoaminergic modulatory systems that the idea of volume transmission is most often proposed. This is so because past studies suggested that the terminals of the axons of these systems are applied closely to neuronal membranes, but that many make no special synaptic relation to target-cell membranes. The diffusion of their transmitters through the intercellular spaces is sufficiently free and the removal mechanisms sufficiently slow that it is easy to envisage "actions at a distance" from the release sites. However, more detailed serial electron-micrographic studies of the terminals of these systems show that many of these apparently nonsynaptic terminals do make small specific synaptic contacts of the classical type with postsynaptic neurons. The wide divergence of these systems within the cortical neuropil insures their action by a mode of "volume transmission," whether by paracrine or synaptic modes, or indeed perhaps by both.

The concept of volume transmission as a second mode of neuronal communication in the cortex has been considered for decades. It is, of course, the necessary mode of the action of the endocrine upon the nervous system. Volume transmissions operate in slow tempo in a spatially random mode—though perhaps with target-cell specificity—and its transmitters commonly act upon postsynaptic cells via second-messenger systems.

Several mechanisms of interaction between neurons other than classic synaptic transmission may be operative in the neocortex. The gap-junction relations so prevalent in the developing cortex may persist in some locations, although such junctions have been very hard to find in the mature cortex. If present, such local modes of interaction are effective only at close proximity. It is important to emphasize that the results of all local neural interactions in the neocortex, classic synaptic or otherwise, are expressed in the impulse trains of pyramidal projection neurons. It is those trains of action potentials that leave one local region and project to another, and it is only those trains that carry signals between spatially separate nodes of distributed systems.

Summary

Synaptic transmission at chemically operated central synapses is accomplished by the release of neurotransmitters from their vesicular stores in presynaptic endings. Axon terminals contain two classes of vesicles: small, electron-translucent ones (40–50 nm) that contain small-molecule transmitters, and larger (100–200 nm), electron-dense vesicles that contain polypeptides or/and monamines and sometimes small-molecule transmitters as well. More than twenty small-molecule transmitters, and an even larger number of neuropeptides, have been identified in nervous systems.

Neurons are secretory cells, and the secretion of transmitters is regulated by a specific signal. An action potential invading the terminal opens by depolarization voltage-gated Ca^{2+} channels packed at the docking sites of the vesicles in the presynaptic terminal membrane. The large, rapid, but spatially localized surge of Ca^{2+} initiates fusion of vesicle and presynaptic plasma cell membranes, and exocytosis of the vesicular contents into the synaptic cleft follows. Synaptic vesicle membranes are recycled and vesicles recharged with transmitter, within the terminal for the small, clear vesicles that contain small-molecule transmitters, but only after retrograde transport to the Golgi apparatus for the large, dense-cored vesicles.

Either or both of two modes of synaptic action follow. In fast or direct transmission, the transmitter binds to a select site in a postsynaptic membrane protein molecule that contains an ion channel. An allosteric change in molecular conformation of the channel protein follows, the channel opens, and rapid ion flow leads to either depolarization and excitation or hyperpolarization and inhibition of the postsynaptic cell—which one is determined by the properties of the receptor and its ion channel, not the transmitter molecule. Alternatively, transmitter-receptor binding may lead to closure of an open ion channel. In slow or indirect transmission, the postsynaptic receptor does not contain an ion channel but a transmembrane link to a specific intracellular G-protein. Activation of this protein by the receptor sets in motion one or more of the several second-messenger systems in the postsynaptic neuron. These molecular chains initiate actions that range from changes in the conductance of ion channels to the initiation of gene expression. More than 40 neuroactive peptides have been identified in neurons, and several of these are co-localized with GABA in the terminals of inhibitory cortical neurons. Peptide function in synaptic transmission is still poorly understood.

The majority of neocortical synapses end on dendrites, which do contain voltage-gated Na^+ channels and can generate Na^+ action potentials as well as slower Ca^{2+} spikes. Nevertheless, the concept of the initial segment as the trigger zone for synaptic transmission has been confirmed for cortical neurons. Dentritic spines appear to function as chemical sequestering devices, segregating within a small volume the postsynaptic surge of Ca^{2+} produced by NMDA receptor activation. Intrinsic properties differ between different classes of cortical neurons; these determine in part the response properties of cortical cells.

A major discovery of recent years is that plasticity is an almost universal property of central synapses (Chapter 6).

Activity-Dependent Changes in Synaptic Strength in the Hippocampus and Neocortex

Two central themes in neurobiology are that synaptic relations between neurons are plastic—they can be changed by experience—and that long-term changes in synaptic strength are important brain mechanisms for learning and long-term memory. These general hypotheses date from Cajal's description of the synapse and elaboration of the neuron theory and have been put in more specific terms by many neurobiologists in the years since (e.g., see Eccles, 1953, chap. 6; Kornorski, 1948; Kandel and Spencer, 1968; Huang et al., 1996). Synaptic changes are thought to depend upon enduring increments in strength of the circuits activated by the initial experience; these increments lead to quasi-permanent changes in dynamic circuit operations that depend for long life upon gene expression, protein synthesis, and changes in synaptic ultrastructure. Many uncertainties surround the questions of how those changes in synaptic effectiveness embed a memory in the distributed systems of the brain, how memories are maintained, sometimes for a lifetime, in the face of recurrent molecular turnover, and how they can be recalled almost instantaneously to conscious experience. The problems of learning and memory have dominated the behavioral sciences for decades, and have been addressed in almost innumerable behavioral studies and in many theoretical and modeling efforts. Several of these provide partially satisfactory descriptions at the behavioral level and have emphasized many important facts about *declarative* memories: among them, that what is recalled is not an isomorphic replication of the original experience but a reconstruction of it, a recategorization

(Edelman, 1989, pp. 109–117). Everyone knows that such recalls are scarcely ever exact reproductions of the original experience, that they may vary from one recall to another, and that they are frequently in error. Surely no one will argue that the changes in synaptic effectiveness described below, conjectured to be the cellular bases of memory, are themselves "memories." It remains for further study to reveal how it is that changes in synaptic effectiveness can change in a permanent way the dynamic properties of widely distributed systems in the brain to allow elaborative recall.

The changes in synaptic effectiveness induced by previous activity vary in the direction of change, cellular mechanisms, and durations. The durations of synaptic changes vary from minutes to hours, days, or weeks, over the range of post-tetanic potentiation (PTP), short-term potentiation (STP), the early and late phases of long-term potentiation (LTP), and long-term depression (LTD). Whether the changes induced in synaptic transmission are a strong facilitation, as in long-term potentiation, or conversely a strong depression, as in long-term depression (LTD), depends upon the frequency of the inducing presynaptic activity, on the degree of changes in Ca^{2+} concentrations, and on the selectivity of the incremented enzymatic cascades that follow in the postsynaptic neurons. The application of the methods of cellular neurophysiology and molecular biology has increased understanding of these processes, but even after thirty years of effort considerable confusion remains, particularly in the specifics of the complex intracellular biochemical changes that intervene between presynaptic input and synaptic change.

I describe in this chapter several of these changes in synaptic transmission because of their importance for understanding cortical function. They are central for such disparate functions as normal development, the recovery of cortical circuits from injury, and the plastic changes in cortical maps induced by increments or decrements in afferent input; moreover, they remain the most likely candidates for the molecular basis of the action of cortical circuits in memory and learning.

The molecular and cellular mechanisms of some forms of nonassociative (habituation and sensitization) and associative learning were discovered by Eric Kandel and his colleagues in the invertebrate sea snail, *Aplysia* (Hawkins et al., 1993). Related long-term changes in synaptic strength have been observed in other invertebrates and in the mammalian hippocampus, neocortex, and cerebellum. Although the mechanisms of synaptic plasticity differ substantially between different synaptic locations in the same nervous system, and between different nervous systems, one or all of several general themes appear at many sites. These are modulations of presynaptic transmitter release, which may take several forms; changes in postsynaptic response; linkage from post- to presynaptic elements by retrograde messengers; and, for the late phase of LTP, the stimulation of gene expression, protein synthesis, and changes in synaptic ultrastructure. Most research on synaptic plasticity in the mammalian brain has been made on the hippocampus because this structure and the circuits in which it is embedded are known on other grounds to be central for the brain mechanisms in learning and memory. The accessibility and remarkable regularity of the synaptic circuits in the hippocampus ease the difficulties of the experimental procedures required. The relevance of these studies for understanding synaptic plasticity in the cerebral cortex is obvious.

The Human Hippocampus Is Essential for the Formation of Declarative Memories

Many studies of patients with enduring loss of memory after disease, ischemia, or surgical brain interventions provide evidence that the hippocampus is essential for the acquisition of new knowledge of people, objects, and events—a form of memory that is susceptible to conscious recall and is called *declarative* (Milner, 1966; Corkin, 1984). There is evidence that the hippocampus may serve as a temporary storage for items of declarative memory, even for days or weeks, before the memory is "consolidated" in other areas of the brain, particularly in the neocortex, after which transfer the long-term memory is accessible even in the absence of the hippocampus (Zola-Morgan and Squire, 1990). *Procedural* memories—how to do things—appear to be embedded and persist without involvement of the hippocampus. An informative case of loss of declarative memory was studied by Zola-Morgan et al. (1986). The patient developed an anterograde amnesia after an ischemic episode during cardiac surgery. He was studied intensively by these authors from the time of that episode until his death five years later. The patient's anterograde amnesia was coupled with a virtually intact memory for events in his life before the ischemic episode. He retained a procedural memory and showed no signs of cognitive defect. Histological study of this patient's brain re-

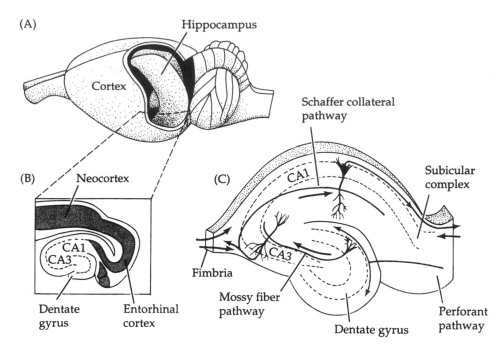

Fig. 6-1 The trisynaptic pathway of the rat hippocampus. (A) Schematic diagram of the rat brain, with a cutaway view showing location of the hippocampus. (B) A horizontal section through hippocampus and cortex. (C) The hippocampal circuit: dashed lines represent layers of tightly packed neuronal cell bodies. Axons enter the hippocampus through the fimbria, the subicular complex, and the entorhinal cortex (via the perforant pathway). (From Kennedy and Marder, 1992.)

vealed a circumscribed and almost complete loss of cells in field CA1 of the hippocampus, bilaterally.

The hippocampus receives input from many areas of the neocortex over relays in the entorhinal cortex, and projects through its intrinsic circuits back to the entorhinal cortex, and via it recurrently to the neocortex (Fig. 6-1). It is over these connections that the hippocampus is thought to impose the long-term changes in cortical circuits upon which the consolidation of learning and memory depend. Activity in the circuits linking the hippocampus with the limbic lobe, the central core systems of the brainstem, and with the thalamic intralaminar system is thought to lend saliency and a certain hedonic color to the operations of the hippocampus.

It is for these reasons that much current research on synaptic plasticity is made on the hippocampus, most commonly in rodents. In what follows I consider that aspect of the field, and then relate it to

Activity-Dependent Changes in Synaptic Strength

several similar studies on the neocortex. First, I describe a simpler change in synaptic efficacy, post-tetanic potentiation.

Post-Tetanic Potentiation

High-frequency trains of impulses in presynaptic axons produce an increase in the local postsynaptic responses of the relevant set of postsynaptic neurons to subsequent testing volleys in the activated axons. This was shown half a century ago by Feng (1941) for the neuromuscular junction, and then by Larrabee and Bronk (1947) for sympathetic ganglionic transmission and by David Lloyd (1949) for the large afferent fibers from muscle that project monosynaptically upon motoneurons of the spinal cord. Lloyd also discovered that a synaptic depression follows low-frequency presynaptic stimulation. Post-tetanic potentiation (PTP) lasts for several minutes, during which time neurons from the subliminal fringe are recruited in the discharge zone of the postsynaptic neuronal population engaged. It is confined to the pathway conditioned by the high-frequency stimulation; no potentiation is observed over converging pathways of presynaptic terminals not tetanized. PTP results from an increased flow of Ca^{2+} ions into the presynaptic terminals of the axons stimulated, saturating the Ca^{2+}-buffering proteins. Each successive action potential in the post-tetanic period elicits an increased Ca^{2+}-dependent transmitter release, and increased postsynaptic response. An additional factor may be that high-frequency volleys of impulses promote invasion of previously "silent" presynaptic terminals. Whether PTP as such plays a role in activity-dependent changes in central neural circuits remains uncertain. The original experimental observations in the central nervous system were made on spinal reflex arcs using conditioning trains of stimuli at high frequencies (300–500/sec) that seldom if ever occur in cortical circuits. It has now been shown that similar changes are produced in polysynaptic circuits activated at lower frequencies (Fig. 6-2).

Long-Term Changes in Synaptic Effectiveness in the Hippocampus

The study of candidate cellular mechanisms of memory began with the discovery by Lomo (1966) that high-frequency stimulation of axons of the perforant pathway afferent to the granule cells of the dentate gyrus produces a long-term potentiation (LTP) of the synap-

Fig. 6-2 The three phases of postsynaptic facilitation: post-tetanic potentiation (PTP) and both short- and long-term potentiation (STP and LTP) can be elicited by high-frequency afferent input to hippocampal CA1 pyramidal cells, as demonstrated in studies with slice preparations. (A) Graph plots the slope of the EPSP versus time in an experiment in which different tetani were delivered, first in the presence and then the absence of saturating concentrations of the NMDA receptor antagonist D-APV. In the presence of the blocker, only post-tetanic potentiation lasting 30–40 sec was elicited. After washout of the blocker, tetanus 2 elicited a transient facilitation of synaptic transmission (short-term potentiation), whereas tetanus 3 caused a maintained long-term potentiation. The tetanic stimuli were delivered at 0.1 Hz. Sample raw data records appear at upper right at the times indicated by small letters. (B) A graph of the EPSP slopes versus time from an experiment in which the same tetani (1 and 2) were applied during different degrees of NMDA receptor blockade. Only PTP was evoked in the presence of 25 μM D-APV; in the presence of 2 μM blocker, the same tetanic stimuli caused STP; when the blocker was washed out, the longer tetanus evoked a sustained LTP. (From Malenka, 1991.)

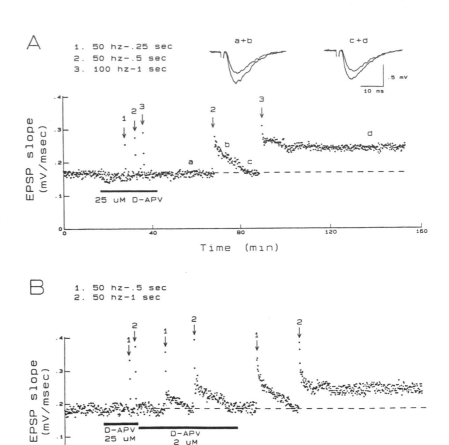

tic responses evoked in those same cells by subsequent testing volleys delivered at low frequencies (see also Bliss and Lomo, 1973; Bliss and Gardner-Medwin, 1973). Scarcely before or since has a single experimental discovery stimulated such an outburst of investigation; since Lomo's brief report, about 2,300 papers have been published on the subject (MEDLINE, 1966–1997). The reasons are obvious. Here is a long-lasting, use-dependent increase in synaptic effectiveness that meets some of the requirements for a cellular mechanism of learning and memory. It is evoked by brief periods of high-frequency stimulation of presynaptic afferents that resembles some patterns that occur in the hippocampus in waking mammals. LTP has since been shown to persist for hours in a hippocampal slice preparation, and

Activity-Dependent Changes in Synaptic Strength

for months in the intact mammal. Moreover, it was discovered in just that region of the brain, the hippocampus, already suspected to be of critical importance in the CNS mechanisms in declarative memory; LTP has since been identified in a number of other areas in the brain.

High-frequency input to the hippocampus produces LTP at each of the three synaptic relays in the hippocampal circuit shown in Fig. 6-1. Glutamate is the transmitter at each of these excitatory synapses; when released, it combines with postsynaptic ionotropic and metabotropic receptors. An experimental observation widely confirmed is that a pharmacological block of the NMDARs blocks LTP at the perforant path–dentate gyrus synapses and at the synapses the Schaffer collaterals make with the pyramidal cells of CA1, but not at the mossy fiber–CA3 synapses. The two NMDA-dependent LTPs have many properties in common, and they differ in mechanism from the non-NMDA-dependent LTP evoked at the mossy fiber synapses. The NMDA-dependent form of LTP is the most widely used experimental model of long-term synaptic plasticity, and it has been observed at synapses in many places in the brain, including the neocortex.

Low-frequency stimulation of the Schaffer collaterals produces a reciprocal effect, a long-term depression (LTD) of synaptic transmission in CA1 (Dudek and Bear, 1992; Mulkey and Malenka, 1992). While the details of the biochemical events leading to these two quite opposite effects are not completely understood, the general outline is clear. They are both NMDA-dependent and are initiated by an influx of Ca^{2+} into the cell. LTP operations, through the resulting increase in Ca^{2+}-calmodulin-dependent protein kinases, lead to phosphorylation of intracellular proteins, including ligand- and voltage-gated channels, and to increases in synaptic response by up-regulation of channel currents. LTD is evoked by the minimal Ca^{2+} influx evoked by low-frequency stimulation of afferents to the NMDARs, which by some unknown, quantitatively sensitive mechanism activates phosphatases and not kinases, with a resulting dephosphorylation of intracellular proteins and decreases in synaptic response.

NMDA-Dependent Long-Term Potentiation at CA1 Synapses

NMDA-dependent LTP is induced at the pyramidal cell synapses in area CA1 of the hippocampus by a few seconds' high-frequency stimulation of the afferent fibers, the Schaffer collaterals. It is expressed in the accelerated slopes and increased amplitudes of EPSPs, which in-

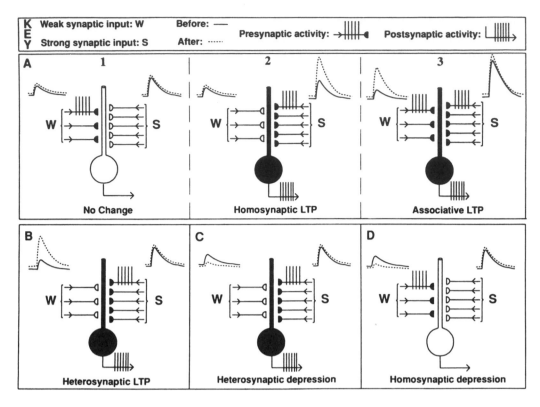

Fig. 6-3 Several varieties of use-dependent synaptic change. Each neuron is shown receiving overlapping weak *(W)* and strong *(S)* synaptic inputs, reflecting the relative number of active afferent fibers. The waveforms above each input illustrate the response produced by a single input afferent volley before (solid curves) and after (dashed curves) high-frequency stimulation of one or both inputs. Filled elements indicate activity during the tetanic stimulation. (From Brown et al., 1990.)

(A) *Associative LTP.* (1) Tetanic stimulation of *W* alone does not cause LTP in either channel. (2) Tetanic stimulation of *S* may produce homosynaptic but not heterosynaptic LTP. (3) Simultaneous stimulation of *W* and *S* causes associative LTP, with enhancement in *W;* LTP may occur also in *S* under these conditions.

(B) *Heterosynaptic LTP.* Stimulation of *S* alone causes LTP in unstimulated *W.* LTP may also occur in *S* under these circumstances.

(C) *Heterosynaptic depression.* Stimulation of *S* alone causes depression in unstimulated *W;* depression may occur also in *S* (not shown here).

(D) *Homosynaptic depression.* Stimulation of *W* causes depression in *W* alone.

crement slowly and persist for several hours in experimental preparations of the hippocampus, and for days in the intact mammal. The CA1 form of LTP requires simultaneous activity of postsynaptic and presynaptic neurons. LTP may be homosynaptic, limited to the set of fibers activated by the conditioning stimulation; or it may be heterosynaptic, as when an "associative" LTP is induced by activation of one set of fibers, combined with low-frequency activity in a converging pathway, and may thereafter be evoked by testing volleys in either channel (Fig. 6-3; see also Brown et al., 1990). This associative property suggests that LTP may be involved in associative learning, and memory, in the CNS.

Mechanisms of Induction and Expression of NMDA-Dependent LTP

The phenomenon at CA1 synapses is illustrated in several figures in this chapter (see Figs. 6-2, 6-5, 6-6, and 6-10). The candidate initiating molecular mechanisms are schematized in Fig. 6-4 (for reviews, see Bliss and Collingridge, 1993; Hawkins et al., 1993; Larkman and Jack, 1995; Malenka, 1995; Huang et al., 1996). The presynaptic axons innervating the dendritic spines of the CA1 pyramidal cells are glutaminergic. The several classes of glutamate receptors with different properties are clustered in the membranes of postsynaptic spines (Seeburg, 1993). The non-NMDA receptors operate with rapid kinetics, and when open they have high conductances for monovalent cations and low Ca^{2+} conductance. The NMDA receptor is a coincidence detector ("associative"), requiring for activation both the presence of glutamate and postsynaptic depolarization, which expels a blocking Mg^{2+}. The channel then binds with glutamate to produce a high-conductance channel for Ca^{2+} (but low for Na^+) into the postsynaptic cell. The time window for this coincidence detection is set by the duration of the NMDA postsynaptic response, about 100 msec. LTP initiating events are cooperative between the nearly simultaneous depolarization of postsynaptic cells (via the AMPA-glutamate receptors) and the induced inward flux of Ca^{2+} into the synaptic spine compartment (by glutamate activation of the unblocked NMDA receptors). Pharmacological blockade of NMDA receptors prevents induction of LTP (Collingridge et al., 1983, and many since then); sequestration of the intracellular Ca^{2+} surge by injection of Ca-chelators prevents the initiation of LTP; and, conversely, direct injection of Ca^{2+} into postsynaptic cells increases LTP (for reviews see Malenka, 1995; Nicoll and Malenka, 1995). There is some evidence that LTP may be influenced by other glutamate receptors. One candidate is the metabotropic receptor, mGluR. These are transmembrane receptors linked by G-proteins to intracellular second-messenger systems, through which they may mediate slow responses to glutamate by modulatory control of both voltage- and ligand-gated channels (O'Connor et al., 1994). mGluRs are widely distributed in the nervous system and may play a modulatory role in LTP (Nakanishi, 1994; Ben-Ari and Aniksztejn, 1995).

The signal transduction chain in LTP leads from Ca^{2+} entry through the adenylyl cyclase–cAMP pathway to activation of several intracellular kinases, and by them to phosphorylation of intracellular and membrane-bound proteins, including channel proteins. These events result in an increased conductance in both the NMDA and AMPA channels and increased postsynaptic response (Fig. 6-4) (Raymond et al., 1993; Roche et al., 1994). Among the kinases are Ca^{2+}/calmodulin-dependent protein kinase II (CaM-KII), protein kinase C (PKC), and tyrosine kinase (fyn). Pharmacological inhibition or blockade of any one of these three reduces LTP, sometimes drastically, but may not eliminate completely its induction by presynaptic volleys (Fig. 6-5; Hvalby et al., 1994). Intracellular injections of CaM-KII via the intracellular recording pipette produced a gradual increase in excitatory postsynaptic currents (EPSCs), a rise that resembled LTP; occlusion experiments between CaM-KII and LTP effects suggested that the two operate by shared mechanisms (Fig. 6-6; Lledo et al., 1995). The exact role CaM-KII and PKC play in the signal transduction chain is still uncertain. CaM-KII has received the most attention: it is present in high concentration in the postsynaptic densities, its intracellular concentration is increased during LTP, and it has the unusual property of autophosphorylation. This latter is of interest, for the increase in Ca^{2+} within cells lasts no longer than 2–3 seconds after the end of the train of impulses inducing LTP. After that time, the self-phosphorylating CaM-KII is independent of Ca^{2+} concentration, and it will therefore phosphorylate target proteins for extended periods of time. A simple sequence proposed for the expression of LTP is the continued phosphorylation of AMPARs by CaM-KII and their continued up-regulation, leading to increased postsynaptic response to an unchanging presynaptic release of transmitter.

Embryological and DNA recombination methods have made it

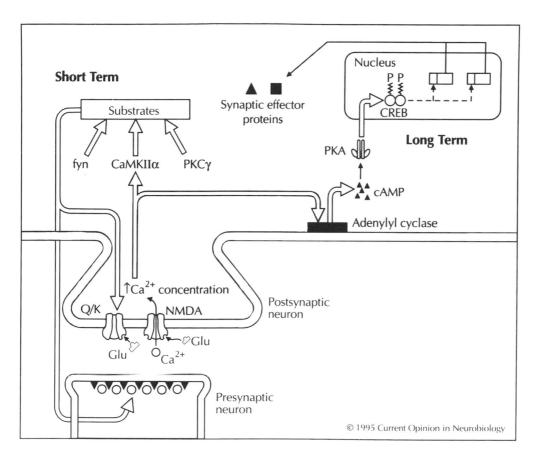

Fig. 6-4 Model of the molecular basis of long-term potentiation at the CA1 synapses in the hippocampus. Activation of the postsynaptic neuron by glutamate *(Glu)* leads to two processes. A short-term process lasts 1 hour or less. It involves CaM-KIIα, PKC, and the tyrosine kinase *fyn* and leads to a retrograde signal (which may be nitrous oxide) that is postulated to act presynaptically to increase transmitter release. The long-term process, initiated by activation of adenylyl cyclase, leads to an increase in cAMP and activation of genes via the transcription factor CREB. It is postulated that the induced gene products result in long-lasting maintenance of synaptic potentiation, perhaps through a structural change. *P,* phosphorylation site; *Q/K,* quisqualate/kainate glutamate receptor. (From Mayford et al., 1995a.)

possible to produce a specific mutation of any gene in the mouse genome. Mice lacking CaM-KII show an almost complete absence of STP, LTP, and LTD. Post-tetanic potentiation is intact in these CaM-KII-deficient animals (Stevens et al., 1994; Silva et al., 1992). Incomplete deficiencies in LTP occur in mice lacking tyrosine kinase (Grant and O'Dell, 1994) or protein kinase C (Abeliovich et al., 1993). Con-

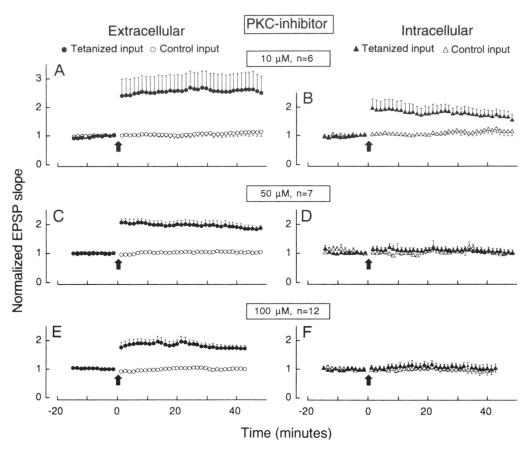

Fig. 6-5 Effects of a protein kinase C (PKC) inhibitor on the induction of long-term potentiation at the hippocampal CA1 synapses. Intracellular and extracellular recordings made through separate electrodes in a rat slice preparation are shown here. Increasing concentrations of the kinase inhibitor in the intracellular pipette (from top to bottom) produced total inhibition of LTP in the tetanized pathway (solid symbols); open symbols show no changes in control pathway. Vertical bars = SEMs; arrows indicate times of stimulation. (From Hvalby et al., 1994.)

versely, when CaM-KII is increased in hippocampal pyramidal cells by linking it to an infecting recombinant vaccinia virus, synaptic transmission is greatly potentiated (Petit et al., 1994). Mayford et al. (1995b) generated transgenic mice expressing a Ca^{2+}-independent, autophosphorylating form of CaM-KII. These mice showed a normal induction of LTP by high-frequency (100/sec) presynaptic input, but a shift from LTP toward LTD at lower frequencies (1–10/sec). The role of frequency in shifting the threshold between LTP and LTD is discussed below.

Activity-Dependent Changes in Synaptic Strength

Tonegawa and associates used the P1-phage-derived Cre/lax P recombination system to produce genetically engineered strains of mice in which the single gene for the NMDAR1 receptor protein of the pyramidal cells of CA1 of the hippocampus has been deleted (Tsien et al., 1996a). It was not possible to produce LTP, LTD, or STP at these synapses using methods that did produce these phenomena at NMDA-mediated synapses in the adjacent perforant pathway–dentate gyrus. The mutant mice had impaired spatial memory (Tsien et al., 1996b). Electrophysiological studies made using many chronically implanted microelectrodes yielded the surprising result that the CA1 pyramidal cells in the spatially impaired mutant mice still demonstrated place-related activity. However, further analyses of the population activity revealed a marked loss of correlation between the

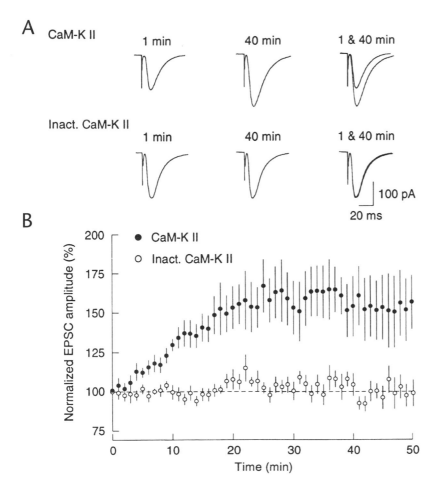

Fig. 6-6 The enzyme CaM-KII potentiates transmission at hippocampal CA1 synapses, as demonstrated by intracellular recordings in guinea pig hippocampal slice preparation. When active CaM-KII was included in the intracellular pipette, there was a gradual and long-lasting increase in EPSC amplitudes. When heat-inactivated CaM-KII was included in the pipette, no change in synaptic transmission was observed. (From Lledo et al., 1995.)

Activity-Dependent Changes in Synaptic Strength

activity of pyramidal cells in the population (McHugh et al., 1996; for review, see Wilson and Tonegawa, 1997). For further discussion of the importance of correlation of activity in neuronal populations, see Chapter 12.

Is a Retrograde Signal Required to Initiate a Presynaptic Change Necessary for the Expression of LTP?

There is general agreement that LTP at CA1 synapses is initiated as a postsynaptic event, perhaps as a result of an acceleration of the opening rate of the non-NMDA channels and an increase in the time they remain open. An interesting and hotly debated question is whether the persistence of LTP depends upon an increased presynaptic release of glutamate, and whether this in turn depends upon a retrograde signal from the LTP-initiating postsynaptic cell to the presynaptic terminal. Alternatively, some investigators conclude that postsynaptic mechanisms are sufficient to account for both the initiation and expression of LTP at this particular junction, the mossy fiber–CA1 synapse. No inherent logic speaks against the action of both mechanisms, but these diverse views have been maintained with considerable vigor.

Several molecules with high diffusion rates have been suggested as putative retrograde signals. Among them are arachidonic acid (Williams et al., 1989) and carbon monoxide, but it is the oxygen radical nitric oxide (NO) that has aroused the greatest interest (Dawson and Dawson, 1995). NO is the "endothelial relaxing factor" that when released from the vascular endothelium diffuses to the adjacent vascular smooth muscle, causing its relaxation and vasodilatation, commonly in response to local hypoxia. Garthwaite et al. (1988) discovered that cerebellar granule cells release NO when their NMDA receptors are stimulated by glutamate, and NO is thought to be the essential retrograde messenger for cerebellar associative LTD (Ito, 1989). Gally et al. (1990; see also Edelman and Gally, 1992) developed the general hypothesis that NO functions as a spatial signal in development and in associative learning: it is believed to diffuse rapidly from its site of origin in active cells to strengthen the potency of synapses simultaneously active within its diffusion domain. The volume of that signal space is limited to about 300 μm diameter by the 1 sec half-life of NO (for reviews, see Bredt and Snyder, 1992; Haley and Schuman, 1994; Hawkins et al., 1993; Schuman and Madison, 1994).

The evidence is not wholly convincing on either side of the disagreement over whether a retrograde signal is necessary for the maintenance of LTP. Many experimental observations fit the NO hypothesis. NO synthase (the endothelial form!) is present in nonspiny, nonpyramidal cells of the cerebral cortex (Bredt et al., 1991) and in CA1 pyramidal cells (Wentland et al., 1994). NO synthase is activated via the glutaminergic, Ca^{2+}-calmodulin sequence, requires NADPH (nicotinamide adenine dinucleotide phosphate hydride) as a co-enzyme, and produces NO from L-arginine with stoichiometric amounts of citrulline. NO is thought to initiate a presynaptic second-messenger cascade that leads to increased transmitter release, perhaps by an increase in the probability of vesicle fusion (Stevens, 1993; Meffert et al., 1996). LTP induction in the postsynaptic CA1 pyramids is linked to an increased transmitter release from the presynaptic axon terminals of the Schaffer collaterals. A complete block of both the endothelial and neuronal isoforms of NO synthase eliminates LTP under many, but not all, experimental circumstances (O'Dell et al., 1994).

Equally cogent arguments speak against the necessity for a retrograde signal. Attempts have been made to clarify the problem by the use of quantal analysis. This method allows a change in synaptic strength to be assigned to one or both of two underlying causes. A presynaptic change is indicated by an increased probability of release of quanta of transmitter. A postsynaptic change is indicated by an increased response to each quantum released, indicated by an increase in the evoked postsynaptic excitatory currents (Bekkers, 1994; Redman, 1990; Voronin, 1994). The results obtained in studies of the CA1 synapses during LTP in different laboratories are conflicting, some finding increased probability of release, some finding increased amplitude of response, others both (Kullmann and Siegelbaum, 1995; Kuhnt and Voronin, 1994). The conflict may arise because the general assumptions that underlie the method and are applicable to peripheral synapses may not hold for central synapses. Some new findings indicate that under normal conditions silent glutaminergic synapses exist on postsynaptic spines; some spines expose only NMDA receptors, others only AMPA receptors, still others neither. It has been suggested that these silent synapses are uncovered during an input that elicits LTP, and that these same synapses then reveal strong NMDA and AMPA responses. The uncovering of silent synapses during the high-frequency afferent input that evokes LTP provides a simple and sufficient explanation for the expression of LTP by a postsynaptic mechanism; it also may account for the apparent increase in the probability of transmitter release during LTP observed by some investigators (Isaac et al., 1995; Liao et al., 1995; Manabe and Nicoll, 1994).

LTP appears to be a complex set of several somewhat different processes; some require a presynaptic mechanism for continued expression that depends upon NO or some other rapidly diffusing retrograde signal. Other types of LTP, or LTP evoked under other circumstances, may depend only upon postsynaptic mechanisms for both induction and expression. How else to account for the variety of conflicting experimental findings in the field than on the basis of a heterogeneity of the very process under study? For example, Manabe and Nicoll (1994) present evidence that there is no increase in transmitter release during the expression of LTP. On the other hand, Malgaroli et al. (1995) used an immunohistochemical method to show a marked increase in presynaptic vesicular recycling during LTP; and Pasinelli et al. (1995) describe an increase in PKC activity in phosphorylating its specific substrates both pre- and postsynaptically during hippocampal LTP. There the matter rests, temporarily!

Can LTP Be Correlated with Procedural Memory or Spatial Learning at the Behavioral Level?

The hypothesis to be tested is whether the experimentally induced plasticity of the LTP type defines processes that are used in the brains of waking mammals for encoding and stabilizing memories (Maren and Baudry, 1995; Martinez and Derrick, 1996). One can scarcely imagine a more difficult experimental task, for it appears likely that several forms of LTP plasticity exist. The match between what can be observed with what is being used in the animal's brain is uncertain. The electrophysiological methods adaptable to the waking animal are limited to the several forms of extracellular recording. The field potentials generated by postsynaptic responses, or the population spike of neuronal discharges, may not be adequate measures of changes in synaptic effectiveness. Moreover, the processes under study are likely to be widely distributed in synaptic systems, and the changes that occur at any local testing site quite small (Barnes, 1995). Some circumstantial evidence has accumulated to support the hypothesis. Rodents with pharmacological blockade of NMDA receptors (Morris et al., 1986; Davis et al., 1992), or with imposed defects in the CaM-KII system (Bach et al., 1995), show selective abnormalities in hippocampal LTP and, simultaneously, deficiencies in spatial learning. Complete saturation of LTP at hippocampal synapses by electroconvulsive shock stimulation produces an enhancement of synaptic responses, an occlusion of induced LTP, and spatial learning deficiencies in the Morris water maze test; these defects persist for weeks (Barnes et al., 1994).

All these compose circumstantial evidence of some importance, but given the weakness of correlated change, they do not establish causal relation. It is also true, however, that no experiments have been published that disprove the hypothetical causal link between LTP and certain forms of learning and memory.

NMDA-Mediated Long-Term Depression

The idea that LTP is an important part of the CNS mechanisms of learning and memory suggests that a complementary process of opposite sign functions at the level of cellular mechanism as a resetting device. A long-term associative depression (LTD) was first identified at cerebellar synapses, where it is regarded as a "memory element" in motor learning (Ito, 1989). Absent such a mechanism, cortical synapses might from time to time saturate at the high end of the excitability range, with a concomitant reduction in flexibility of response. Moreover, LTP and LTD are thought to be important, use-dependent mechanisms, responsible for the strengthening or pruning of synapses in early postnatal life. LTD is then more readily evoked and of greater amplitude, dropping the postsynaptic responses from a peak of about -50 percent to about -20 percent of control values from birth to adulthood in mice (Dudek and Bear, 1993). Input-specific, homosynaptic LTD has been described for both hippocampal and neocortical synapses (for reviews, see D. J. Linden, 1994; Linden and Connor 1995; Bear and Malenka, 1994). The records of Fig. 6-7 show the frequency dependency of LTD; it is best evoked by afferent stimuli delivered at 1/sec for many hundreds of stimuli (Dudek and Bear, 1992; Mulkey and Malenka, 1992). NMDA antagonists or intracellular injection of Ca^{2+} chelators both block LTD completely. LTD is presumably initiated by a low-intensity surge of Ca^{2+} through NMDA channels, which leads in this case to activation of intracellular phosphatases and dephosphorylation of intracellular substrate proteins,

Fig. 6-7 The effect of frequency of input upon the direction of postsynaptic change, studied in hippocampal slice preparations. The local field potentials plotted here were evoked by trains of impulses in Schaffer collaterals projecting to CA1 pyramids. Volleys at 3/sec (A) produced prolonged synaptic depression; those at 10/sec only transient depression (B); and those at 50/sec produced long-term potentiation of the synaptic responses (C). (From Dudek and Bear, 1992.)

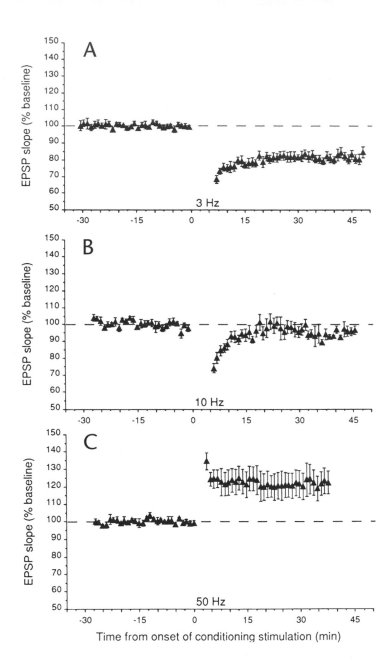

Activity-Dependent Changes in Synaptic Strength

including channel proteins (Mulkey et al., 1993). The link from Ca^{2+} entry to phosphatase activation is still uncertain. There is some evidence that mGluRs also play a role in the modulation of LTD (Bolshakov and Siegelbaum, 1994). When LTP is produced in a population of synapses, that same stimulation produces a low-level heterosynaptic LTD at the synapses of neighboring populations of cells. This long-range effect depends upon the spread of some signal between neurons, but the evidence suggests that it is not nitric oxide (Scanziani et al., 1996).

Frequency Control and the Sliding Threshold Hypothesis

The discovery of a homosynaptic form of LTD at hippocampal CA1 synapses led to the realization that LTD and LTP have many properties in common; they are in a sense reciprocals. Either one can be induced at the same synapses upon the same postsynaptic neurons by volleys of impulses in the same presynaptic fibers, volleys that differ only in frequency. High frequencies (5–50 Hz) evoke LTP, low (1–3 Hz) evoke LTD. Each is initiated by a surge of Ca^{2+} through NMDA channels, in synchrony with membrane depolarization. If that surge is sufficiently intense, the kinase pathway leading to phosphorylation of target proteins like ionic channels is activated, and LTP results. If the Ca^{2+} surge is below that threshold, the phosphatase pathway is activated, leading to the dephosphorylation of target proteins, and LTD results (Fig. 6-8). Some links in these signal pathways are still uncertain; e.g., the phosphatases are not Ca^{2+}-dependent, and an intervening step through calcineurin may occur.

Bienenstock et al. (1982) predicted on theoretical grounds that the frequency of transition from LTD to LTP is not fixed but is shifted by immediate past history of the synapses (Fig. 6-9). That is just what Bear and his colleagues have now demonstrated (Bear, 1995; Gold and Bear, 1994; Dudek and Bear, 1993; see also Bear and Malenka, 1994). If LTP is induced, LTD can then be induced at frequencies somewhat higher than in the unconditioned state, and vice-versa. Mayford et al. (1995a,b) have demonstrated this same threshold flexibility in a different way. They produced transgenic mice that express a Ca^{2+}-independent form of CaM-KII that functions continuously as if phosphorylated. This produces a state of high postsynaptic responsiveness. The frequency transition threshold is much higher in these mutant mice than in normals, for LTD can be produced by frequen-

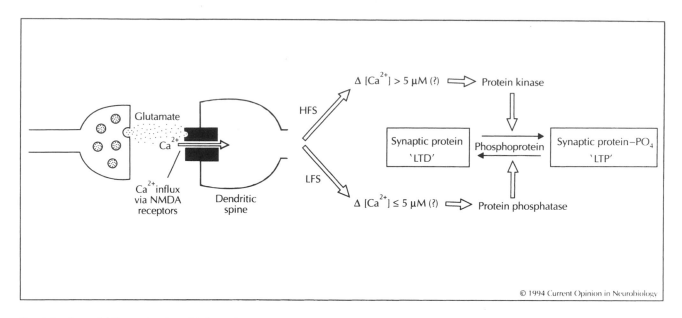

Fig. 6-8 A model illustrating how high- and low-frequency stimulation of the same afferent inputs might produce the opposite effects of LTP and LTD in the postsynaptic cells. During high-frequency stimulation *(HFS)*, Ca^{2+} concentration reaches high levels in the postsynaptic spines, preferentially activating protein kinases leading to phosphorylation of synaptic proteins and, e.g., increased channel conductance. During low-frequency stimulation *(LFS)*, much lower levels of intracellular Ca^{2+} are reached, preferentially activating protein phosphatases, which dephosphorylate the synaptic proteins. (From Bear and Malenka, 1994.)

cies in the range of 4–12 Hz, which routinely evoke LTP in normal animals.

Other Factors Influencing LTP

The induction of LTP at CA1 synapses requires high-frequency stimulation of presynaptic afferents. At low frequencies, GABA-mediated postsynaptic inhibition holds the pyramidal cell membrane potentials hyperpolarized, so that NMDA receptors remain blocked by Mg^{2+} (Davies et al., 1991). Higher-frequency stimulation elicits $GABA_B$-mediated autoinhibition of GABA release from presynaptic terminals, and excitatory action via the AMPA Glu receptors drives the postsynaptic membrane potentials to levels of depolarization that relieve the Mg^{2+} block of the NMDA channels.

Activation of the NMDA receptor is enhanced or enabled by the co-transmitter glycine (Thomson, 1989; Oliver et al., 1990) and by modulatory synaptic transmitters such as norepinephrine and acetylcholine. Activation of the NMDA receptor evokes expression of immediate early genes that elicit the transcriptional activity of late-onset genes leading to protein synthesis and structural change at synapses (Morgan and Curran, 1989; Armstrong and Montminy,

1993; Worley et al., 1990; Buchs and Muller, 1996). There is some evidence that a form of LTP can also be elicited by activation of the metabotropic glutamate receptor, without the STP component and without accompanying NMDA activation (Bortolotto and Collingridge, 1993; Bear and Malenka, 1994).

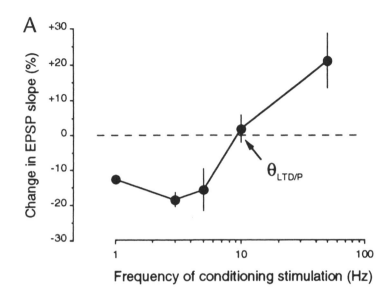

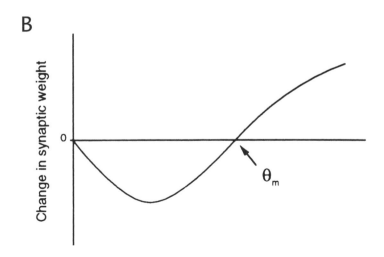

Fig. 6-9 A comparison of theory and experiment. (A) Changes recorded in the mean effect ($\pm$ standard error) of 900 conditioning volleys in the Schaffer collaterals, at different frequencies, upon the synaptic responses of CA1 pyramidal neurons of the rat hippocampus. The transition from LTD to LTP occurs at about 10/sec. (B) According to the theory from Bienenstock et al. (1982), the weights of synapses are assumed to modify according to this function of the postsynaptic response. At the modification threshold, Θ_m, the function changes from negative to positive. The value of Θ_m is not fixed but varies continuously as a function of the postsynaptic response. (From Bear, 1995.)

Short-Term Potentiation at CA1 Synapses

Studies of hippocampal CA1 synapses reveal that a short-term potentiation (STP) may be evoked without LTP by certain patterns of presynaptic stimulation. STP differs from LTP by its independence of protein kinase activity (for review see Malenka and Nicoll, 1993). STP when seen alone decrements to control values in about 30 min; but when LTP is also induced it may be superimposed upon the slower rise of the LTP. The experiment illustrated in Fig. 6-2 (Malenka, 1991) indicates that each of three phases of synaptic enhancement can be evoked under different circumstances. PTP is evoked in isolation when NMDA receptors are blocked. STP and LTP are evoked by different patterns of presynaptic activity, with NMDA receptors unblocked. Malenka (1991) proposed that it is the magnitude of the postsynaptic surge of Ca^{2+} per se that controls the time course of synaptic change, and that LTP is induced as a threshold event governed by that level. Kullmann et al. (1992) demonstrated a form of STP produced by Ca^{2+} entry through voltage-sensitive Ca^{2+} channels independently of synaptic activity, but that synaptic activity was required to convert STP to LTP. These and other results indicate that LTP depends upon both a threshold level of Ca^{2+} in the postsynaptic cell and at least in some cases upon another process evoked by presynaptic input. However, it has recently been shown that late LTP depends upon protein synthesis (as does long-term memory), for the late phase of LTP is prevented if transcription is blocked during a critical time period shortly after presynaptic stimulation (Nguyen et al., 1994; Huang et al., 1996).

Non-NMDA-Dependent LTP at Hippocampal CA3 Synapses

LTP at the mossy fiber–CA3 synapses is produced by high-frequency afferent input, as is LTP at CA1; otherwise the two phenomena are quite different (Nicoll and Malenka, 1995). The mechanisms for induction and expression of LTP at the CA3 synapses are located in the presynaptic terminal, and the increase in synaptic effectiveness is independent of events in the postsynaptic cell. NMDARs, for example, are thinly distributed in this area (Monaghan and Cotman, 1985), and blockage of those few receptors leaves LTP unaffected. Injection of Ca^{2+}-chelators or kinase inhibitors into the postsynaptic cells are equally without effect on induced LTP at this synapse. The critical observations are, first, that LTP is accompanied by an increase in presynaptic glutamate release; and, second, that removal of Ca^{2+} from the local extracellular environment blocks LTP completely. How entry of Ca^{2+} into the presynaptic terminal initiates increased transmitter release is still not understood completely. The evidence available suggests a chain of events that links Ca^{2+} entry to Ca^{2+}-calmodulin-activated adenylyl cyclase. The resulting increase in cAMP concentration then activates protein kinase A (PKA) (Weisskopf et al., 1994). The direct evidence stops there, but it seems likely that PKA facilitates synaptic vesicular mobilization, transport, docking, and terminal fusion, to accomplish increased glutamate release. The late phase of LTP depends upon protein kinase activity and protein synthesis; it can be evoked by the appropriate pattern of stimulation at each of the three monosynaptic excitatory pathways in the hippocampus.

Derrick et al. (1991) discovered that LTP at the mossy fiber synapse is blocked by naloxone, which indicates that opioid receptors are involved in LTP at this synapse. LTP produced at other synapses on these same cells by volleys in the commissural afferents is not affected by naloxone.

Long-Term Changes in Synaptic Effectiveness in the Neocortex

Studies of synaptic plasticity in the neocortex followed quickly upon the discovery of LTP and LTD in the hippocampus and cerebellum. Cortical LTP and LTD are of great interest, for the property of plasticity is believed essential for the strengthening or pruning of synaptic contacts in the postnatal development of the neocortex (Chapter 9). There is now evidence of a temporal correlation in cortical development between the modification of thalamocortical synapses by peripheral sensory perturbations during an early postnatal period and the presence of a readily evoked LTP at those same synapses later (Fox, 1995). Crair and Malenka (1995) have demonstrated this temporal correlation at the thalamocortical synapses in the rat somatic sensory cortex, where, during the critical period of the first four postnatal days, the normal barrel structure of the cortex can be altered by removal of a contralateral mystacial vibrissa (see Chapter 7). Kirkwood et al. (1995) found a similar correlation in the visual cortex of rodents during that critical period in which the binocular connections are forming, and discovered that both the critical period and the parallel presence of a readily evoked LTP can be prolonged in dark-reared animals.

There is now compelling evidence that this same capacity for activity-dependent changes in synaptic effectiveness persists into adult life in broadly distributed classes of cortical synapses. Synaptic change of this type is one candidate cellular basis for such complex cortical operations as those involved in learning, in the consolidation of long-term memories, in the embedding of new motor patterns, and in perception itself (Singer, 1995).

Experimental studies of synaptic plasticity in the neocortex have been made in both the *in vitro* cortical slice preparation and in several areas in the intact, waking mammal (for reviews see Tsumoto, 1992; Teyler et al., 1990). EPSPs are recorded intracellularly (e.g., Baranyi et al., 1991; Keller et al., 1990), or field potentials are recorded with extracellular microelectrodes (Aroniadou and Teyler, 1991, 1992). LTP is induced by electrical stimulation of the subjacent white matter, of a cortical area projecting to the one under study, or of the relevant thalamic nucleus. Cortical LTP resembles hippocampal LTP in some properties, but it differs in others. It may be homosynaptic or associative. In some locations cortical LTP is NMDA dependent, as it is at CA1 synapses; at other locations it is independent of NMDA receptor activation, as LTP is at CA3 synapses. Like hippocampal LTP of either type, it depends upon the postsynaptic surge of Ca^{2+}. LTP is easily produced only in layers II/III, and it is obtained more readily and at greater amplitude after GABA blockage, which indicates that under normal circumstances LTP is under inhibitory regulation. It is influenced by adrenergic or muscarinic agonists, and thus may also be controlled by the corticipetal modulatory systems from the basal forebrain and the central brainstem core.

LTP is more readily evoked in some cortical areas than in others. Castro-Alamancos et al. (1995, 1996) compared the synaptic plasticity expressed in the vertical pathways in the somatic sensory and motor cortical areas in the rat. LTD could be generated with ease in the networks of the somatic sensory granular cortex, but it could be generated in the motor cortex only if GABA-mediated inhibition were reduced (Chen et al., 1994). Undoubtedly, the distribution of the various forms of plasticity will be found to vary between different cortical areas. For example, a long-lasting synaptic enhancement can be produced after NMDA blockade at some cortical locations but not at others. NMDA-dependent LTP and LTD have been demonstrated

Activity-Dependent Changes in Synaptic Strength

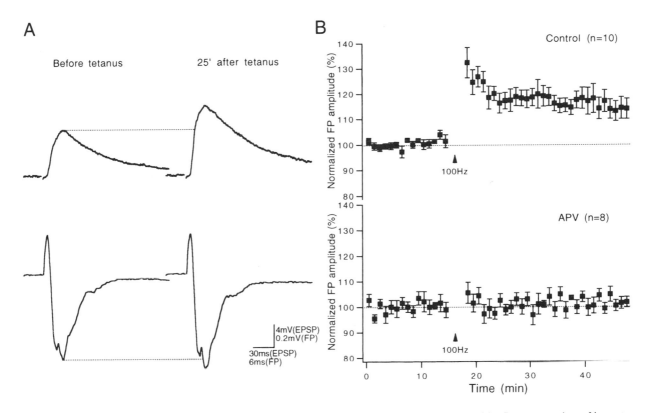

A

Before tetanus   25' after tetanus

4mV(EPSP)
0.2mV(FP)
30ms(EPSP)
6ms(FP)

B

Control (n=10)

Normalized FP amplitude (%)

100Hz

APV (n=8)

Normalized FP amplitude (%)

100Hz

Time (min)

Fig. 6-10 Demonstration of long-term potentiation (LTP) of synaptic transmission in a slice from human inferior temporal cortex. (A) 100 Hz stimulation induced LTP in both intracellularly recorded EPSPs (upper traces) and evoked field potentials (lower traces). The EPSPs and field potentials were averaged over 5 min recording periods immediately before and 25 min after the tetanus. (B) Time courses of the averaged field-potential responses evoked in the absence (upper half) and presence (lower half) of 50–100 μM APV, a blocker of the NMDA glutamate receptors. (From Chen et al., 1996.)

in slices of surgically resected human inferior and middle temporal cortex (Figs. 6-10 and 6-11; Chen et al., 1996).

Singer and his colleagues studied these phenomena in slices of the kitten visual cortex, where LTP and LTD can be induced in sequence by differences in the frequency of presynaptic input (Artola et al., 1990; Artola and Singer, 1993; Brocher et al., 1992; Artola, 1994). They concluded that the different outcomes depend upon quantitative differences in postsynaptic depolarization and in the amplitudes of the postsynaptic Ca^{2+} surge. At a low level of depolarization and low-amplitude CA^{2+} surge, synaptic depression results; with a stronger depolarization and higher-amplitude Ca^{2+} surge, potentiation results. The first is inferred to be related to the threshold of voltage-gated Ca^{2+} channels, the second to NMDA receptor activation. These observations fit well with the sliding threshold hypothesis described above, which includes the proposition that quantitative differences in Ca^{2+} concentration lead to differential activation

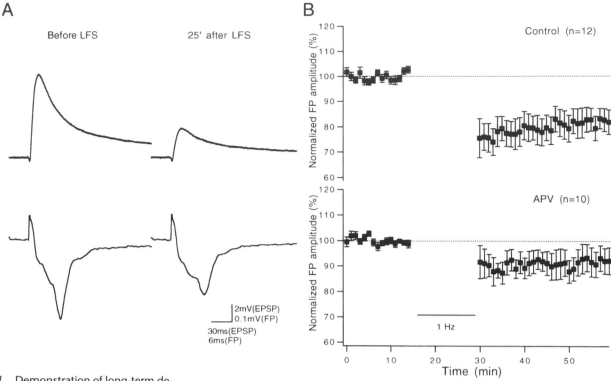

Fig. 6-11 Demonstration of long-term depression (LTD) of synaptic transmission in a slice from human inferior temporal cortex. (A) Low-frequency stimulation (1 Hz for 15 min) induced LTD of both intracellularly recorded EPSPs (upper traces) and evoked field potentials (lower traces). The EPSPs and evoked field potentials were averaged over 5 min recording periods immediately before and 25 min after conditioning stimulation. (B) Time courses of the average field potential evoked in the absence (upper half) and presence (lower half) of 50–100 μM APV, a blocker of the NMDA receptors. (From Chen et al., 1996.)

of different Ca^{2+}-dependent second-messenger systems (Lisman and Harris, 1993; Malenka and Nicoll, 1993) and thus to either LTP or LTD.

Summary

It is now three decades since Lomo discovered that high-frequency stimulation of afferents to the hippocampal dentate gyrus elicits a persisting increase in synaptic strength, now called long-term potentiation (LTP). This change is expressed as an acceleration in the onset slopes and increases in amplitudes of EPSPs of postsynaptic cells. It may be homo- or heterosynaptic, may have associative properties, and may persist for *weeks* in the mammalian brain. The intensity and duration of LTD and LTP are correlated with the degree of expression of immediate early genes (Abraham et al., 1994). LTP has been studied most intensively at CA1 hippocampal synapses, and the activity-

Activity-Dependent Changes in Synaptic Strength

dependent model derived from this research guides study of synaptic plasticity in the neocortex.

LTP at CA1 synapses is produced by nearly synchronous activation by the excitatory transmitter glutamate of both voltage- or ligand-gated NMDA receptors and ligand-gated non-NMDA receptors. The strong postsynaptic CA^{2+} surge through the former activates second-messenger systems leading to phosphorylation of membrane proteins, gene expression, protein synthesis, and changes in synaptic ultrastructure. Maintenance of some forms of LTP are thought to depend upon an increased presynaptic release of transmitter per impulse. This is presumed to require a retrograde signal, for which the rapidly diffusing gas nitric oxide (NO) is a candidate. This model of LTP is not universally applicable, and several postsynaptic mechanisms have been identified through which LTP can be expressed for long periods. There is a growing conviction that several forms of plasticity exist, of which the standard model of LTP is one. What they all have in common is the postsynaptic surge of Ca^{2+}. A salient feature of the CA1 model of LTP is that it depends upon virtually synchronous pre- and postsynaptic events, release of glutamate by presynaptic impulses, and postsynaptic depolarization. There is also evidence that under some circumstances the mGluRs and the voltage-gated Ca^{2+} channels make important contributions to LTP.

LTP is accompanied by ultrastructural changes at synapses and is now regarded as one of the cellular mechanisms of learning and memory. If so, it is now necessary to link those changes in central synapses to the activity of neural circuits and to determine how the synaptic change can be "embedded as memory" in a neural circuit in such a way that subsequent input signals that may resemble the initiating ones only partially elicit a construction of the full pattern of activity—the memory.

The discovery of LTP and its tentative link to memory mechanisms led to the idea that there might exist a similar mechanism of opposite sign. Long-term depressions (LTD)—well known for cerebellar synapses—have now been identified at hippocampal and neocortical synapses; a two-level setting mechanism exists. The influence upon it of inhibitory mechanisms, and of the corticipetal modulatory systems, lends a delicate nuance to regulation of the operation. The remarkable fact is that patterns of input evoking LTP and LTD differ only in quantitative parameters. Both depend critically upon the postsynaptic Ca^{2+} surge and the degree of postsynaptic depolarization. When both are strong, LTP results; when weak, LTD. The different levels of Ca^{2+} are thought to set in motion different second-messenger cascades, leading to protein kinases and phosphatases that compete in the phosphorylation-dephosphorylation of membrane proteins (Malenka and Nicoll, 1993). The frequency at which a threshold shift from LTD to LTP occurs is not set; rather, frequency varies depending upon the immediate past history of the synaptic system.

These mechanisms for strengthening or weakening synaptic potencies are thought to be important in the "self-organization" of synaptic networks in the developing cortex (Chapter 9).

The Columnar Organization of the Neocortex

The basic unit of the mature neocortex is the *minicolumn,* a narrow chain of neurons that extends vertically across the cellular layers II–VI, normal to the pial surface. Each minicolumn contains about 80–100 neurons, except for the striate cortex in primates, in which the number is about 2.5 times larger. Minicolumns contain all the major phenotypes of cortical neural cells (Chapter 3), which are heavily interconnected in the vertical dimension. The minicolumn is produced by the iterative division of a small cluster of progenitor cells in the neuroepithelium, via the intervening ontogenetic unit in the cortical plate of the developing neocortex (Chapter 8). It is uncertain whether the Cajal-Retzius cells should be included in this unit, for they derive from the primordial plexiform layer. My general hypothesis is that the minicolumn is the smallest processing unit of the neocortex.

Cortical columns are sometimes called *modules,* and I shall use these terms interchangeably. They are formed by many minicolumns bound together by dense, short-range horizontal connections. The neurons of a column have certain sets of static and dynamic properties in common, upon which others that may differ are superimposed. The binding of minicolumns into columns is determined during cortical ontogenesis by both cell-autonomous and secondary influences, described in Chapter 9. The pattern of growth into the neocortex of afferent systems in an intermittent, tangential distribution is of critical importance. Columns vary from 300 to 500 μm in diameter between species whose brains differ in volume by three factors of ten. Cortical expansion in evolution is achieved by expanding cortical surface area, with little change in thickness. This expansion is generated by an increase in the number of cortical columns, not in individual column size (see Chapter 2). Neuroepithelial proliferation, vertical gliophilic migration, and radial organization occur in all mammalian forms. The primitive cortex of reptiles is generated similarly (Goffinet, 1984).

Columnar organization allows for intermittently recursive mapping, a consequence of which is that several variables can be mapped to the two-dimensional surface of the neocortex. This is clearly so for the primary sensory receiving areas of the brain, and appears likely to be so for all areas in which systematic maps have been observed.

A cortical column is a complex processing and distributing unit that links a number of inputs to a number of outputs via overlapping internal processing chains. A partial segregation of cortical efferent neurons with different extrinsic targets exists: efferents of layers II/III project to other cortical areas, those of V/VI to subcortical structures. This suggests that the processing operations leading to those different output channels differ in some fundamental way.

The modular organization of the neocortex has been documented in studies of sensory, motor, and homotypical cortical areas under many experimental conditions, including that of the waking, behaving monkey. I present some of the relevant evidence in that which follows, particularly for the somatic sensory and other heterotypical areas. I know of only one dissent (Slimp and Towe, 1990).

Physiological Studies of Somatic Sensory Cortical Areas

Electrophysiological Studies of the First Somatic Sensory Cortex

Evidence for the columnar organization of the neocortex was obtained in single-neuron electrophysiological studies of the somatic sensory cortex in anesthetized cats and monkeys (Mountcastle et al., 1955; Davies et al., 1955; Mountcastle, 1957; Powell and Mountcastle, 1959). Microelectrode penetrations made normal to the pial surface encounter neurons in each cellular layer with similar properties of place and modality. Penetrations parallel to the pial surface and crossing the vertical axis of the cortex pass through blocks of tissue, 300–500 μm in size, in each of which neurons with identical properties are encountered. Sharp transitions are observed from a block with one set to the adjacent block with different properties (see

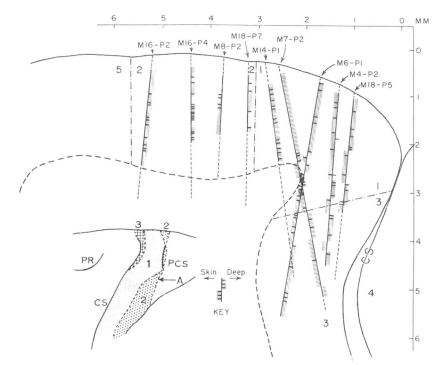

Fig. 7-1 Reconstructions of the tracks of several microelectrode penetrations made into the postcentral gyrus of anesthetized monkeys. All were placed within 1 mm of the plane marked *A* on the inset drawing, which shows the cytoarchitectural areas of the monkey somatic sensory cortex of the postcentral gyrus. Penetrations made perpendicular to the cortical surface and passing down parallel to its radial axis encountered neurons all of the same modality type. As the penetrations were made more anteriorly in areas 1 and 3, where the vertical axis of the cortex rolls, block alternations of groups of neurons with different modality properties between groups were encountered more frequently. In area 3 on the posterior bank of the central sulcus, the electrodes passed across modality-pure cortical columns. (From Powell and Mountcastle, 1959.)

Figs. 7-1 and 7-2). The defining property for place is the peripheral receptive field, the zone on the body surface within which an adequate stimulus evokes a response of the cortical cell. *Modality* is used here in a special sense to describe the nature of those adequate stimuli and the rate of adaptation to steady stimuli. The modality of a set of cortical neurons can frequently be equated with a particular set of primary afferent fibers: the quickly adapting cutaneous neurons of the somatic sensory area in the monkey with receptive fields on the glabrous skin of the hand are driven by input in the quickly adapting Meissner afferents, the slowly adapting cortical neurons by input in the slowly adapting Merkel afferents, Pacinian cortical neurons by that in Pacinian afferents. Several less precisely defined sets of neurons in the somatic cortex are activated by receptors that lie in the deep tissue beneath the skin.

In some cortical areas the defining properties for columns are set by afferent inflow, like those of place and modality defined above. In other cases, properties constructed by intracortical processing predominate. The degree to which afferent inflow or intracortical con-

Fig. 7-2 The cutaneous receptive fields of neurons studied in microelectrode penetrations made normal to the pial surface of the postcentral somatic sensory cortex in anesthetized monkeys. The receptive fields encountered in each penetration are nearly superimposed, with some variation in shape and total area. The central loci of maximal sensitivity were virtually identical for the fields of neurons in a single penetration. (From Powell and Mountcastle, 1959.)

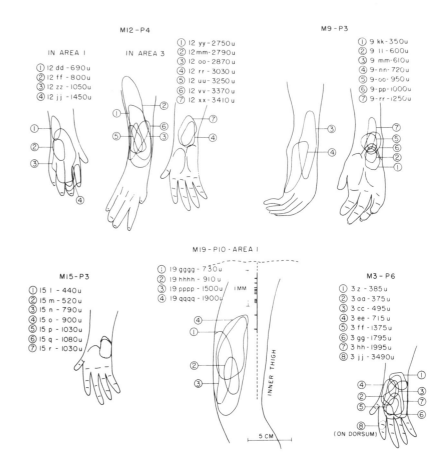

structions dominate in setting column-defining properties varies greatly between cortical areas. It is only in a region like the koniocortex of area 3b that the static properties set by inflow predominate. The directionally selective columns of areas 1 and 2, for example, are determined by a combination of the static properties of place and mode, combined with a result of intracortical processing.

It was a major discovery that there are four separate somatotopic maps of the body form in the postcentral somatic sensory area in primates, one each in areas 3a, 3b, 1, and 2 (Kaas, 1991). It is important to emphasize that the cortical maps of the body surface are not continuous representations but collections of regions, each of which is devoted to an afferent inflow from some body part. As Fig. 7-3 shows, however, some adjacent cortical regions map widely separated body parts, and some adjacent body parts are mapped to separated cortical zones.

Place Specificity Is a Defining Characteristic of Columns in the Somatic Sensory Cortex

The minicolumn-columnar organization of the somatic sensory cortex for place has been confirmed in experiments in cats (e.g., McKenna et al., 1981) and in microelectrode mapping experiments in monkeys by Favorov, Whitsel, and their colleagues (Favorov, 1991; Favorov et al., 1987; Favorov and Whitsel, 1988a,b). First the "minimum receptive fields" were mapped in anesthetized animals in microelectrode penetrations, some made parallel and others orthogonal

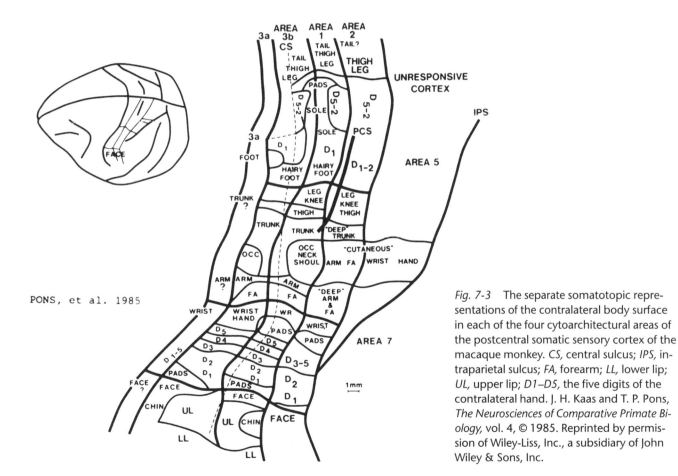

Fig. 7-3 The separate somatotopic representations of the contralateral body surface in each of the four cytoarchitectural areas of the postcentral somatic sensory cortex of the macaque monkey. *CS,* central sulcus; *IPS,* intraparietal sulcus; *FA,* forearm; *LL,* lower lip; *UL,* upper lip; *D1–D5,* the five digits of the contralateral hand. J. H. Kaas and T. P. Pons, *The Neurosciences of Comparative Primate Biology,* vol. 4, © 1985. Reprinted by permission of Wiley-Liss, Inc., a subsidiary of John Wiley & Sons, Inc.

Fig. 7-4 Near-radial penetrations made into the somatic sensory cortex of anesthetized cats. The receptive fields of the neurons encountered were mapped at intervals of 100–200 μm along the electrode tracks. Radial cords of cells indicated by thin lines, recording sites (on the cat's paw) by filled circles. (A) All the receptive fields are located at a single skin site. (B) Here two sectors of cells were encountered with nearly identical receptive fields in each but an abrupt shift between sectors. (From Favorov and Diamond, 1990.)

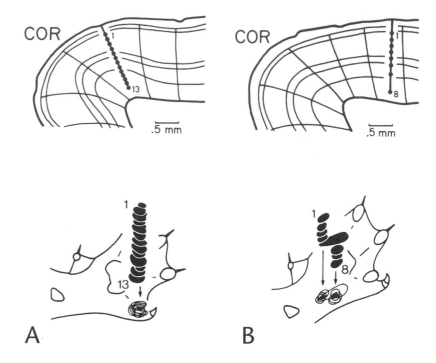

to the plane of the cortex. The maximum receptive fields were determined for each neuron whose action potential could be isolated, in similarly directed penetrations, in unanesthetized animals. General anesthetic agents decrease the sizes of receptive fields in layers above and below area IV in the somatic sensory cortex. Therefore, in some experiments the two methods were combined. The maximum receptive fields were determined in unanesthetized animals upon microelectrode insertion. The animal was then anesthetized and the minimum receptive fields determined upon withdrawal.

Fig. 7-4A shows the superimposition of the minimum receptive fields determined in a penetration made normal to the surface plane of the cortex. Fig. 7-4B gives the result for a penetration in which an abrupt shift in receptor field locus occurred in mid-course. This spatial shift indicates movement of the electrode from one column to an adjacent one, with differently located receptive fields. The transitions occur upon electrode movement of 40–50 μm. Three transitions were observed in a penetration made across the vertical axis of the cortex, and abrupt shifts in receptive field accompanied the transitions from one column to another (Fig. 7-5).

The maximum receptive fields observed were always larger and more varied than the minimum fields, but all ranged about a common central locus (the "hot spot"). When the two methods were combined as described above, the common zone for the maximum fields identified upon penetration (in the unanesthetized state) was identical to that of the minimum fields determined upon withdrawal (in the anesthetized state).

Favorov and Diamond (1990) made many penetrations in closely spaced grids. The results defined the shape of the cortical column as quasi-hexagonal, usually surrounded by six other columns, and doubly convex in the long dimension, with widths of 300–400 μm (Fig. 7-6). This form resembles the description of the rodent somatic sensory cortex by Senft and Woolsey (1991c) as Dirichlet domains. Such a column contains about 80 minicolumns of 50–60 μm diameters; the minimum receptive fields of neurons in the minicolumn of a column shift about the columnar common locus, without topographic progression.

A nerve-regeneration experiment in monkeys provides further evidence for the minicolumnar composition of cortical modules (Kaas et al., 1981). In an initial recording experiment, microelectrodes were passed tangentially across the hand area of the postcentral somatic

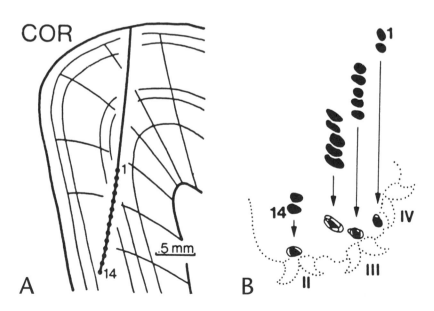

Fig. 7-5 Locations of the cutaneous receptive fields of neurons observed in a microelectrode penetration made nearly tangentially through the somatic sensory cortex of an anesthetized cat. Fields were mapped every 100 μm along the track. (A) Histological reconstruction of the electrode track; locations of recordings indicated by filled circles. The electrode trended from layer 5 to layer 3 in the region of recording. (B) There were three abrupt shifts in the receptive field locations separating four sectors, in each of which the fields were identical. (From Favorov and Diamond, 1990.)

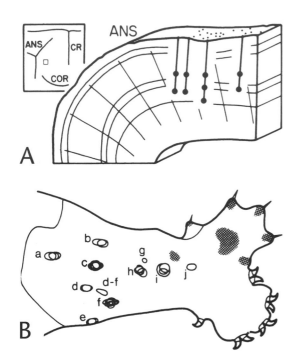

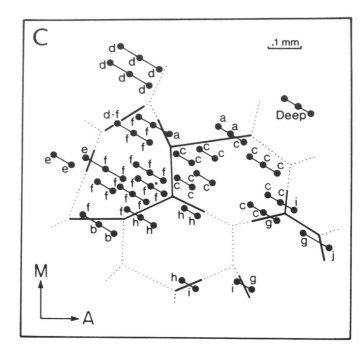

Fig. 7-6 Results of a study in which 25 microelectrode penetrations were made into the somatic sensory cortex of an anesthetized cat reveal the topographic units (columns) of this cortex. (A) Side view of cortex, showing locations of penetrations with four reconstructions; inset, area of study enclosed in the rectangle. (B) Outlines of the 62 minimum receptive fields of neurons recorded in the ten penetrations *a–j*. (C) Surface view of cortex, showing positions of the recording sites (filled circles), connected in each penetration. Each recording site is labeled according to the discrete cluster in (B) to which its field belongs. The solid lines indicate boundaries of columns, across which there is an abrupt shift in receptive field locations. (From Favorov and Diamond, 1990.)

cortex. Over a considerable distance, neurons of the same modality type were observed with overlapping fields (Fig. 7-7, *left*). The median nerve was then sectioned and resutured. After some time allowed for re-innervation of the skin, the recording experiment was repeated (Fig. 7-7, *right*). Now, instead of a smooth progression of overlapping receptive fields, zones of cortex of 40–60 μm dimension were traversed within which receptive fields were identical, but with sharp shifts in receptive field location between adjacent zones. This was attributed to the misdirection of re-innervating peripheral nerve bundles; i.e., such a bundle innervating a new and abnormal location

The Columnar Organization of the Neocortex

of skin imposed that new receptive field upon the entire minicolumn of neurons to which it projected. This experiment reveals a minicolumn of a dimension comparable to that of the embryologic units described in Chapter 8 as the forerunners of minicolumns in the adult cortex.

Modality Specificity Is a Defining Characteristic of Columns in the Somatic Sensory Cortex

Each set of modality-specific primary afferent fibers entering the dorsal column–medial lemniscal system engages synaptically with populations of neurons it thus endows with those same modality properties. Those mode-specific populations are successively linked from the dorsal column nuclear complex to the ventrobasal complex of the thalamus, and from thence to the somatic sensory area of the

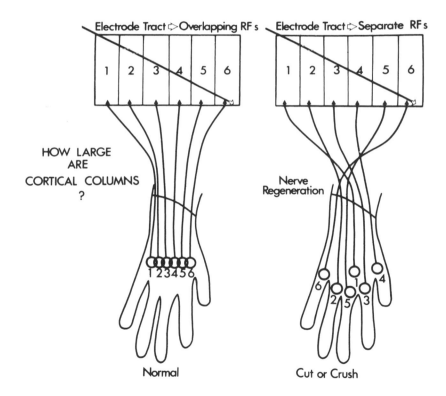

Fig. 7-7 A nerve-regeneration experiment in the monkey provides evidence for columnar organization of the somatic sensory cortex and an estimate of the smallest identifiable element, the cortical minicolumn. *(Left)* A recording microelectrode was passed nearly parallel to the pial surface of the cortex of the postcentral somatic sensory cortex, through a region of neurons with the same modality properties. Neurons in adjacent minicolumns are related to adjoining and overlapping peripheral receptive fields *(RFs),* and the transitions between minicolumns pass unnoticed. *(Right)* Results obtained in the same animal in a similar experiment after section and resuture of the contralateral medial nerve. There is a misdirection of the regenerating bundles of nerve fibers now innervating the glabrous skin of the hand. Sudden displacements of the locations of the receptive fields occur at intervals of 50–60 μm, revealing the minicolumns and their transverse size. (From Kaas et al., 1981.)

cerebral cortex (Mountcastle, 1984). This general conclusion is drawn from many extracellular microelectrode recording experiments in cats and monkeys, made under a variety of experimental conditions. It is unlikely that a subthreshold convergence has been missed, for the modality specificity of somatic cortical neurons is unchanged when they are depolarized to the peri-threshold level by the excitatory transmitter glutamate administered iontophoretically close to the cell under observation. No cross-modal convergence is revealed after blocking of GABA-mediated inhibition (Dykes et al., 1984; Alloway and Burton, 1986, 1991). Divergence and convergence occur at each level for place but not for modality. Cross-modal convergence occurs in other ascending components of the somatic afferent system, and in their forebrain targets as well. Modality specificity at the postcentral level in primates is expressed in modality-pure columns. Modality specificity is the second defining property for columns in this cortical area.

Each of the four postcentral maps receives its major input relayed largely from one or two of the modality-specific sets of primary afferent fibers. Area 3a neurons are driven largely from muscle afferents. Area 3b and 1 each receive input from both rapidly and slowly adapting sets of cutaneous afferents; and area 2 largely from joint afferents, although area 2 also contains a complete representation of the cutaneous surface of the hand. If a single area receives input from more than one set of primary afferents, neurons of the different modality properties are segregated within the area. For example, the rapidly and slowly adapting cutaneous neurons of both 3b and 1 are segregated to different cortical columns. Sur et al. (1984) mapped these postcentral areas in several species of monkeys to correlate modality, place, and cortical area. They emphasized the projection of the two cutaneous afferent classes to both areas 3b and 1, for they found that microelectrode penetrations made normal to the cortical surface in 3b and 1 encountered either the rapidly or the slowly adapting class throughout the cortical depth. The two modality classes were each clustered in bands oriented in the antero-posterior direction, intersecting the medio-lateral line of the representation of the body form (see also Sretavan and Dykes, 1983). The receptive fields of the rapidly and slowly adapting neurons in different modality zones are similar within the same topographic zone (see Fig. 7-8). This intermittently recursive mapping of modality on place is further illus-

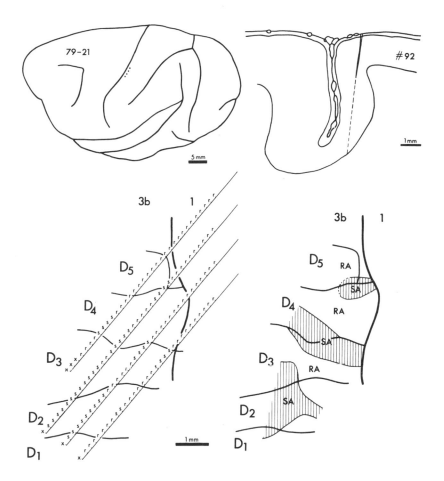

Fig. 7-8 Distribution of recording loci in the postcentral gyrus of an anesthetized macaque monkey at which slowly adapting *(SA)* or rapidly adapting *(RA)* responses were evoked by stimulation of the contralateral fingers, *D1–D5,* shown below on the right. Points of entry of four microelectrode penetrations are shown on the outline drawing of the brain, and a partial reconstruction of one of the electrode tracks on the section drawing at the upper right. The receptive fields for the neurons observed for three rows of recording sites across the *RA* and *SA* bands in the representation area of the third digit of the contralateral hand are shown at lower left: *r* = rapidly adapting; *s* = slowly adapting. The receptive fields of the two classes of neurons recorded in the bands overlap. (From Sur, Wall, and Kaas, 1984.)

trated in the right-hand side of Fig. 7-8. Columnar organization based on place and modality specificity has been shown also for the second somatic area in anesthetized cats (Carreras and Andersson, 1963; Alloway and Burton, 1985) and in both anesthetized (Whitsel et al., 1969) and waking monkeys.

Metabolic and Blood Flow Studies of the First Somatic Sensory Cortex

Local mechanical stimulation of the body surface evokes modular patterns of increased metabolic activity in the contralateral somatic sensory cortex in both cats and monkeys, indicated by the 2-deoxyglucose uptake method (Juliano et al., 1981). The pattern consists of multiple and separated elongated regions (0.5 × 1.5 mm), as if several adjacent columns were activated by the peripheral stimuli, for these metabolically defined modules are larger than those defined electrophysiologically. These linked sets of modules are bordered by zones of decreased uptake as a result of intracortical inhibition, for the metabolically labeled zones spread and fuse when GABA-mediated intracortical inhibition is blocked with bicuculline (Juliano et al., 1989). Correlated metabolic and electrophysiological studies indicate that identical stimuli evoke both the patch of increased metabolic activity and the activity of neurons within it (Juliano and Whitsel, 1987). The increase in metabolism is not uniform within a module; it occurs in narrow, translaminar columns separated by narrow zones of decreased activity, with a spatial period of 18–33/mm (Tommerdahl et al., 1993). This demonstrates active minicolumns in the sensory cortex and supports the general idea that cortical modules are composed of groups of minicolumns.

A radially oriented periodic variation of 2-deoxyglucose uptake around the background level was also observed in regions of the somatic cortex not activated by the peripheral stimuli used. The spatial variation was similar to that observed in optical density measurements of Nissl-stained sections of the sensory cortex, a reflection of the vertical cording of neuronal cell bodies in this region.

Physiological Studies of Other Heterotypical Cortical Areas

The Columnar Organization of the Visual Cortex

The primary visual cortex of mammals, variously called the striate cortex, area 17, or V-1, is the most intensely studied structure in the mammalian brain. This tide of research was set in motion in the early 1960s by the work of several investigators, especially by that of David Hubel and Torsten Wiesel. Hubel and Wiesel established in their first experiments, and elaborated fully in many that followed, that columnar organization in the primate V-1 is defined by the neuronal properties of ocularity and place imposed by the geniculate input, and by orientation specificity generated mainly by intracortical processing. Neurons in V-1 are preferentially driven by stimuli delivered to one eye or the other, from a particular locus in the visual field, and are selectively sensitive to short, straight-line visual stimuli at particular, limited angles of orientation. These properties are more or

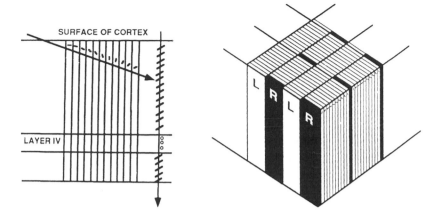

Fig. 7-9 *(Left)* Organization of the striate cortex for orientation preferences (from the work of Hubel and Wiesel). For penetrations made perpendicular to the surface of the cortex, the preferred orientation remains almost constant, except for layers IVa and IVc. For penetrations made nearly parallel to the cortical surface, the preferred orientations rotate linearly with distance in sequence, forming orientation slabs of 0.5–1.0 mm thickness, in which a full 180 degree rotation of orientation preferences is repeated. Linearity is broken at longer intervals by reversals in the direction of rotation. *(Right)* The Hubel and Wiesel model, generated from the inference that slightly rotated orientation preferences may be organized in stacks of parallel slabs, with spacing between slabs of about 700 μm. K. Obermayer and G. G. Blasdel, "Geometry of orientation and ocular dominance columns in monkey striate cortex," *Journal of Neuroscience* 13(10): 4115–4129 (1993).

less constant from neuron to neuron encountered in microelectrode penetrations made normal to the pial surface. By contrast, these properties change from locus to locus in long, tangential penetrations made nearly parallel to the pial surface (Fig. 7-9, *left*). The neurons studied in such tangential penetrations vary systematically in ocularity and orientation selectivity. The latter appears to shift with electrode movements as small as 20 μm. A full sequence of 180 degrees is covered in distances that vary from 500 to 750 μm. A set of such minute orientation columns was termed an *orientation hypercolumn*.

The property of ocular dominance of these same neurons varied in such a way as to reveal adjacent ocular-dominance columns. A pair of such columns contains neurons grading systematically from full dominance by one eye to full dominance by the other, with all gradations in between; it was defined as an *ocular-dominance hypercolumn*.

Hubel and Wiesel conjectured from measures of the tangential dimensions of the two classes of hypercolumns and the point spread that a set composed of one, full orientation column for each eye would be adequate to process all the input from a local region in the visual fields, with minimal overlap in the region of the visual field served by adjacent sets. These findings, summarized in their review of 1977 (Hubel and Wiesel, 1977), are illustrated by the model shown in Fig. 7-9.

Since that time the columnar sets in primate V-1 have been studied intensively; indeed, 14 different methods have been used to identify the ocular-dominance columns! The most startling results have

Fig. 7-10 *(Above)* Contour plot of orientation preference and ocular-dominance bands in the macaque monkey striate cortex, determined by the method of optical imaging. The iso-orientation lines (gray) are drawn at intervals of 11.25 degrees in the orientation rotation sequence. Black lines indicate the borders between the ocular-dominance columns. *(Below)* Contour plot of a part of the results in another monkey. The singularities tend to be at the center of the ocular-dominance columns. The linear zones occur at the edges of those columns, where the short iso-orientation bands within the linear zone tend to intersect the borders of the ocular-dominance columns at angles of about 90 degrees.

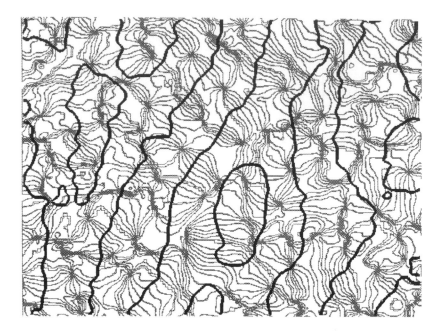

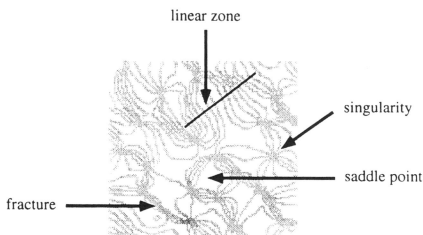

linear zone

singularity

saddle point

fracture

been obtained with optical imaging, particularly in experiments like those of Blasdel, in which both the orientation and ocular-dominance columns were identified in the same local region of the visual cortex (Blasdel, 1992a,b; Obermayer and Blasdel, 1993). In their map (Fig. 7-10), it is clear that in some locations the lateral progression of change in orientation preference occurs in a linear way, while elsewhere the changes are markedly nonlinear. The orientation columns

The Columnar Organization of the Neocortex

form orientation slabs that measure 0.5–1.0 mm in the iso-orientation direction, and in which a full 180 degree rotation of orientation preference is repeated in about 550 μm. These linear regions occupy about 50 percent of the cortical surface and are preferentially located at the edges of the ocular-dominance columns, which they intersect in nearly orthogonal directions. This intersection creates a module in which the several functional properties of V-1 neurons are mapped in a reiterative manner, the original "ice-cube" model of Hubel and Wiesel.

Three types of nonlinear changes in orientation preferences were identified in Blasdel's experiments. *Singularities* are point-like discontinuities created when orientation preferences change continuously through 180 degrees around them. These points tend to be located in the centers of the ocular-dominance columns. *Fractures* are local discontinuities at which orientation preferences change abruptly; such sudden local changes were identified by Hubel and Wiesel in their electrophysiological experiments. Finally, *saddle points* are small, patch-like areas within which orientation preferences appear to change very little. Saddle points are usually located at the center of four singularities (Fig. 7-10). It is still uncertain what role these regions of nonlinear orientation changes play in the function of the visual cortex.

Understanding of the functional architecture of primate V-1 was complicated by the discovery that local zones of above-average metabolic activity occur intermittently along the ocular-dominance columns. These dots or blobs were revealed by 2-deoxyglucose (Hendrickson and Wilson, 1979) or cytochrome oxidase staining (Wong-Riley, 1979; Horton and Hubel, 1981; Horton, 1984). They are local zones of about 150 μm diameter most prominent in layers II and III, arranged along the centers of the ocular-dominance columns at a repeat interval of 500–550 μm; the parallel rows are about 350 μm apart (Fig. 7-9). Blob regions receive a direct input from the intercalated layers of the lateral geniculate; the interblob regions receive only intrinsic cortical input. Neurons in the blobs are sensitive to particular colors and are not strongly orientation-specific; neurons in the interblobs are the reverse. Blob cells respond differentially at low spatial frequencies (1.1 ± 0.8 cycles/degree), interblob cells at high spatial frequencies (3.8 ± 0.2 cycles/degree) (Tootell et al., 1991). The blob and interblob regions differ in intrinsic and extrinsic connectivity and in the distribution of a number of molecular markers.

The problem of the functional organization of primate V-1 attracted interest from neural modelers; a critical review of a number of these has appeared (Erwin et al., 1995). For reviews of this organization, see LeVay and Nelson (1991) and Peters (1994). Zeki (1993) has provided a scholarly survey of the cortical mechanisms in vision, with particular emphasis upon motion sensitivity and color vision. One important result of these and many other studies is the emphasis put on the idea that the striate cortex functions in the main as a *distribution center* for several aspects of vision: color, directionality, orientation, etc. (Shipp and Zeki, 1985; Hubel and Livingstone, 1987; Livingstone and Hubel, 1983).

The Columnar Organization of the Auditory Cortex

The earliest electrophysiological studies of the auditory cortex of carnivores revealed that sound frequencies are mapped in an orderly tonotopic way to several cortical areas (Woolsey and Walzl, 1942; Tunturi, 1950). Tunturi discovered in the dog that the afferent cochlear fibers serving a narrow range of frequencies project to a band of cortical tissue "no wider than 200 μm and 5–7 mm in length extending across the gyrus." This remarkable discovery was made using the gross electrode, evoked potential method! The isofrequency bands have since been identified with single-neuron methods in cat, monkey, and other mammals (Brugge and Merzenich, 1973; Merzenich and Brugge, 1973; Ahissar et al., 1992; Brugge et al., 1969; Morel et al., 1993). These bands are stacked in a linear array to form a sequential representation of sound frequencies that runs, in the cat, from low to high in the posterior-to-anterior direction (Fig. 7-11).

The functional properties of auditory cortical neurons are not uniform along the isofrequency bands. Neurons with different sensitivities to binaural stimulation (EE = excitatory/excitatory or EI = excitatory/inhibitory, from the two ears) are spatially segregated along each isofrequency band. Each binaural class forms an antero-posteriorly directed band that crosses the isofrequency bands orthogonally, thus specifying by intersection cortical modules each of which contains neurons with particular combinations of frequency selectivity and binaural response (Fig. 7-11) (Imig and Adrian, 1977; Middlebrooks et al., 1980). It is the binaural summation columns that send and receive callosal fibers (Imig and Brugge, 1978). These binaural neurons signal the azimuth location of sound sources in the contralateral hemisphere (Middlebrooks and Pettigrew, 1981; for review see Wong, 1991).

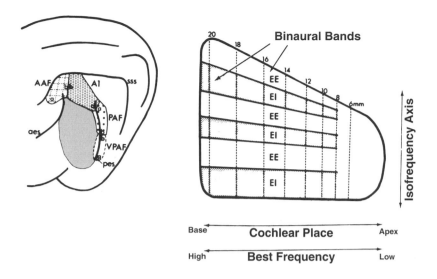

Fig. 7-11 *(Left)* A map of the auditory sensory areas in the neocortex of the cat. *AAF,* anterior auditory field; *A1,* primary auditory field; *PAF,* posterior auditory field; *VPAF,* ventral posterior auditory field. These four fields are tonotopically organized. The darkly shaded field is an auditory responsive area in which no tonotopic organization has been defined. *Aes,* anterior ectosylvian sulcus; *pes,* posterior ectosylvian sulcus; *sss,* suprasylvian sulcus. *(Right)* A schema of the organization of the primary auditory cortex in the cat. The isofrequency bands run in the vertical direction and are crossed by the binaural bands in a nearly orthogonal manner. Modes of binocular interaction: *EE,* excitatory from both ears; *EI,* excitatory from one ear, inhibitory from the other. (From Merzenich et al., 1982.)

Every cellular study of the auditory cortex in cat and monkey has provided direct evidence for its columnar organization. Microelectrode penetrations made normal to the pial surface encounter successively neurons from layer II through VI that have similar spectral sensitivities and binaural response properties, as well as other functional attributes described below. Penetrations made in the tangential direction, parallel to the pial surface, encounter successive blocks of cells whose properties change abruptly as the electrode passes from one group to the next. These changes occur in step-like fashion, and the blocks of cells may be as narrow as 50–100 µm.

A number of other functional properties also vary along the isofrequency bands. The degree of frequency tuning itself is not uniform, but sharpest in the mid-region of the bands and somewhat broader for neurons located either medial or lateral to the central zone (Schreiner and Sutter, 1992; Heil et al., 1992a,b). Auditory cortical neurons are sensitive to frequency-modulated stimuli, particularly if the FM sweep is centered at the best frequency of the cell; they are differentially sensitive to the direction and speed of the FM sweep (Mendelson et al., 1993; Mendelson and Grasse, 1992; Schreiner et al., 1992) and to periodicity pitch (Eggermont, 1991). All these properties appear to be distributed periodically along the isofrequency bands, but how these spatial variations relate to the periodicity of the binaural response columns is uncertain.

The frequency sensitivity of auditory cortical neurons is determined by the primary afferent input from the cochlea. The other properties of auditory cortical neurons are constructed by neuronal processing within the several stages of the ascending auditory system and in its cortical targets.

The Columnar Organization of the Motor Cortex in Primates

The layer V neurons of origin of the pyramidal tract fibers are clustered into groups distributed intermittently in the horizontal dimension at periods of 300–500 μm. In the human motor cortex, the somata of the pyramidal and nonpyramidal neurons are clustered into columnar aggregates about 300 μm wide, separated by 100 μm cell-sparse zones (Meyer, 1987). Forty percent of neurons in clusters project to a given motoneuron pool in the spinal cord, the remainder to the motoneuron pools of muscle groups active in similar movements. The recurrent axon collaterals of pyramidal cells project vertically into a 300–500 μm zone that extends through the cellular layers. These connections provide a strong excitatory drive to adjacent neurons and, via inhibitory interneurons, an inhibitory effect on surrounding columns. The vertical projection of the bundles of pyramidal cell dendrites and the axons of the double bouquet cells contribute further to the vertical pattern of intrinsic connectivity (Keller, 1993). Other collaterals of the pyramidal cells of III and V project horizontally through the cortex for 2–3 mm. They end in terminal clusters in columns thought to have spinal cord linkages similar to those of the layer V pyramids of the column of origin (Aroniadou and Keller, 1993; Huntley and Jones, 1991a). The projections to the motor cortex from the thalamic ventrolateral (VL) nucleus and from other cortical areas terminate in intermittently distributed patches, thus contributing also to columnarity.

The question of the relation of muscles to movements in the motor cortical representations has until recently remained unresolved, in spite of more than a century of electrical stimulations of the motor cortex in many primates, including man. It appears that the problem is not whether muscles or movements are represented, per se, but how sets of neurons related to particular muscles are combined in groups that from time to time form different combinations, and thus generate the variety of different movements in which any muscle participates. Several lines of study have contributed to the suggested solution, particularly those in which the motor cortex was explored with penetrating microelectrodes. This method allows at-choice delivery of weak electrical stimuli to local groups of neurons (intracortical microstimulation, ICMS), or the recording of the responses of those same cortical cells to sensory stimuli. The discoveries made with ICMS are due largely to the work of Asanuma and his colleagues (Asanuma and Rosen, 1972; Asanuma, 1975). Their main findings are the following.

1. ICMS at threshold elicits contractions of single muscles at about 40 percent of stimulation sites; at others, somewhat more intense ICMS is required and elicits contractions of small groups of muscles.

2. The cortical area within which ICMS produces a particular local movement is confined to a narrow zone of columnar shape extending through the cellular layers (Fig. 7-12). Muscle- and group-specific columns are interspersed in the tangential dimension.

3. Neurons in a column receive afferent input from deep receptors located in the zone of movement, and from cutaneous afferents whose receptive fields are arranged spatially to be activated if the evoked movement brings them against an object (Rosen and Asanuma, 1972; Asanuma, 1981).

4. It is the tangential intermingling of columns related to different single muscles and different small muscle groups that suggests how movements are represented. They are thought to be driven by the grouping together, from time to time, of active columns related to muscles and muscle groups involved in one particular movement, and in different groups to produce related movements. What mechanism or afferent input selects the particular groups appropriate for a specific movement is unknown.

Extensive studies have been made of the motor cortex in waking monkeys as they execute one of a variety of motor tasks, a research program initiated by the late Edward Evarts in the 1960s. In general, the aim of these studies has been to seek correlations between the activity of motor cortical neurons and movement parameters. Little attention was paid to the question of columnar organization. How-

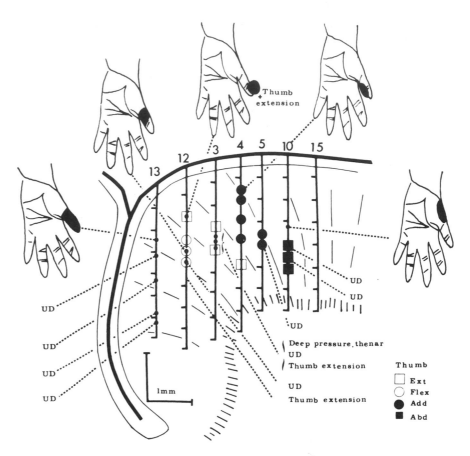

Fig. 7-12 Results of an experiment with intracortical microelectrode stimulation (ICMS) in the precentral motor cortex of a monkey that revealed some aspects of the input-output relation for the contralateral thumb and the columnar organization of this cortical area. Several microelectrode tracks (indicated by solid lines and numbers) passed through efferent zones projecting to various thumb muscles. Short horizontal lines indicate sites at which weak currents did not evoke motor responses. Locations where movements were produced and receptive fields of the cells studied at those locations are marked by solid dots or squares and connected by dashed lines to figurines showing the receptive fields. (From Asanuma, 1975.)

ever, Georgopoulos has shown that motor cortical neurons active during directed projections of the arm and hand discharge optimally for a particular direction of movement (Georgopoulos et al., 1993). He made an observation important in the present context, that the preferred directions for neurons in any single penetration are similar

The Columnar Organization of the Neocortex

to one another in microelectrode penetrations made normal to the pial surface and crossing the cortical layers.

Physiological Studies of Homotypical Cortical Areas

A striking feature of homotypical cortical areas is that the defining parameters for columns are constructed within intracortical processing systems. These properties are complex, and rarely do the sensory-input-linked properties that define modules in sensory areas like 3b or V-1 appear unchanged in homotypical areas. The plasticity of cortical synapses suggests that homotypical defining properties may be changed by experience (e.g., with learning and memory), and there is preliminary evidence that this is indeed the case.

Modular organization of homotypical cortex depends in part upon the fact that connections between such areas are distributed intermittently in the transverse cortical dimension, at both source and target. They terminate in columns 200–500 μm wide, most densely in the supragranular layers, separated by zones of equal width in which terminals from that source are scarce. The cells of origin in the source area are similarly distributed in intermittent patches in layers II and III. This mode of inter-areal connectivity is described further in Chapter 10, where it serves as an important base for the idea of distributed systems.

I consider briefly four areas of homotypical cortex in which modular organization has been documented in electrophysiological experiments in waking monkeys: the posterior parietal cortex, the medial temporal area, the inferotemporal cortex, and the frontal association cortex. In the posterior parietal cortex (area 7a—now divided into several sub-areas), neurons with similar properties are arranged in vertical modules extending across the cellular layers, interdigitated with other sets of neurons with different properties (Mountcastle et al., 1975). These cortical areas do not reflect any single sensory input, nor are they linked in any unconditional way to peripheral effectors. Neuronal properties in them were discovered in combined electrophysiological and behavioral experiments in monkeys trained to emit acts chosen on the basis of both the defects in behavior produced by lesions of the area and the connectivity of the area. The properties of the modular sets in the posterior parietal cortex differ greatly, but they have one thing in common: they are all related to the animal's actions in immediately surrounding space, or

Fig. 7-13 Results obtained in a microelectrode penetration made into the posterior parietal cortex of a waking, behaving monkey as he executed a series of tasks relevant for parietal lobe function. The electrode passed down the intraparietal sulcus and area 7 lining the posterior bank of the intraparietal sulcus. Five blocks of neurons with different functional properties were encountered: *VS,* visual neurons; *VT,* visual tracking neurons; *R,* reach neurons; then *VT* again; and finally *R* again. The electrode traversed different distances in the columns it passed through. (From Mountcastle, unpublished experiment.)

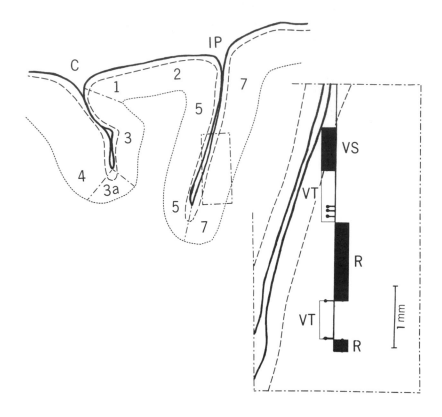

his perception of, and attention to, objects or events within that space. Different neuronal sets are active during (a) the fixation of gaze upon and attention to an object of interest, (b) slow-pursuit tracking of the object, (c) projection of the arm toward the object, (d) manipulation of the object, and (e) visual stimulation, but with visual properties not seen in any tributary visual areas. This set of visual neurons provides a dynamic image of the flow fields in the spatial surround, of the animal's movement through those fields, or of the movement of objects through them. Microelectrode penetrations made normal to the surface of the inferior parietal lobule have a high probability of encountering neurons of only one of these classes, as the electrode moves across the cellular layers. Electrode penetrations made parallel to the plane of the pia encounter successive blocks of neurons, first of one class and then another (Fig. 7-13). How these several modular sets are interdigitated in area 7a is still unknown.

The medial temporal area (MT) is a small area of distinctive myeloarchitecture in the posterior bank of the superior temporal sulcus of the monkey. It was discovered by Zeki (1974), who showed it to be specialized for processing information about the movement of visual objects and about their direction of movement. Zeki labeled it V-5— the fifth-order prestriate visual area; it receives input from both V1 and V2. The homologue of monkey V-5 has been identified in the human brain by the method of positron emission tomography (Zeki et al., 1991). A patient with bilateral and nearly symmetrical brain lesions that include this area has been studied in detail (Zihl et al., 1983). This woman has no experience or knowledge of objects in motion, but she perceives them accurately when they are stationary. Her defect is specifically selective for visual motion; other aspects of vision, and of motion perceived through other senses, appear reasonably intact.

Neurons of monkey MT with similar axes of motion preference are arranged in vertical columns set in slabs in which a full rotation of 180 degree in the axis of motion is represented in 400–500 μm of cortex (Albright et al., 1984). Axis-of-motion columns are intersected by a second set, in which the two opposite directions of motion along each axis are represented in two adjacent columns, as shown in Fig. 7-14. Each MT column is specified by the intersection of the two parameter sets, each of which is constructed by intracortical processing.

It is well known that the homotypical inferotemporal cortex is critical for object vision, for its removal renders a monkey severely handicapped in learning a visual discrimination or recognition task. Gross and his colleagues discovered that many neurons in this area respond selectively to the shapes of objects. In their earliest experiments they observed a few cells best activated by such shapes as the outline of a monkey's hand, or the view of monkey or human faces (Gross et al., 1969, 1972). This intriguing discovery has attracted the interest of many investigators, and we now have a detailed knowledge of this class of cortical neurons (e.g., see Perrett et al., 1985, 1992). A study by Tanaka is of particular interest in the present context (Tanaka, 1992, 1996; Tanaka et al., 1992). Tanaka was able to reduce the outlines of complex effective stimuli, like faces, to the features critical for neuronal activation, and he confirmed that most of the cells in the anterior part of the inferotemporal cortex require moderately complex features for their activation. Neurons with similar or closely related selectivities are clustered in columns that extend

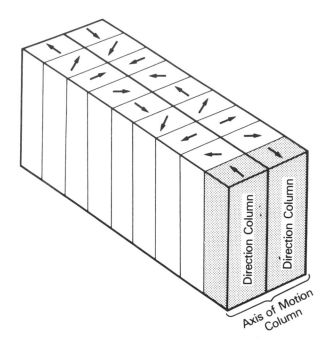

Fig. 7-14 Three-dimensional model of co-lumnar organization for direction and axis-of-motion sensitivity of neurons in prestriate area MT in the macaque monkey. Vertical dimension represents depth in the cortex. The long axis of the figure represents two complete revolutions of *axis*-of-motion columns; the two *directions* of motion along each axis are represented in adjacent columns. Movements of the electrode in this latter direction reveal neurons with 180 degree reversals in preferred direction of motion, with no change in the preferred axis of motion. (From Albright et al., 1984.)

across the cellular layers (Fujita et al., 1992), and neurons with different selectivities are arranged in a mosaic like that shown in Fig. 7-15.

Studies of the patterns of termination of the corticocortical connections to and from the frontal association cortex (Walker's areas 9, 10, and 46; see Chapter 10) reveal a clear columnar organization, described first by Goldman and Nauta in 1977. The terminals of connections from other cortical areas in the same hemisphere and those from homologous areas in the contralateral hemisphere are interdigitated in the frontal target areas in alternating, 500 μm wide columns that span the full thickness of the cortex (Goldman-Rakic and Schwartz, 1982). Friedman and Goldman-Rakic (1995) found that these columns can be individually activated during specific behaviors; they are thought to serve specific functions.

The Anatomical Basis of Columnar Organization

When the general hypothesis of columnar organization was first proposed (Mountcastle, 1957), it was met with disbelief by almost all neuroanatomists. Zeki (1993, p. 87) put it just right:

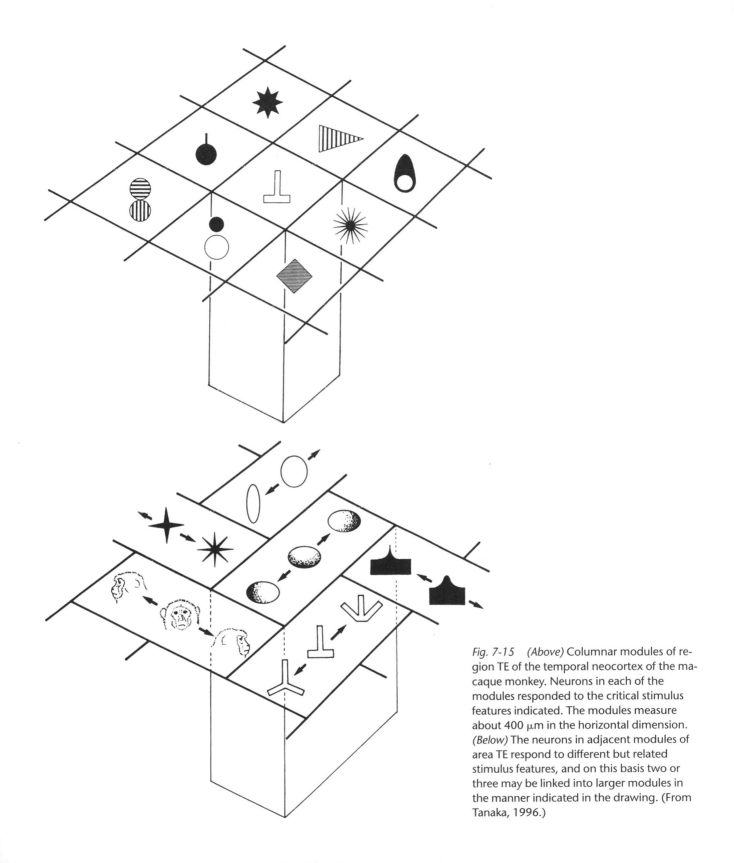

Fig. 7-15 (Above) Columnar modules of region TE of the temporal neocortex of the macaque monkey. Neurons in each of the modules responded to the critical stimulus features indicated. The modules measure about 400 μm in the horizontal dimension. *(Below)* The neurons in adjacent modules of area TE respond to different but related stimulus features, and on this basis two or three may be linked into larger modules in the manner indicated in the drawing. (From Tanaka, 1996.)

> When confronted with a difficult problem which goes against their way of thinking, scientists often begin by shutting their eyes firmly to the evidence and pretending that it does not exist. The next stage consists of accepting the evidence but pretending that it is not important or that it can be adequately explained by the known facts. The third and final stage consists of admitting the evidence and its significance, but pretending that it has all been said before.

This was so even though the general pattern of vertical connectivity linking neurons across cortical layers had been described by Lorente de No nearly two decades earlier in his studies of what we now know is the somatic sensory cortex of the mouse (Lorente de No, 1922, 1938). The classical idea of laminar organization of the cortex was dominant, and suggestions for functional specificity for each of the cellular layers were frequently made—e.g., that the supragranular layers are specialized for "psychic" functions. I included in my original description evidence that columnar specificity is dynamic in nature, is maintained by pericolumnar inhibition, and might not be revealed by the anatomical methods then in use. These ideas were largely ignored, and perhaps properly so, for the large sets of cortical inhibitory interneurons had yet to be identified.

It was for these reasons that after completing a study of the postcentral gyrus of the monkey (Powell and Mountcastle, 1959; Mountcastle and Powell, 1959a,b), in which we confirmed and extended the observations made earlier in the somatic sensory cortex of the cat, I turned to other interests, leaving time and new methods to reveal the anatomical evidence for columnar organization. That evidence is now compelling (Jones, 1983); I review some of it briefly in what follows.

Columniation by Afferent Projections

The physiological observations that generated the hypothesis of the columnar organization of the somatic sensory cortex suggested two sets of anatomical facts then unknown. They implied, first, that the terminations of afferent systems to the cortex be disposed in focal clusters of 0.5–1.0 mm dimensions, and that each cluster subtend a bundle of place- and mode-specific primary afferent fibers feeding input to the system. Second, it was necessary to postulate that this thalamically imposed focus of activity is relayed in the vertical direction in columns limited in the x-y dimension by the input cluster, and that it engages neurons in all the cellular layers, including both intrinsic interneurons and efferent pyramidal cells. Moreover, the physiological observations suggested that intracortical pathways exist over which the activity in one column can suppress that in its immediate neighbors.

New anatomical methods used intensively during the last two decades have yielded descriptions of the two anatomical arrangements required by the columnar hypothesis. It is largely due to the productive efforts of Jones and his colleagues that we have a rich fund of knowledge concerning the afferent systems to, and the intrinsic connectivity within, the postcentral somatic sensory cortex of the monkey (for review see Jones, 1981). It is now clear from many correlated anatomical and physiological studies that the lemniscal afferent system is modularized from the level of dorsal root entry to that of the postcentral gyrus. Bundles of axons from cells of thalamic modules project to columnar zones of termination in layers IV and IIIb of the postcentral cortex, forming clusters separated by zones in which terminals are much less dense. Such clustering obtains also for the ipsilateral corticocortical and transcallosal systems. The apical zones of the postcentral pattern in which the hands, feet, and face are represented are not connected transcallosally to the other hemisphere. Within those regions of the somatotopic map that are connected, callosal afferents terminate in 0.5–1.0 mm sized patches (Jones et al., 1979). These and the terminal patches of the ipsilateral corticocortical systems overlap to some still undefined degree the clusters of terminals of thalamic afferents in IV and IIIb, but they extend also into the more superficial layers. In many other cortical areas the terminal zones of these two systems are interdigitated (see Chapter 10). Convergence does occur, for the pyramidal cells of IIIb that emit callosal fibers receive direct synaptic input from thalamic afferents (Hendry and Jones, 1983).

The focal zones of terminations of these systems (e.g., the callosal) are arrayed in mediolateral strips that cross in a quasi-orthogonal way the general anterior-to-posterior representations of each body part across areas 3b, 1, and 2 (Jones et al., 1979). The intersections specify a module by place, mode, and interhemispheric connection, although the meaning of the latter for function is still obscure. The specification of a module by the intersection of such strips appears to be a general cortical property, for it occurs in both the auditory and visual cortices as well as in the postcentral somatic sensory cortex. The specificity of afferent projections in the modular mode is even more spectacular in the motor system. There are separate channels for afferents of cerebellar, pallidal, and sustantia nigral origin through separate thalamic nuclei to the motor cortex. Moreover, in the ventrolateral nucleus there are separate rods of neurons driven from the dentate, interpositus, and fastigial nuclei, without overlap; these project separately to adjacent columns in the motor cortex. How those adjacent columns thus differ functionally is unknown.

An important generality can be inferred from these anatomical results and many related physiological observations: *the effective unit of operation in such a distributed system is not the single neuron and its axon, but bundles or groups of cells and their axons with similar functional properties and anatomical connections.*

Columniation by Intrinsic Connectivity

The local excitatory interneurons of IV and IIIb (the spiny nonpyramidal or stellate cells) are one of the principal postsynaptic targets of afferents from the thalamic ventroposterior nucleus. The axons of these interneurons project vertically into narrow bundles of 100–200 μm dimension that run across all the cellular layers and terminate upon the dendrites and dendritic spines of pyramidal cells, as well as upon inhibitory interneurons. They extend the local patch of thalamic terminals into a translaminar column. As a general rule, all other intrinsic excitatory synaptic actions are imposed via the recurrent collateral branches of pyramidal cell stem axons. These reentrant circuits create a bidirectional excitatory system, for pyramidal cells of the supragranular layers innervate in this way pyramidal cells of the infragranular layers, and vice versa. The collaterals of any single stem axon avoid its cell of origin but project profusely within the restricted zone of the local columnar population of pyramidal cells, with the exception described below. The recurrent collaterals also terminate upon inhibitory interneurons, providing one mechanism for pericolumnar inhibition.

Other recurrent collaterals of the stem axons of pyramidal cells of III and V in each of the cytoarchitectural fields of the postcentral cortex project horizontally for long distances within their own area (see Chapter 3). They generate local, column-like foci of terminal boutons, which occur at horizontal intervals of about 800 μm. These projections are linking pathways between columns with similar modality properties but different receptive fields. The functional aspects of this projection are still uncertain (but see Chapter 12).

The specific thalamocortical afferents also terminate directly upon the dendrites of pyramidal cells of III, V, and VI, and provide candidate pathways for monosynaptic transcortical actions through the somatic sensory cortex (Hendry and Jones, 1983). The disynaptic IPSPs evoked in pyramidal cells by thalamocortical volleys indicate that the thalamocortical afferents also terminate directly upon local inhibitory interneurons (Agmon and Connors, 1991).

The GABAergic, inhibitory double bouquet cells are present in all layers, but are most dense in II and III. They project their axons into the vertical bundles of the cortex described below, and they terminate upon both pyramidal cells and inhibitory interneurons (DeFelipe et al., 1989a, 1990). They impose a strong, vertically directed stream of inhibition and may also exert a vertically directed disinhibition of those pyramidal cells upon which the inhibitory interneurons postsynaptic to them project. Other classes of inhibitory interneurons form local control loops. The large and small basket cells and the chandelier cells exert powerful inhibitory controls upon pyramidal cell bodies and initial axon segments, respectively. The horizontal projections of the myelinated axons of the large basket cells, which extend for 1–2 mm, provide another pathway for pericolumnar inhibition. The peptide cells terminate upon the somata and dendrites of pyramidal cells, but little is known of their function.

The layer I circuits are the least well known of all cortical systems (cf. Chapter 3). How they may affect the formation or operation of columns is unknown, and what role they may play in more global cortical function is equally mysterious. It is usually said that, since Cajal-Retzius cells are the first to appear in the embryonic cortex, the layer I circuits are important in cortical histogenesis. Four facts seem certain:

1. The Cajal-Retzius pathway is the first one completed in the developing cortex; it is glutaminergic and excitatory and is first driven by modulatory afferents from the central core of the brain stem.

2. The pyramidal cell apical dendrites that reach layer I divide there and turn horizontally, and many run for distances that exceed the dimension of modules.

3. Afferent signals reaching layer I in the mature cortex evoke synaptic responses in apical dendrites of sufficient strength to elicit action potentials in the pyramidal cell somata.

4. The small neurons in the lower edge of layer I in the mature cortex are GABAergic, but little more is known about them.

Dendritic Clusters and Axon Bundles Group Cortical Neurons into Modules of Minicolumnar Size

The apical dendrites of pyramidal cells that ascend through the cortex are not homogeneously distributed in the tangential dimension. The dendrites of 3–20 large pyramidal cells of layer V form clusters that ascend together through IV. They are joined in the supragranular layers by the successive addition of the apical dendrites of pyramidal cells of II and III, and all ascend farther, many sending their terminal arrays to I (Fleischauer et al., 1972; Peters and Walsh, 1972). The apical dendrites of pyramidal cells of VI are grouped into separate bundles that do not join the clusters but reach only to IV, where they end within the terminal bushes of thalamocortical fibers (Escobar et al., 1986). Further knowledge of the clusters and bundles has come from the quantitative studies of Peters and his colleagues on the neocortex of rodents, cats, and primates (Peters and Payne, 1993; Peters and Sethares, 1996; Peters and Yilmaz, 1993). These investigators propose that each dendritic cluster is the center of a module of pyramidal cells like those of Fig. 7-16. These clusters, about 30 μm in diameter, occur with center-to-center spacing that varies from 20 to 80 μm; the wider spacings occur in the larger brains of the macaque monkey and man. Dendrite clusters appear early in ontogenesis, as the cortical plate is forming and before it receives any afferent axons. The clusters have been described in a wide range of mammalian brains and in every cortical area examined in detail. The dendrites within a cluster are frequently separated only by an intercellular cleft. Gap junctions occur between them during cortical ontogenesis, but linkages of this sort are rare in the mature cortex.

Dendritic clusters appear to represent the mature development of the ontogenetic units of the developing cortex (Chapter 8); they fit the observed sizes of minicolumns. Such a minicolumn may not itself be a uniform processor, for it contains pathways that differ in their patterns of synaptic input and in the targets of projecting ax-

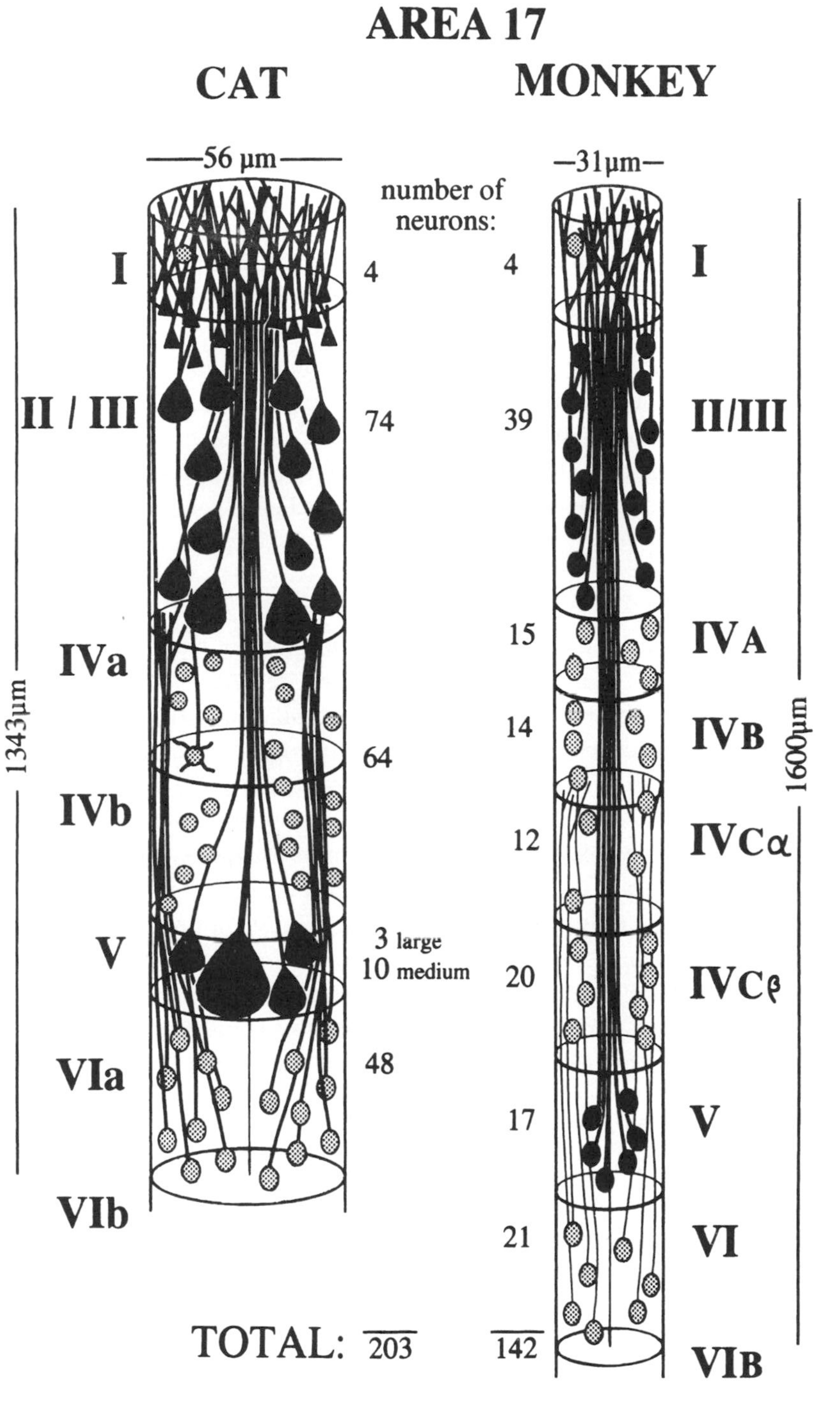

AREA 17

CAT **MONKEY**

—56 μm— number of neurons: —31μm—

1343μm

	CAT	MONKEY	
I	4	4	I
II / III	74	39	II/III
IVa		15	IVA
IVb	64	14	IVB
		12	IVCα
V	3 large 10 medium	20	IVCβ
VIa	48	17	V
VIb		21	VI
			VIB

1600μm

TOTAL: $\overline{203}$ $\overline{142}$

Fig. 7-16 The pyramidal cell modules in cat and monkey visual cortex, drawn to show the relative thickness of the cerebral layers, the numbers of neurons in each layer, and the dendritic clusters. The inhibitory interneurons (16–20 percent of the total) are not shown in these diagrams. Cells of layer IV shown without dendrites are spiny stellate cells, the excitatory interneurons (lightly shaded). The dendrites of the pyramidal cells of layer VI (also lightly shaded) project vertically only to layer IV. A. Peters and E. Yilmez, "Neutral organization in area 17 of cat visual cortex," *Cerebral Cortex* 3 (1993): 49–68. Reprinted by permission of Wiley-Liss, Inc., a subsidiary of John Wiley & Sons, Inc.

ons. This argument assumes that cortical outputs to such diverse targets as the contralateral hemisphere or the thalamus differ in some quality. However, there is to my knowledge no direct experimental evidence for this assumption. There is some evidence that the structure of the dendritic bundles may differ between cytoarchitectonic areas (Viebahn, 1990).

Fig. 7-16 does not show all the connectivity that contributes to the modular columnarity of the minicolumns. The ascending axonal branches of the excitatory spiny nonpyramidal cells are intertwined in the dendritic clusters, as are the axonal branches of one set of inhibitory interneurons, the double bouquet cells.

The transverse diameter of the cortical minicolumn has been measured in 15 studies in mice, rats, rabbits, cats, and monkeys, with a variety of methods. The mean transverse diameter from these studies (mean of means) is 56 μm ($\pm$ 4 μm standard error).

The Special Case of the Rodent Somatic Sensory Cortex

A striking feature of the trigeminal component of the somatic afferent system in rodents is the modular arrangement of its neurons at each of its levels, in the brainstem, in the thalamus, and in layer IV of the somatic sensory cortex. The cortical modular structures are called *barrels*. They occur throughout the map of the body in the cortical sensory area (Welker, 1971), but are most robust in a posteromedial subfield devoted exclusively to representation of the large mystacial vibrissae (whiskers) on the contralateral face. The modules are arrayed spatially to mimic in a one-to-one relation the spatial distribution of the whiskers on the facial skin. Several methods have been used to show the strong relation between each vibrissa and a single corresponding barrel. The finer hairs of the facial fur between the large vibrissae are represented outside this special barrel field.

The barrels were observed long ago by several neuroanatomists and described by Lorente de No in 1922. T. A. Woolsey (1967) and Woolsey and Van der Loos (1970) observed in Nissl- and Golgi-Nissl-stained sections that each unit consists of a cell-rich wall packed with neuronal somata surrounding a relatively cell-poor interior. This central zone is filled with groups of axon terminals that synapse upon the dendrites of the wall neurons. Modules are separated from one another by narrow septa of constant width. Dendritic clusters and radial glia are denser in the walls and septa than in the barrel hollows

(Crandell et al., 1990; White and Peters, 1993). Neurons above and below each of the layer IV barrels are aligned to it in a columnar manner.

Rodents palpate their often dark and narrow surrounds by moving their mystacial whiskers back and forth at frequencies in the range of 8 to 10/sec. The barrage of impulses generated when the moving whiskers encounter objects provides a population signal of the spatial landscape immediately surrounding the head. This system has served as a model for experiments that range from development to cortical transplantation. It has been particularly useful for studies of the intrinsic organization of the cortex and of induced plasticity (for review, see Woolsey, 1990). Evidence that the barrels of IV are the centers of functional columns has come from studies of intracortical neuronal connectivity, from electrophysiological studies of the intact cortex, and from measures of the changes in metabolism induced by stimulation of a single vibrissa (Jones and Diamond, 1995).

Intracortical Connectivity

The neuron phenotypes and the intrinsic circuitry of the rodent barrel cortex resemble those described above for the primate somatic sensory cortex, except for the differences in neurite distribution in layer IV that produce its barrelled appearance (Simons and Woolsey, 1984). Neuron somata are more numerous in the walls than in the hollows of the barrels; their dendrites and the axon terminals of afferent fibers pack the neuropil of the hollows. Verticality in processing is set initially by the restricted distribution of the axonal arbors of whisker-specified sets of thalamocortical fibers that terminate in IV and lower III. It is maintained by the vertical distribution of the axons of the spiny and nonspiny nonpyramidal interneurons of IV, and by the narrow radial distributions of the axons and dendrites of the double bouquet cells, which compose the radial bundles so obvious in sections reacted immunocytochemically for calbindin (DeFelipe et al., 1990). Axonal collateral projections link pyramidal cells of II to III, and those of III to V and VI. The latter are linked reciprocally to the supragranular layers by retrograde axonal collaterals. Horizontal connections to near- and far-neighbor barrel columns are made by pyramidal cell axon collaterals at both supra- and infragranular levels.

Electrophysiological Studies

Application of the method of single-neuron analysis to the intact rodent somatic sensory cortex has provided compelling evidence for the hypothesis of columnar organization. The results of every study have met the criteria for identity of place and mode given above. All neurons of a barrel column are activated by movement of a single, matched, principal whisker on the contralateral face; the pyramidal cells all have similar directional selectivities. Many neurons are also activated by deflection of adjacent whiskers, creating an excitatory surround receptive field. Eighty-five percent of neurons in IV respond to stimulation of only a single whisker; multi-whiskered neurons increase in prevalence at successive levels of intracortical processing, particularly in Va, where they are 65 percent of the total (Armstrong-James, 1975; Simons, 1978). The excitatory input to a barrel column from near- or far-neighbor whiskers is generated intracortically through parallel column-to-column relays from near- and far-neighbor columns (Armstrong-James and Fox, 1987; Armstrong-James et al., 1991, 1992; Armstrong-James and Calahan, 1991). The modular structure of the rodent trigeminal system can be modified by changing in a differential way the input from the sensory periphery, or its linking connections to the cortex, during a critical period in development that extends to the fifth postnatal day. The mature properties of the barrels and barrel neurons are established by the seventh postnatal day.

The barrel column system is well disposed for analysis of the dynamic aspects of intracortical processing. Neuronal cell types and their intracortical connections are reasonably well known. A single barrel column can be activated discretely by a brief deflection of its principal whisker, and the responses to near- and far-neighbor whiskers are easily observed. When experimental conditions are held constant, measurements of latency, response magnitude, receptive field, and directional selectivity for neurons in different laminae can be assumed—as a first approximation—to have been made at the same time. The results allow construction of a diagram of the sequential flow of neural activity within the column.

An elegant experiment of this sort has been made by Armstrong-James et al. (1992) in the rat. The experimental design emphasized the early responses to stimulation of the principal whisker, and that late activity evoked by stimulation of near- and far-neighbor whiskers reaches the column by intracortical projection from *their* principal columns. The direct early responses are stronger than the delayed responses to transcortical input, except in Va, where the two are nearly equal. The temporal order in which neurons in different layers are activated is summarized in Fig. 7-17. Layer IV is activated first, as expected, but is soon followed by neurons of Va. Activity is relayed upward from layer IV to III to II (panels B and C of Fig. 7-17), just as the first transcortical activity reaches Va. Frames D, E, and F of Fig. 7-17 show the late activation relayed from neighbor columns. This horizontal spread occurs only after the initial, early activation of neurons in layers II, III, IV, and Vb; layer Va is an exception. The general result is that cortical activity evoked by a brief afferent volley is first relayed vertically within the relevant column, and only after 3–4 msec is there a limited transcortical spread to closely adjacent columns.

Welker et al. (1993) have extended these studies to the barrel cortex of the mouse and added important new information. They identified two classes of cells in layer IV: (1) those with thin spikes that respond at shortest latency and are assumed to be those of the nonspiny, nonpyramidal inhibitory neurons; and (2) those with regular spikes that respond at longer latencies, presumably those of the spiny nonpyramidal excitatory neurons. The surprising conclusion was reached that the activation of the column by a brief afferent volley is initially inhibitory, accounting for in-field and surround inhibition, quickly followed by activation of the excitatory neurons of IV and then sequentially by activation of neurons of the supragranular layers. Whether this general pattern of activity applies to other areas of the neocortex, or to other species, remains for further experiment to reveal. It is important to emphasize that the translaminar flow pattern determined by latency measurements obtains only when the column is activated by a brief, synchronous volley of impulses. Under normal circumstances—in a rodent using its whiskers to locate objects—the intracolumnar channels and their output neurons will be occupied by ongoing, time-varying patterns of activity for which the time relations determined by latency measurements are meaningless. Analyses of these ongoing patterns of activity can be made by recording in waking, behaving animals, and preferably with multiple microelectrodes in the manner used by Nicoletis et al. (1993) in their experiments on the ventrobasal complex.

Fig. 7-17 Intracolumnar and pericolumnar flow of activity in a barrel of the somatic sensory cortex of anesthetized adult rats, evoked by brief deflection of the related contralateral whisker. Cellular discharges were recorded with extracellular microelectrodes. (A) Cells in layer IV are activated at a mean latency of 8.5 msec. (B–F) Sequential activation of laminae and sublaminar units at the mean latencies after panel A (superpositioned numbers). (B and C) Cells within the column in layers II and Vb are activated 2.4 msec after those of layer IV, simultaneously with layer Va cells in near-neighbor columns; there are no significant differences in the latencies of these responses. Activity then spreads to near-neighbor layers II–IV (D) and to VI within the first column. The next cells activated are the far-neighbor layer Va cells (E) and the last group are the far-neighbor cells of II, III, and IV (F). (From Armstrong-James et al., 1992.)

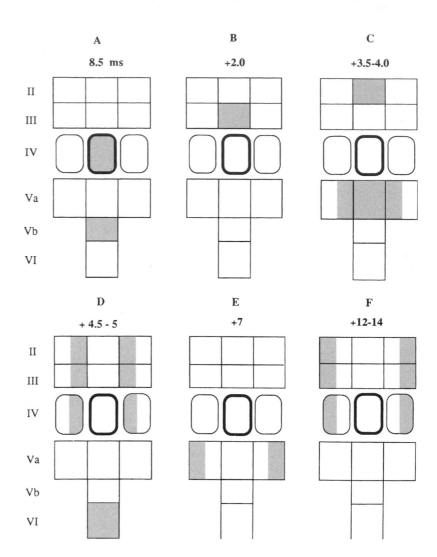

Metabolic Studies

Several investigators have used the 2-deoxyglucose radiographic labeling method to highlight single, active barrel columns in the rodent somatic sensory cortex. When all large vibrissae save one are clipped, stimulation of the remaining whisker evokes increased activity and labeling that is largely but not completely confined to the single relevant column in the contralateral somatic sensory cortex. Such a labeled column has a cylindrical shape and extends across all the cortical layers, but is centered upon the barrel in layer IV (Hand,

1981; Chmielowska et al., 1986; Durham and Woolsey, 1985; Kossut et al., 1988). McCasland and Woolsey (1988) used a high-resolution form of this method to demonstrate a patchy inhomogeneity within each such labeled column. Patches in a barrel are in spatial register with similar patches in cortical layers above and below layer IV. Each cylindrical stack is thought to consist of a single minicolumn or a small group of minicolumns. This finding is similar to that made by Tommerdahl et al. (1993) in cats and monkeys, described above. Some variation in the spatial pattern of these minicolumnar patches was seen in barrel columns matched between individuals and in homologous columns in the two hemispheres of the same individual.

A Comment on Secondary Histogenesis of the Barrels

I consider in Chapter 9 the question of cortical ontogenesis and the relative influences of cell-autonomous and subsequent events in specifying neocortical areas. How the barrels of layer IV of the rodent S1 cortex are specified is of special interest in the present context. The barrel field reaches its mature form by postnatal days 5–7. The terminals of the whisker-specific sets of thalamocortical afferents to S1 from the ventrobasal complex are present in the cortex from the day of birth. The terminal arbors are distributed in the incipient IV in tangential, overlapping gaussians centered at the center of the prospective barrel (Senft and Woolsey, 1991a,b). These distributions change rapidly, with exuberant growth of local axonal terminal branches in their centers and pruning of branches in the region of peripheral overlap of the gaussians, the future septa. This distribution was found by Senft and Woolsey (1991c) to be fitted by Dirichlet domains, superimposed upon the labeled septa in a tangential section of layer IV from a mature cortex. Dirichlet domains (solutions to the first boundary value problem) are complex polygons that form in many systems around nucleating centers, just as the centers of developing barrels nucleate around the densest portion of the terminal arborizations of thalamocortical afferents.

Several molecules are markers for barrels. Acetylcholinesterase defines the barrel outlines during a transient phase in development. The monaminergic afferents from the brainstem with serotonin, noradrenaline, or dopamine as transmitters also reach the cortex early and influence its further development. For example, transgenic mice lacking the gene for monamine oxidase express excessive amounts of serotonin in the somatic cortex and do not develop the characteristic barrel structure (Cases et al., 1996). Other more permanent markers (cytochrome oxidase, succinic dehydrogenase, glycoconjugates, and cytotactin) are expressed in S1 before the first appearance of the cellular arrangements of the barrels (Schlagger and O'Leary, 1993).

A Central Core System Projecting to the Cortex without Columnar Organization of Its Terminations

When considering the validity of the concept of columnar organization of the cerebral cortex, it is important to set the idea in proper perspective. No one has ever suggested that the neocortex consists of isolated cylinders held together by an impervious cement! Indeed, in 1957 I took care to emphasize, on the basis of the evidence then available, that this mode of organization might apply only to the first 100 msec or so of activity after an afferent entry. The question was left open whether during continuing intracortical processing neural activity patterns might be formed, dissolved, and reformed sequentially into a number of different spatial arrays. This caveat has become less necessary with a host of new discoveries. For example, I consider the fact that the horizontal projections of collaterals of intracortical pyramidal cell axons link together distant modules with overlapping sets of properties one of the strongest proofs for columnar organization.

Other systems engage the cortex in quite different ways, the most obvious being the cortical projections of the central core systems; a good example originates in the locus ceruleus. Molliver and his colleagues (Wilson and Molliver, 1991a,b) used an immunofluorescent method to trace this system in detail. The nucleus emits two separately identifiable ascending tracts that reach the cortex. They pass upward through the subthalamus; the medial component reaches the cortex via the cingulum bundle, the lateral via the external capsule. The special aspect of the system is that, from these two local points of entry, fibers pass tangentially through the gray matter to reach every cortical region and every cortical layer (see Fig. 3-6). In Molliver's montage reconstructions, the neocortex sits in a space encompassed in three dimensions by a web of fibers spaced at intervals of 30–40 μm. These fibers are now known to terminate in classical synapses, but an added volume conduction of transmitter is not ruled out. Surely no one can doubt that the system has the capacity to influence directly every cell in the neocortex. *Not a sign of columnar organization!*

Any single cell of the locus ceruleus projects upon a very wide area of cortex and sustains an immense and divergent axonal field. Single neurons of the system may even innervate both the cerebral and cerebellar cortices. It is known that the locus ceruleus receives a wide convergent sensory input. The system is commonly believed to have a controlling and level-setting influence upon the cerebral cortex, considered as a whole. Its importance in sleep mechanisms may be only the most obvious of these controls, and others of a more subtle nature may operate also.

Summary

The idea of the columnar organization of the neocortex is part of the more general hypothesis of the modular organization of nervous systems, a widely documented principle of design for both vertebrate and invertebrate brains (Liese, 1990). That is, the large entities of brains we call cortical areas or subcortical nuclei are composed of smaller units. These local neural circuits, repeated iteratively within each larger structure, may function independently, or they may act together when combined in groups whose composition may vary from time to time. Such modules may differ in cell type and number, in internal and external connectivity, and in mode of neuronal processing between different large entities; but within any single entity, like the neocortex, they have a basic similarity of internal design and operation. Modules are grouped into entities by a set of dominating external connections, or by replication of an intrinsic function over a topographic representation. These unifying factors are most obvious for the heterotypical sensory and motor areas of the neocortex. Modules in homotypical areas are commonly specified by properties generated by intracortical operations. The set of all modules of a cortical area may itself be fractionated by different extrinsic connections for different modular subsets. Linkages between them and subsets in other large entities form distributed systems. The neighborhood relations between connected subsets of modules in different entities result in nested systems that serve distributed functions (Mountcastle, 1978). A cortical area defined in classical cytoarchitectural terms may belong to more than one and sometimes to several such systems (Chapter 10). Columns within a single cytoarchitectural area with some common properties may be linked by long-range, intracortical connections (see Chapter 3).

The Ontogenesis of the Neocortex

The three-dimensional structure of layers and columns in the neocortex is generated from a two-dimensional array of progenitor cells lining the lateral ventricular and subventricular zones early in embryonic life. The genomic content of cells is unchanged during development. The progression of events from cell birth to mature neuronal phenotype, and the specification of neocortical areas, is determined by the temporal order in which certain genes are expressed, often in combinations that change with time. A major goal in developmental neurobiology is to determine the interactive roles of intrinsic and extrinsic molecular and cellular influences that control the sequence of events from cell birth to cortical area specification.

Several features of cortical ontogenesis apply to all neocortical areas, and in general to all mammals. Cortical neurons are generated in the pseudostratified, columnar epithelium lining the ventricular walls of the developing forebrain, in its ventricular and subventricular zones. They migrate from the locus of generation to their final positions in the cortex; migration begins with the first asymmetric division. Neurons differentiate further after migration and become arranged in cortical layers, where they form efferent and receive afferent extrinsic connections characteristic of the layer (Chapter 3). They also develop translaminar intrinsic connections that form the network basis of the columns of the mature cortex. Glial cells are also produced within this epithelium and migrate to the neocortex: they may thereafter continue to proliferate, but neurons rarely do so. Progenitor cells in many parts of the nervous system are multipotent, and the traditional view has been that the neural epithelium of the telencephalon contains at an early stage only a single class of progenitor cells. New methods for marking and following cells during embryogenesis indicate how "environmental" factors determine neuronal cell fate in many parts of the nervous system. To what degree this is true also for the specification of glial and neuronal cell lines in the cerebral cortex is a question now under intensive study. Some major phenotypic characteristics are specified early in development. For example, from about embryonic day 40 in the macaque monkey, just before neurogenesis of the cortex begins, both neural and glial precursor cells are present in the ventricular and subventricular zones of the germinal epithelium (Levitt et al., 1983). Thereafter both cell lines are observed in germinative cell cycles in the ventricular and subventricular zones throughout the period of active neurogenesis. This conclusion is supported by the results of experiments in rats in which cells were tagged with a replication-defective retroviral marker and later identified by ultrastructural criteria (Luskin et al., 1993).

The earliest event in the formation of the neocortex is the generation of the preplate, which is composed of a superficial sublayer of the earliest corticipetal nerve fibers and the earliest generated neurons. These are the Cajal-Retzius cells and a lower layer of cells that will become the subplate. Subsequent waves of migrating neurons form the cortical plate in an inside-to-outside temporal sequence, the future layers VI to II of the mature cortex. The cortical plate is inserted into the preplate, splitting it into three layers. The outermost is the marginal zone, the future layer I (Marin-Padilla, 1984). The second is a thick and partially transient band called the subplate (Fig. 8-1; Marin-Padilla, 1978; Kostovic and Molliver, 1974; Kostovic and Rakic, 1980, 1990; Kostovic et al., 1989, 1991; Shatz et al., 1988; Bayer and Altman, 1991). The third band in the lower intermediate zone consists of neurons that migrate in a tangential direction and end as interstitial cells in the white matter, as demonstrated in rats by DiDiego et al. (1994). Both these and the surviving subplate cells form the population of interstitial cells in the white matter of the mature cortex.

Neurons migrating to the neocortex move along radial glial fibers that form palisades between the neural epithelium and the developing cortical plate (Rakic, 1972; see Fig. 8-2). The time of generation of

Fig. 8-1 The developmental history of the earliest-generated cells (black dots) of the cat visual cortex. By embryological day E30, after the last round of symmetrical division and the onset of asymmetrical division, some cells have migrated from the ventricular zone *(VZ)* to the marginal *(MZ)* and intermediate zones *(IZ)*. By E40, latter-generated and migrating cells have split the first population into the marginal zone above and the subplate *(SP)* below. These migrating cells form the cortical plate *(CP)* and generate the lower five layers of the cortex, from below upward; layer I is formed from the marginal zone. At birth, postnatal day P0, some cells remain in the subplate. Some surviving cells of the subplate remain in the white matter *(WM)* in the adult; they are GABAergic and fast-spiking, but their function is unknown. M. B. Luskin and C. J. Shatz, "Studies of the earliest generated cells of the cat's visual cortex," *Journal of Neuroscience* 5(4): 1062–1075 (1985).

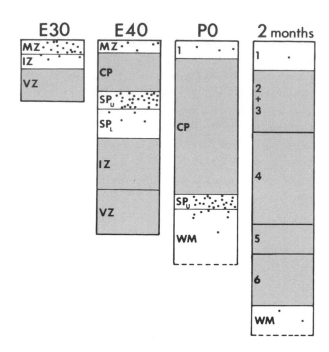

a neuron determines its final laminar or vertical position in the mature neocortex (Rakic, 1974). The *x-y* spatial position of origin of a neuron in the neural epithelium determines the final tangential position of the cell in the mature neocortex, for the majority (85–90 percent) of neocortical neurons. Neurogenesis begins at about E40 and ends at about E100 in the 165-day gestational period of the macaque monkey; it extends from E11 to E17 in the 22-day gestational period in the mouse; migration continues in the mouse until the day of birth (Caviness et al., 1995; Takahashi et al., 1996a,b). It is likely that humans acquire their full complement of neocortical neurons during the middle trimester of gestation. Projection and intrinsic neurons differentiate in sequence from deep to superficial layers, just as they are sequenced in migration. The pyramidal cells lead the intrinsic interneurons in the emission and growth of neurites and in achieving synaptic contacts (Jones, 1990a).

The methods of cellular and molecular neurobiology are now used to study several questions central to cortical neurogenesis. Are single cells in the neural epithelium capable of generating both neurons and glia? How do neurons migrate over distances of several millimeters? What is the force producing migration? At what stage in development are neural stem (i.e., self-renewing) cells committed to a given neuronal progenitor cell with restricted potential? What are the interactions between genetic signals, cell birthday, positional information, and environmental influences in determining final laminar and tangential positions and cell phenotype? Is there plasticity in neurogenesis? What are the roles of cell-surface molecules in migration and composition of the neocortex?

It is important to emphasize that the concept of cell *lineage* refers to the normal presumptive fate of a cell if left undisturbed. The *develop-*

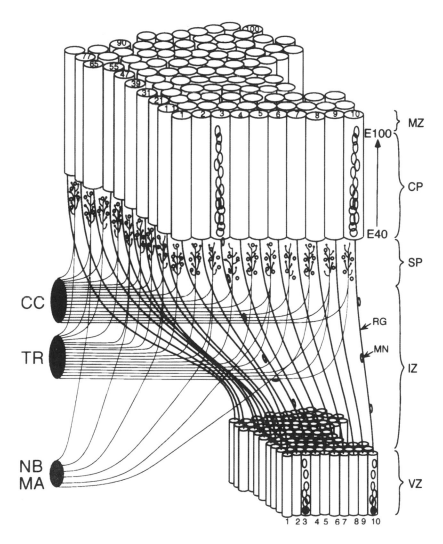

Fig. 8-2   A three-dimensional illustration of the developmental events occurring during early stages of corticogenesis in the monkey. The drawing illustrates radial migration, the predominant mode of neuronal movement that in primates produces the columnar organization of the adult cortex. After their last division, cohorts of migrating neurons *(MN)* traverse the intermediate zone *(IZ)* and the subplate *(SP),* where they may interact with afferents arriving sequentially from the nucleus basalis *(NB),* from the monamine nuclei of the brain stem *(MA),* from the thalamic radiation *(TR),* and from several ipsilateral and contralateral corticocortical bundles *(CC).* Newly generated neurons bypass those generated earlier, which are situated in the deep cortical layers, and settle at the interface between the developing cortical plate *(CP)* and the marginal zone *(MZ).* Eventually they form a radial stack of cells that share a common site of origin but are generated at different times. Although some, presumably neurophilic, cells may detach from the cohort and move laterally, guided by an axonal bundle, most are gliophilic, have affinity for glial cell surfaces, and obey the constraints imposed by transient radial glial scaffolding *(RG).* This cellular arrangement preserves the relation between the proliferative mosaic of the ventricular zone *(VZ)* and the corresponding map within the SP and CP, even though the cortical surface in primates shifts considerably during the massive cerebral growth in the mid-gestational period. (From Rakic, 1995a.)

mental potential of a cell, by contrast, describes what a cell might do under different conditions: in cell culture, after transplantation to a new environment, or after chemical labeling. An experimental demonstration of a wide developmental potential need not correspond to the path a cell would take during normal development (Price, 1993).

Generation of Cells in the Proliferative Ventricular Zone

The neuroepithelium of the cerebral vesicle consists in its earliest stages of a single line of columnar epithelial cells, each of which stretches over the short distance from the ependymal surface of the

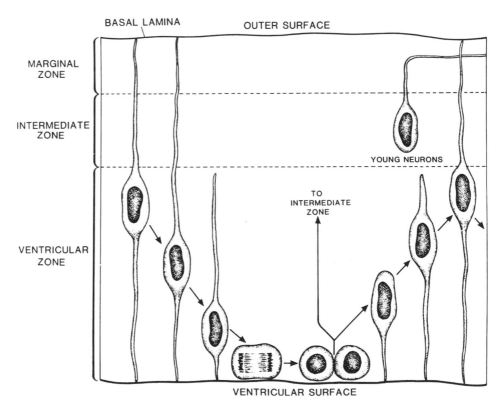

Fig. 8-3 The cycle of cell division in the germinal neuroepithelium, shown in sequential drawings from left to right. At this early stage the neural and glial precursor cells extend from the inner to the outer surfaces of the neural tube. The three subphases of interphase (G1, S, and G2) occur with the nuclei in mid-position in the cell. At the onset of prophase, they withdraw their processes and assume a globular form, and the nuclei move toward the ventricular surface. After cell division the daughter cells again extend processes to the outer surface and begin new cycles. (From Purves, 1988; after Sauer, 1935.)

The Ontogenesis of the Neocortex

neural tube to the pia, attached by endfeet to both surfaces (Sidman and Rakic, 1973; Meller and Tetzlaff, 1975). The phases of the germinal cell cycle are shown in Fig. 8-3. The three subphases of interphase (G1, S, and G2) occur with the nuclei in the midposition in the cells. When cells enter the prophase of mitosis they withdraw their processes and assume a globular form, and their nuclei move toward the ventricular surface. After cell division is complete, the nuclei of daughter cells move away from the ventricular surface and the cells once again extend processes to each surface and initiate new cycles (Sauer, 1935; Sauer and Walker, 1959). A cell cycle in the mouse lasts about 12 hours. For a summary, see Fig. 8-4 (Takahashi et al., 1996a,b).

The stem cells in the earliest stages (E10 in the mouse) produce daughter cells capable of generating either neural or glial cell lines. There follows a rapid shift from this state of pluripotentiality to one of cell-line specificity, so that at E16, just before asymmetric mitosis and the initiation of cell migration, the population of progenitor cells in the neural epithelium consists largely of those capable of generating either neurons or glial cells, but not both (Parnavelas et al., 1991; Price et al., 1992). Indeed, it is likely that phenotype specificity is further restricted at this stage, which means that just before the onset of migration the majority of progenitor cells can each generate either pyramidal neurons, nonpyramidal neurons, astrocytes, or oligodendrocytes, but only one of these (Parnavelas et al., 1991). This conclusion is strengthened by the discovery of Mione et al. (1994) that cells of the rat neuroepithelium, dated as early as E14 by retrovirus labeling, compose non-overlapping populations of transmitter-specific phenotypes with immunoreactivity to GABA or glutamate. They are committed progenitor cells for the pyramidal (glutaminergic) and nonpyramidal (GABAergic) neurons of the mature cortex.

The discovery of the inside-to-outside sequence of formation of the cortical plate was made by Angevine and Sidman (1961) in the mouse, using the ^{3}H-thymidine labeling method. This general pattern of migration and cortical plate formation has since been observed in a number of mammalian species, including carnivores (Luskin and Shatz, 1985; Jackson et al., 1989) and nonhuman primates (Rakic, 1971, 1972, 1974). The pattern of timing and settling is particularly prominent in fetal human brains of different ages, suggesting that a similar pattern is present in humans (Sidman and Rakic, 1973; Krmpoti'c-Nemani'c et al., 1984).

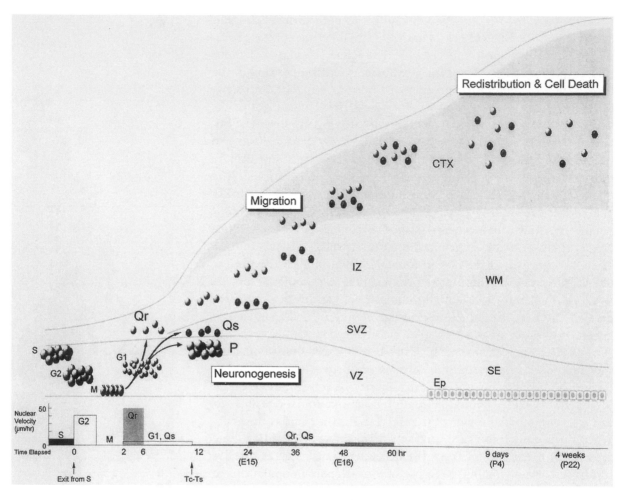

Fig. 8-4 Schematic diagram of neuronogenesis in the pseudostratified ventricular epithelium and migratory behavior for a small cohort of neocortical neurons generated in the cerebral wall of the rat. The group of cells is pictured as arising over an interval of 1–2 hours on E14. The cohort separates after mitosis into a *Q* fraction that leaves the cell cycle and a *P* fraction that continues to cycle (labeled *Neuronogenesis*). The *Q* fraction separates into rapidly exiting (*Qr*, light spheres) and slowly exiting (*Qs*, dark spheres) subpopulations. After transit from the ventricular to the subventricular to the intermediate zone, the two subpopulations migrate *(Migration)* at the same rates until the leading *Qr* fraction is slowed on entering the cortex *(CTX)*; after that the two populations overlap and are indistinguishable. They come to lie deeper than neurons arising at later dates and are moderately reduced in numbers by cell death. After migration is complete, the intermediate zone *(IZ)* and subventricular zone *(SVZ)* are replaced by the cerebral white matter *(WM)* and subependyma *(SE)*, and the PVE within the ventricular zone *(VZ)* is replaced by a cuboidal ependymal ventricular lining *(Ep)*. A temporal profile of these events at the bottom of the diagram provides the nuclear velocities for cells in the proliferative cycle in S, G2, N, and G1 phases, and VZ exit and migration velocities of the *Q* fractions registered on the ordinate. The diagram is schematic for both scaling and time. T. Takahashi, R. S. Nowakowski, and F. S. Caviness, Jr., "Interkinetic and migratory behavior of a cohort of neocortical neurons arising in the early embryonic murine cerebral wall," *Journal of Neuroscience* 16(18): 5762–5776 (1996).

The Radial Unit Hypothesis and the Ontogenetic Unit of the Neocortex

The pathways followed and the temporal sequence of events in the fetal monkey brain have been elucidated in a series of experiments by P. Rakic (Rakic, 1972, 1974, 1975, 1977, 1978, 1982), which have culminated in the radial unit hypothesis (Rakic, 1988a, 1990a,b). The general idea is as follows. Migration of immature neurons from the germinal epithelium to the cortical plate is mainly radial and mainly gliophilic. Following the last mitotic division, immature neurons of the ventricular and subventricular zones in rats attach to an adjacent set of glial guide fibers (Gadisseux et al., 1990). Neurons generated serially in time at the same locus in the germinal epithelium migrate sequentially along the same or adjacent sets of glial guide fibers, and settle in the inside-to-outside pattern in a radial column. Neurons of this radial column form an *ontogenetic unit,* the fundamental building block in the developing neocortex (see Fig. 8-2; Rakic, 1988b, 1995a); the basic columnar organization of the neocortex reflects its mode of generation (Mountcastle, 1978). The ontogenetic unit is oriented normally to the pial surface. Early in development, the radial guide fibers along which neurons migrate are short and arranged in palisades radial to the cortical surface. As the brain and the cortex enlarge, and as incipient sulci and gyri appear, the palisades curve in long, sweeping arcs, often several millimeters in length, but they remain parallel to each other in a precise topological relation between loci in the *x-y* dimension of the germinal epithelium and the *x-y* dimension of the cortical plate (Gadisseux et al., 1989).

The hypothesis best supported by the available data is that surface area, and thus the size, of any neocortex is determined by the number of its ontogenetic units, a number set by the number of symmetric divisions of progenitor cells in the neural epithelium before migration begins. One extra symmetric division will double the number of ontogenetic units, and thus double the surface area of the neocortex. The number of cells in each ontogenetic unit is determined by the number of asymmetric divisions of its progenitor cells, beginning with the first division at the onset of migration. One additional asymmetric division will add only one cell from each of the several progenitor cells in the relevant polyclone in the neuroepithelium. Expansion of the neocortex in evolution is thought to depend upon mutational change in the number of symmetric divisions in regional zones of the neuroepithelium. The increased number of ontogenetic units interacts with other factors in the creation of new cortical areas and their evolution through natural selection (Rakic, 1995b). Areas may vary in size between conspecifics and even between the hemispheres of the same brain. The surface area of the cortex in mammals varies by nearly three orders of magnitude, while cortical thickness varies only over a ratio of 1 to 4 between mouse and human.

A Mosaicism Exists in the Ventricular Zone

The proliferative units of the ventricular zone (VZ) in the monkey consist of 3–5 stem cells gradually increasing to 10–12 stem cells, groups separated by glial septa (Rakic, 1988a,b). A similar patchy aggregation of cells is clear in the VZ of embryonic rats at days E12–E13 (Altman and Bayer, 1990). The rate of neuron production varies between adjacent zones in the neuroepithelium (Reznikov et al., 1984; Rakic, 1990a). For example, it varies by more than 2 to 1 between the VZ zone producing neurons for area 17 and that producing neurons for area 18 (DeHay et al., 1993), a difference reflected in the mature cortex by a comparably larger number of neurons per unit area of cortical surface in area 17 than in any other cortical areas. There is a heterogeneous expression of oncogenes within the VZ; the peptides coded are concentrated in repetitive clusters of radial glial fibers, which form a transient columnar organization within the VZ during the period of maximal neuron production (Johnston and Van der Kooy, 1988). During the early phase of histogenesis, the progenitor cells are coupled together by gap junctions into local clusters of 15–90 cells (Lo-Turco and Kriegstein, 1991).

The idea that cortical parcellation is to a certain degree set at the level of the ventricular zone is supported by studies in transgenic (Soriano et al., 1995) and chimeric mice (Natkatsuki et al., 1991). Soriano and his colleagues traced the expression of beta-galactosidase (β-gal) in a line of transgenic mice, β-2NZ3′2. The descendants of the β-gal[+] cells in these mice migrated radially and then remained as polyclones in the local domains of the neocortex. No labeled polyclones were observed distributed in the orthogonal direction, perpendicular to the radial columns. Finally, Tan and Breen (1993) used transgenic mice with *lacZ*-encoded β-galactosidase together with inactivation of one X chromosome to produce a functional genetic mosaicism. On the thirteenth day of the 22-day gestation period of the mouse, they observed a highly ordered distribution of the genetically different cells in the ventricular zone, with alternating columns of X-inactivated and non-X-inactivated cells. Occasionally these columns were a single cell wide, but more commonly they extended to widths of several cells. These observations indicate that early in gestation there exists a tangentially distributed mosaic-like arrangement within the ventricular zone of groups of cells with different properties.

The Radial Astrocytic Glial Cells Form a Transient Scaffold for Neuronal Migration

Shortly before neuronal migration begins, the replicating glial cells of the germinal epithelium enter a period of mitotic arrest and extend processes upward to terminate in endfeet on the basal lamina of the pia. The processes of several glial cells cluster in a fascicle in the developing monkey brain (Schmechel and Rakic, 1979b). The glial fascicles maintain a strict topographical relation between the ventricular zone and the developing cortical plate. After formation of the preplate, the glial fascicles appear to shorten and to reach only to the lower edge of the subplate. As the neuronal layers of the cortical plate are added, guide fibers extend farther upward through the incipient infragranular layers, and are thus positioned to deliver neurons to successively more superficial supragranular layers (Gadisseux et al., 1992, in the rat). The processes of mitotic arrest, process extension, and fasciculation of astrocytic glial cells have been observed in cell culture, but only after neurons are added to the previously pure glial cell cultures; the changes then begin within a few minutes (Hatten, 1985). This change to a radial form is controlled by an extrinsic soluble factor present in the embryonic forebrain (Hunter and Hatter, 1995). At the end of neuronal migration, the glial guide cells defasciculate and withdraw their extended processes. Many then die, but others reenter the mitotic cycle and produce many generations of astrocytes that occupy the developing, and later the mature, neocortex (Schmechel and Rakic, 1973, 1979a,b, in the monkey; Culican et al., 1990, in the mouse; Misson et al., 1988, 1991, in the rat; Voight, 1989, in the ferret). Still other astrocytes of the germinal epithelium do not leave the mitotic cycle and do not enter the intermediate phase of the radial guide cells; they are located mainly in the subventricular zone and produce astrocytes that themselves migrate to the neocortex, particularly to its supragranular layers (Gressens et al., 1992a,b, in the mouse).

Rakic has proposed that the proliferative zone at the surface of the ventricle contains a protomap of the developing neocortex. This map provides for the neocortex a number of cytological, synaptic, and biochemical characteristics that constrain cytoarchitectural differentiation and that differ between different species. This idea is compatible with the observations that many aspects of the organization of the neocortex depend in part upon the influence of invading sets of cortical afferents.

The Dual Pattern of Migration

The migratory course taken by the minority of neurons not following the direct radial pathway to the developing cortical plate has until recently been a matter of some uncertainty. O'Rourke et al. (1992) used time-lapse confocal microscopy to observe migration in living slices of developing rodent cortex; 87–90 percent of the cells observed moved radially along glial guide fibers, as expected. However, the remainder turned aside from this path in the intermediate zone to move tangentially for distances that varied from cell to cell, before resuming radial migration. The problem has been studied further by a number of investigators using as a cell vector a replication-incompetent retrovirus labeled with a reporter gene, *E. coli* β-galactosidase *(lacZ)*, whose produce can be identified histochemically (Cepko, 1989; Cepko et al., 1990; Price et al., 1987; Sanes, 1989b; Luskin, 1996). The virus particles are injected into the ventricles of the living rat embryo, where they are incorporated into the DNA of dividing cells and appear undiluted in 50 percent of their descendants. They can be identified at any later time by histochemical methods. Luskin et al. (1993) found that clonally related neurons were predominantly arranged radially along the migratory pathway and that after migration the neuronal clones remained radially arranged, whereas cells of glial clones were dispersed tangentially. This pattern is particularly explicit in the convoluted monkey cortex, where the majority of clonally related cells, which come from long distances, become arranged in a remarkably radial fashion (Kornack and Rakic, 1995).

Walsh and Cepko (1988, 1992, 1993), in similar experiments injected a library of about 100 genetically identifiable retroviruses, in increasing dilution in different experiments, into rats. They observed what they interpreted to be widely dispersed clonal derivatives in the cortical plate. Assuming that the probability that a single virus infected more than one progenitor cell was very low, they concluded that at least some members of single clones migrate to widely separated areas of the neocortex. Their assumption was criticized on statistical grounds by Guthrie (1992) and by Kirkwood et al. (1992), who calculated that the probability of infection of two or more progenitor cells by a single virus was much higher than Walsh and Cepko had supposed.

Walsh and his colleagues have repeated the experiment in rats, now combined with a method for identifying cell phenotype (Reid et al., 1995). They observed that the laterally displaced clones were not produced by tangential migration between the germinal epithelium and the cortical plate, but by a lateral displacement of some progenitor cells within the ventricular zone, an observation made in rats with other methods by Fishell et al. (1993). This lateral migration of progenitor cells within the ventricular zone was followed by the radial migration to the cortical plate of the neurons produced by asymmetric divisions of each progenitor cell at its new location.

This method has now been used to follow the fate of clonally related cells in the primate cortex, where laminar and columnar organization is more pronounced. Kornack and Rakic (1995; Rakic, 1995a,b) injected into the ventricle of fetal monkeys a mixture of two replication-incompetent, *lacZ*-labeled retroviruses. One of these preferentially labeled the nuclei, the other the cytoplasm, in 50 percent of descendant cells. Two modes of neuronal migration were discovered. In the radial pattern clonal groups of neurons occurred in strict radial alignments extended across several cortical laminae; the layer of destination depends upon the stage of corticogenesis at which injections were made. The results provided further evidence that the several phenotypes observed in mature cortical minicolumns are each derived from one of a small group of progenitors forming a polyclonal group in the ventricular zone. All migrating neurons reach a vertically aligned distribution after migrating along a common glial pathway. Other neuronal clonal groups were arrayed in a horizontal pattern in rows, each row within a stratum of a single cortical layer, parallel to the pial surface. Each neuron in such a row was separated from the next in line by 40–150 μm. The horizontal pattern was spatially limited, and in no instance was a wide tangential dispersion observed. Kornack and Rakic propose that the radial arrays are produced by successive asymmetric divisions of progenitor cells: the neurons of the vertical arrays are produced sequentially. Neurons in the horizontal rows, by contrast, are produced from stem cells that after symmetric division move laterally for set distances within the ventricular zone, and then produce by asymmetric divisions neurons that migrate radially to their common laminar positions. The full implications of this new discovery have not yet evolved. It is likely that the radial arrays compose the ontogenetic units or minicolumns of the mature cortex. It is not yet known which cell types compose the horizontal arrays, nor what their functional significance may be in the adult cortex.

The Mechanisms of Neuronal Migration

The development of the nervous system and its patterns of connectivity are controlled and modulated by interactions between neuronal, glial, and morphoregulatory molecules present in, and on, the cell surfaces and in the extracellular matrix. The processes controlled include induction, histogenesis, compartmentalization, axonal projection, synapse formation, and neuronal migration. These molecules are of several different types: cell adhesion molecules that modulate interactions between one cell and another (CAMs); substrate adhesion molecules that modulate interactions between cells and the extracellular matrix (SAMs); and molecules important in axonal projection, the selection of target cells for axonal terminals, and synapse-junction formation (SJMs) (Edelman, 1983, 1984; Edelman et al., 1985, 1990; Sanes, 1989a; McMahon, 1990; Liesi, 1990). The idea that complementary recognition molecules play a role in the formation of neuron-neuron connections has long been accepted in neuroscience, but only received its first formal statement in the chemosensitivity hypothesis of Sperry (1963). Sperry postulated a very large number of chemical attractants and receptors to account for neural connectivity—one for each connection. This hypothesis proved untenable either in this original or in a modified gradient form (Meyer and Sperry, 1973), because it required an incredibly large number of interactive sets of molecules. It has been replaced by the hypothesis that a number of mechanisms modulate the responses of morphoregulatory genes, and thus the appearance and distribution of the relevant cell-membrane molecules (Edelman, 1987, 1988, 1992). These latter may number dozens, and with several modes of modulation a very large number of permutations is possible. The modulatory mechanisms include control of the density and spatial distributions of the cell-membrane molecules, control of the temporal pattern of their synthesis, and sequential modification of their chemical structures, particularly of the extracellular domains of the cell-surface molecules. More recently, it has become clear that the formation of connections in mammals involves the dynamic modification of connections by functional activity.

The Cellular and Molecular Mechanisms in Neuronal Migration

Postmitotic neurons migrate along glial guide fibers from the ventricular and subventricular zones to the developing cortical plate over distances that vary from 100 μm in some places in small mammalion cortex to more than 5,000 μm in monkey and human cortex. This migration is a special example of the contact guidance of cell movement common in developing organisms. The processes involved are neuron-glia recognition and adhesion and neuron movement.

Adhesion between neuron and glial cells is thought to be due to complementary binding between cell-surface molecules (Rakic, 1985; Rakic et al., 1994). Ng-CAM, for example, is a ubiquitous cell-adhesion molecule expressed in neurons that promotes neuron-glial adhesions in many locations (e.g., Grumet et al., 1984). Deletion of the exon responsible for Ng-CAM produces migratory defects in mice (Tomasiewicz et al., 1993). Rakic suggests that cell movement is accomplished by the transfer of cell-adhesion molecules and membrane segments into the membrane of the leading process, thus expanding that process in the migratory direction (Fig. 8-5A). Membrane segments are at the same time withdrawn from other processes that are less firmly adherent to adjacent cells (Fig. 8-5B–C). It is surmised that the cell nucleus is moved in the direction of the leading process by the action of intracellular contractile proteins, but there is no direct evidence for this proposal.

Knowledge of the cellular and molecular mechanisms of neuronal migration in the brain has been advanced by studies of the cerebellum and hippocampus. Important results have come from the co-culture method developed by Hatten and her colleagues and used in mice (Hatten, 1985, 1993). Neurons and glial cells are separated from fetal cerebellum—or other brain structure—and cultured together in small volumes. Neurons attach themselves to astroglia in these cul-

Fig. 8-5 Hypothesis of a mechanism for neuronal migration. (A) Schematic drawing of a cross-section through a migrating neuron *(N)* and its leading process *(LP)* as it moves along a radial glial shaft *(RG)* through a region densely packed with other cells and their processes. Membrane segments formed near the nucleus are transported toward the tip (arrows) within the leading process via rough and smooth endoplasmic reticulum and vesicles, and inserted (*) at the leading surface of the advancing filopodia. The leading process continues to grow along the surface of the radial glial cells, while the filopodia opposed to other surfaces withdraw (crossed arrows). (B) A possible mechanism for the advancement of filopodia *(F₁)*, alignment of the glial shaft *(RG)*, and regression of filopodia *(F₂)* that contact less adhesive cell surfaces. (C) Illustration of the theory that a higher rate of endocytosis in the filopodia opposed to less adhesive surfaces *(F₂)* results in withdrawal of the process while a net increase in exocytosis at the growing filopodia *(F₁)* produces a selective outgrowth of the leading process, and thus migration. (From Rakic, 1985.)

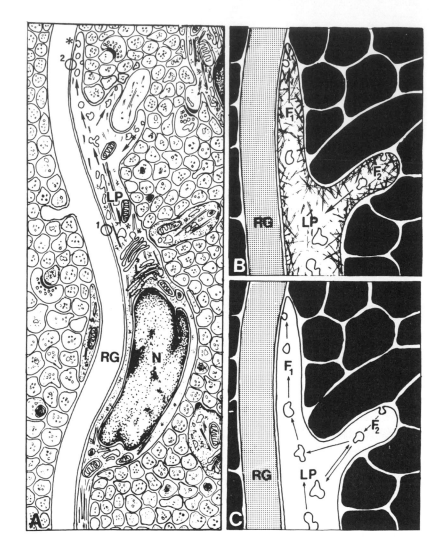

tures within ten minutes of the combination of the two cell types, and project their leading neuronal processes along the extended processes of the glial cells. Migratory movements are saltatory in nature, at average rates of 12–33 μm/hr. The leading process of the migrating neuron resembles an axonal growth cone (Mason et al., 1988; Devoto, 1990). A specialized "interstitial" junctional complex forms between the soma of the migrating neuron and the underlying glial fiber; here the intercellular cleft is widened to 20–30 nm. The cleft contains filamentous material described as passing between the two adjacent cells (Hatten, 1990; Stitt et al., 1991); whether this material is a contractile protein has not yet been determined. Migration is slowed and disordered when antibodies to astrotactin are introduced into the co-culture medium (Edmondson et al., 1988; Fishell and Hatten, 1991). Antibodies to a number of known neuron-neuron ligands did not affect neuronal migration along glial fibers in the in vitro cultures: N-CAM, L-1, NILE, Tag-1, and N-Caherin were tested. Astrotactin is expressed only in neurons of the central nervous system (Hatten and Mason, 1990), and only in migrating neurons; it is found in the migrating zones in the neocortex, but not in the developing cortical plate, where N-CAM is identified. A number of other large molecules may also play a role in neural development (Sanes, 1983, 1989a): (1) promoters of neurite outgrowth, like laminin, fibronectin, collagen I and II, tenascin; and (2) a variety of cell adhesion molecules described above: N-CAM, a neuron-neuron ligand; Ng-CAM, a neuron-glia cell adhesion molecule; cytotactin, which may be similar to tenascin and protein J-1 (see Sheppard et al., 1991). It is clear that "the extracellular matrix mediates adhesion, guides cellular migration, and promotes neurite outgrowth in the periphery" (Sanes, 1989a).

What Are the Stop Signals for Neuronal Migration?

It has been suggested that the molecular signal to stop migration comes from neurons that have already reached the drop zone, and that migration is terminated by recognition of a layer-specific positional cue. Certain molecules are inhibitory or suppressive for growth cone extension and may function as stop signals for axonal projections (Schwab et al., 1993). A second hypothesis, considered by Hatten and Mason (1990), is that ingrowing afferent fibers may produce the stop signal. They observed in culture that when a migrating neuron meets an axonal growth cone it is attracted to it and may stop migrating. There is some evidence that many afferent fibers to the developing cortex do not "wait," but reach the migrating neurons as soon as the latter approach the drop zone. Thus, the stop signal may arise from the axonal growth cones themselves. In either case, a neuron-neuron ligand like N-CAM seems a good candidate for the stop signal. Moreover, a subclass of migrating neurons emits callosal axons *before* reaching their targets in what will eventually be layer III of the fetal monkey cortex (Schwartz et al., 1991), thus providing an-

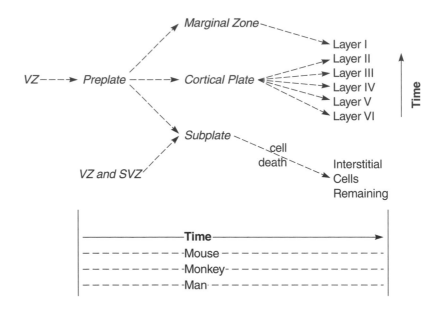

Fig. 8-6 Schema of processes in generation of the neocortex.

other class of input axons to migrating neurons of the opposite hemisphere.

Cell Lineage and the Specification of Neuronal Cell Phenotype in the Neocortex

At early stages of development of the neural plate and tube, single stem cells have the potential to generate all the cell lines found in the mature nervous system. These multipotent neural crest cells produce line-specific progenitor cells that form only neurons or glia (Stemple and Anderson, 1991). The question is whether cell-specific or pluripotential cells, or a mixture of the two, exist in the relevant portion of the ventricular epithelium of the telencephalon at the onset of neurogenesis and migration, and which cell phenotypic characteristics are established at the onset of migration. The relative influence of cell-autonomous and environmental factors in producing phenotypic clones varies greatly from one species to another and from one location to another in the same mammalian brain. Combinatorial gene expression in a cell is controlled by transcriptional regulatory proteins that may themselves be controlled by signals from adjacent cells or from the local intercellular milieu, and/or by mechanisms intrinsic to the cell itself.

The Ontogenesis of the Neocortex

The potential of early stem cells to produce progeny with different phenotypic characteristics narrows in the course of neuronal histogenesis, which produces the variety of neuronal and glial cell types in the mature mammalian nervous system. The general result is that by the time an undifferentiated postmitotic neuron begins migration from the ventricular zone to the cortical plate, its laminar destination and phenotypic fate have been specified to a considerable degree. There is some evidence that cells with some of the properties of stem cells exist in the dentate gyrus of the embryonic and adult mouse brain, where they produce new granule neurons, and in the subependymal layer of the lateral ventricle, where they produce granule cells that migrate to the olfactory bulb (Lois et al., 1996; Luskin, 1996; Luskin et al., 1997; Weiss et al., 1996). It is not known whether stem cells exist in the neocortex of this or any other species.

Neuron phenotypic properties include: the form and size of the cell body and the lengths and distributions of its neurites; the targets of the cell axon both extrinsic to, and within, the cortex; the sources of afferents to the cell, and the locations and densities of their synaptic endings upon the cell surface; and the transmitter molecules expressed in the mature neuron. Obviously, some of these phenotypic properties result from secondary events in cortical histogenesis. Among many phenotypic molecular markers are the transmitter agents, receptor molecules, transmembrane channel proteins, and cell-surface antigens synthesized by the cell. The temporal sequences and the spatial distributions of these markers in, or upon, the cell are major modulating influences during development. Cell-layer position is determined by the cell's place in the temporal chain of progeny production in the ventricular and subventricular zones, and is associated with distinctive phenotypic characteristics. However, it is unlikely that position per se is the factor specifying those characteristics. Likewise, for the large majority of cortical neurons, the final position in the tangential domain of the cortex is determined by the tangential position of its progenitor in the ventricular neuroepithelium.

The lineage of neurons in the developing telencephalon has been studied by following the fate of cells and their progeny during development with methods of cell tagging described in an earlier section. Important discoveries have been made in transplantation experiments, in which cells or tissues taken at one stage of development are moved to new locations within the same donor or to the same or different locations in other conspecific individuals in the same or different stages of development. These test the commitment of the cell to its fate at the time of transplantation, and whether its phenotypic properties can be changed by signals from its neighbors in its new host environment. In this regard, absent more direct evidence, no logical necessity obtains for the conclusion frequently drawn that if a change in the local environment causes changes in expressed phenotypic characteristics of a transplanted neuron, then the environmental influence acts with equal potency during normal development. Price has emphasized this difference between the "presumptive fate" of a cell and its "developmental potential" and concluded that its developmental potential is likely to be broader than its normal fate (Price, 1993). New facts of importance have also come from study of mutant strains of animals.

Cell Lineage Studied with Methods of Cell Tagging

Cell-tag experiments have succeeded, for those locations and in those species in which a tag can be injected into a single progenitor cell, in tracking the fate of a cell over time. This method is not technically possible for cells in the ventricular zone of the developing telencephalon of the mammal. An alternative is to inject into the maternal blood stream, or into the cerebral ventricles of mammalian embryos *in utero,* substances that are incorporated into newly synthesized DNA of progenitor cells and their progeny and that can be identified later by histological methods. Both ^{3}H-thymidine and 5-bromdesoxyuridine have been used in this way, but with each the intensity of the tag signal fades with successive cell divisions. The use of replication-incompetent retroviruses engineered to contain the *E. coli* β-galactosidase *(lacZ)* gene as a tag has the advantage that the tag is replicated in each cell division with undiminished intensity. Success with this method in study of cell lineage requires that it be combined with an independent method for identifying final cell types.

Luskin et al. (1993; Parnevelas et al., 1991) studied cortical cell lineage and migration by combining the retroviral tag method with ultrastructural identification of cell types in the rat postnatal cortex. They injected the viral tag on E15–E16, when neurogenesis is just beginning, and searched for cells labeled with the *lacZ* gene product by electron microscopy at 1–4 months of age. Their results were remarkably uniform, for 25 of the 27 clones they identified were cell type specific, consisting exclusively of either pyramidal neurons, nonpyramidal neurons, astrocytes, or oligodendrocytes. The members of the neuronal classes were distributed radially, usually across several layers, while the cells of glial clones were frequently distributed widely in the tangential dimension of the cortex. This observation indicates that a single neuronal progenitor cell going through successive asymmetrical divisions produces in a temporal sequence postmitotic neurons destined for different cortical layers, neurons that in the adult brain are of an identical cell type (e.g., pyramidal or nonpyramidal) but also possess other phenotypic characteristics that differ. Moreover, in parallel cell culture experiments in which dissociated cells from embryonic brains of rats were labeled at E12–E13 with the retroviral tag, 99 percent of 176 clones identified were cell type specific. Price and his colleagues (1991; Price and Thurlow, 1988), in similar experiments with the retroviral tag method, identified two sets of progenitor cells existing in the germinal epithelium of rats at the time of onset of cortical neurogenesis. They describe a radial migration of neurons, combined with a postmigration lateral movement within the cortical plate, a tangential dispersion much smaller than that described by Walsh and Cepko. The earliest cells produced by a clonal group are located a bit posterolateral to those generated later, reflecting the mild lateral-to-medial neurogenic gradient (Moore and Price, 1992).

The proto-oncogenes of the *myc* family, *C-myc, N-myc,* and *L-myc,* encode a class of regulatory proteins important in determining cell lineage, and thus serve as natural cell tags. *C-myc* is restricted to dividing cells, and the expression of *N-myc* and *L-myc* is correlated with cell line differentiation to neuronal and glial cell lines, respectively. Bernard et al. (1992) found in rodents that single cells obtained from the ventricular zone on E10–E12 express all three genes, but that by E14 progenitor cells express *C-myc* and either *N-myc* or *L-myc,* but not both. This change occurs well before the last mitotic division and cell migration, which lends support to the idea of a temporal evolution within the developing ventricular zone from pluripotential to cell-line-specific progenitor cells by the onset of migration.

Cell Lineage Studied in Transplantation Experiments

A frequent strategy in studies of development is to test whether changes in the local environment of the cell—e.g., by transplantation or local lesion—alter cell fate. McConnell obtained samples of ^{3}H-thymidine-labeled cells from the ventricular zone of embryonic ferrets at the stage in cortical neurogenesis when neurons destined for layers V and VI were being generated (McConnell, 1988, 1990, 1991; McConnell and Kaznowski, 1991). The samples were injected into the ventricular zones of host embryos at either the same stage of development (isochronic experiments) or at a more mature stage, when neurons destined for layers II and III were being generated (heterochronic experiments). Samples obtained 24 hours after thymidine labeling, well after final mitosis, migrated to layers V and VI, as directed by the donor embryo. If samples were taken 4 hours after thymidine labeling, in the S or the early G2 phases of the cell cycle, many of the transplanted cells followed the directive of the host brain and migrated to layers II and III. The laminar fate of a neuron is determined during a short period in the cell cycle, probably in the S phase. Cells that migrated to layers V and VI in the isochronic experiments emitted projections to the thalamus, as expected for normal cells of layer VI. It is not known whether the donor cells that migrated to layers II and III in the heterochronic experiments emitted projections to other cortical areas, as would be expected of normal layer II–III neurons.

The interpretation made of these experiments is that the laminar destination of a neuron is set by local environmental factors in the ventricular zone at the time of last mitosis, just before migration begins, and that the property of laminar destination can be changed by changes in the local environment before the last S phase. It is unknown whether other cell characteristics (e.g., cell type, whether pyramidal or nonpyramidal) were also changed for cells that migrated to unusual locations in the heterochronic experiments.

Study of Mutants Reveals That Laminar Position Per Se Does Not Determine the Phenotype Properties of Cortical Neurons

Genetic mutants with abnormalities of cortical organization provide insight into the factors that determine cortical neuronal phenotypes. The *reeler* mouse exhibits an autosomal recessive mutation, located on chromosome 5, that results in many defects in brain structure, including a systematic inversion of the laminar positions of neuronal cell types in the neocortex, the pyriform cortex, and the hippocampus (Caviness, 1976, 1982; Caviness et al., 1988; Drager, 1981). The *reeler* mutation is most severe in the homologous form; it affects the mechanism of migration of neurons from the neural epithelium to the developing cortex. *Reeler* mice display major disturbances in posture and locomotion and defects in simple behavioral tasks. However, the mutant mice from the strains used experimentally grow and reproduce normally. There is a regular cytoarchitectonic organization of the cortex, with layers inverted: the extrinsic patterns of connectivity are normal (Simmons et al., 1982; Simmons and Pearlman, 1983), the visual field is represented in the usual topographic order in area 17, and many visual cortical neurons have normal receptive field properties (Drager, 1981; Lemmon and Pearlman, 1981; Simmons and Pearlman, 1983). This last finding is remarkable, for the geniculo-cortical fibers penetrate the cortical plate directly after leaving the geniculate and travel to the visual cortex beneath the pia arachnoid, from whence they penetrate the visual cortex and find their appropriate targets, mainly in a layer IV that is somewhat more diffuse than normal.

The defect in *reeler* mouse development occurs in the migration pathway. Neurons are produced in normal sequence, but glial bundle formation is defective (Mikoshiba et al., 1983). Cells cease migration when they encounter the primordial plexiform-subplate layer. Neurons arriving in later waves do not penetrate beyond the first arrivals, the results bring the laminar inversion of the mature *reeler* cortex. One defect appears to be an abnormality in the terminal branching pattern of the radial glial fibers, which do not defasciculate in their transcortical segment in the *reeler* as they do in the normal mouse (Pinto-Lord et al., 1982). Neurons reaching this point retain surface contact with the glial fibers and do not penetrate between those fibers and adjacent postmigratory neurons.

The molecular defect in the *reeler* mutant is the absence of a wild-type gene that encodes for an extracellular protein, reelin, expressed only in fetal and early neonatal life. Antibodies localize this protein in all brain structures that show defective development in *reeler;* in the neocortex it is localized uniquely to the surface of the earliest-generated neurons, the Cajal-Retzius cells (Ogawa et al., 1995; D'Arcangelo et al., 1995; Hirotsune et al., 1995). The protein and perhaps the Cajal-Retzius cells themselves are thus inferred to play important roles in regulating the final critical step in the migration of cortical neurons, the movement by those generated earlier to reach their appropriate position in the sequential inside-to-outside sequence of cortical formation (for review, see Rakic and Caviness, 1995).

Caviness discovered that the cortical neurons in *reeler* mice retain their expected phenotypic characteristics, though they are widely displaced from their normal laminar locations (Caviness et al., 1988). They achieve normal cell morphologies, efferent projections, and afferent inputs to be expected if they had reached their normal laminar locations. For example, the pyramidal cells normally located in layer II/III are positioned in *reeler* mutants in the deepest infragranular layers and send and receive transcallosal axons, as they would be expected to do in their normal layer II/III locations.

Two general conclusions are reached. First, in spite of the remarkably abnormal laminar positions, cortical neurons in *reeler* mutants express phenotypic characters determined intrinsically by their genetic programs and their positions in the temporal sequence of cell production in the neuroepithelium. Second, the success of afferent systems in finding their appropriate targets in the wildly disordered *reeler* cortex suggests that the molecular mechanisms controlling axon-target relations may include cell-type-specific diffusible molecules, as well as families of cell and substrate adhesion molecules.

Secondary Events in Cortical Histogenesis and the Specification of Cortical Areas

Neocortical histogenesis flows continuously through several overlapping phases. After reaching their settle points at the end of migration, cortical neurons differentiate into distinctive phenotypes, develop axons and synaptic terminals linking them with other intrinsic cortical neurons and with neurons in other brain structures, generate molecular transmitter mechanisms for signaling across those synaptic linkages, and synthesize receptor molecules that allow them to respond to signals from other neurons. A gradual change in the density and spatial distribution of membrane channels leads to the electrophysiological properties of mature cortical neurons. The ontogenetic units mature into minicolumns, which later are grouped into columns. Cytoarchitectural areas are specified and the connections within and between them established.

No single factor or process governs the growth of axons into the neocortex or the navigation of the efferent axons of cortical neurons toward their targets. Mechanical constraints, specific membrane-bound molecules in the extracellular matrix, diffusible attractant or repellent molecules produced by target neurons, the interchange of trophic molecules between pre- and postsynaptic cells, and the influence of afferent systems growing into the cortex—all compose a complex system guiding axons to their general target areas. Once neurons reach the target area—when corticothalamic fibers reach a particular nucleus, for example, or thalamocortical fibers reach a particular cortical layer—processes of a different nature come into play in the selection and stabilization of the fine pattern of synaptic relations.

Cooperation and competition between axons for synaptic space on postsynaptic cells are determined by the patterns of activity in them and in the postsynaptic cells. There is some suggestion that this activity-based mechanism may itself depend upon the expression of molecules with both trophic and tropic properties from one or both of the synapsing cells within the microspace of a forming synapse. The degree of selective specificity that obtains in the projections of certain sets of afferents upon local zones of postsynaptic cells suggests that just such a micromolecular mechanism exists. Postmigratory events are more variable than earlier ones, and selection by patterns of activity plays upon that variability to produce the modifiable pattern of microconnectivity of the mature neocortex. The neocortical microstructure in some areas in any individual brain may differ from time to time; modifiability of brain microstructure is fundamental to current theories of learning and memory, and basic for the theory neuronal group selection (Edelman, 1987). This combination of intrinsic (cell-autonomous) and extrinsic factors influencing the specification of areas and connections means that these factors exert their influence over a wide range of times. Timing is particularly variable during the long period of ontogenesis in the primate, in contrast with the temporally compressed ontogenesis in rodents, which extends for several days into the postnatal period.

The events leading from the end of migration to the mature neocortex are major subjects of study in current developmental neurobiology. These center around a number of questions. How are cortical neurons specified by projection type? How do their axons reach their appropriate target structures? How are detailed patterns of synaptic contacts within those structures made, maintained, and modified? Do gap junctions play a role in shaping local neocortical circuits? How are cortical areas specified?

Chemoaffinity Mechanisms Guide the Direction of Axonal Growth

Emerging axonal growth cones of neurons of a developing brain structure enter a permissive extracellular environment composed of a variety of molecules. These molecules provide the cones an adhesive substrate, inducement for axonal extension, and directional signals toward appropriate targets; or, through contact inhibition, they may repel them from other targets (Dodd and Jessell, 1988). Axonal growth cones recognize in the environment some chemotropic molecules bound to cell surfaces; others are encountered in the extracellular matrix; still others are synthesized and released by intermediate and target cells and then diffuse freely for limited distances in the extracellular space. Whether fixed or diffusing, these molecular cues are thought to activate via axonal membrane receptors intracellular mechanisms leading to growth cone extension, or retraction, and axonal branching—perhaps by controlling the polymerization of actin or by modifying the structure of other cytoplasmic proteins within the growth cone (Sheetz et al., 1992), and by regulating the concentration of intracellular Ca^{2+}. It is not known how growth cones detect and react to the spatial gradient of diffusing attractants or repellents, but several examples have been described in submammalian forms—e.g., the retinotectal system in the chick (Baier and Bonhoeffer, 1992)—and in the mammalian spinal cord (Placzek et al., 1990) and pons (Heffner et al., 1990). Several families of proteins have been identified that act to repulse growth cones, such as the semiphorins and netrins. Some members of these families act locally from their transmembrane locations, while others are secreted and may act at a distance after diffusion (Kolodkin, 1996). When the repulsive actions of these proteins are blocked by specific antibodies, axons may grow across a spinal cord transection, in adult rats, and establish functional connections (Bregman et al., 1995). Moreover, in certain systems pioneering axons may provide cues for followers. It is clear that several factors are important in the guidance of central axons to their final synaptic targets, and it is likely that they achieve the final precision characteristic of cortical connectivity by a convergent specification by several variables that change independently with time.

Several classes of adhesive glycoproteins are present on the surfaces of neurons and in the extracellular matrix (ECM) of the nervous system. Among them are three large families: the immunoglobulins, the cadherins, and the integrins. Each family includes some cell adhesion molecules (CAMs) that are widely distributed in nervous systems and others that are more specific for certain structures or cell populations. The most widely distributed member of the immunoglobulin family is a large glycoprotein, N-CAM, which is present on the surfaces of neurons from the time of induction; it links neurons together in a homophilic, non-Ca^{2+}-dependent manner (Edelman, 1983, 1984; Edelman et al., 1985). The N-CAM on axonal surfaces is highly sialylated during the period of axonal growth, and the arrival of the growth cone in the local target regions is correlated with the selective elimination of some sialic acid residues, after which the N-CAM molecule is more adhesive. The highly sialylated form of N-CAM promotes both neurite adhesion and growth; the latter is thought to depend upon linkage to the fibroblast factor receptor and a second-messenger pathway leading to increased intracellular Ca^{2+}. The removal of sialic acid residues increases N-CAM stickiness and decreases its growth promotion (Doherty and Walsh, 1994).

Unlike N-CAM, the ten identified members of the cadherin family of cell adhesion molecules derive from different genes. N-cadherin is present on most neurons and links cell-to-cell surfaces in a homophilic Ca^{2+}-dependent manner. Integrins are expressed on axonal cone membranes and mediate the adherence of neurons to the glycoproteins of the ECM, such as laminin, and may change their ligand-binding properties at different stages of development. Axon growth cones may react adaptively to differences in the molecular environment as they grow from origins to targets.

Many experiments in mammals support the chemoaffinity idea, especially those in which explants of fetal or neonatal neocortex and dorsal thalamus are cultured adjacent to but not touching one another, in serum-free media. Thalamocortical axons grow out from a thalamic explant containing, e.g., the premature lateral geniculate nucleus, and they invade an adjacent explant of visual cortex. If the latter is immature (P0), the thalamocortical fibers grow through the cortex to the pial surface. If the cortical explant is more mature (P6/7), the invading thalamocortical fibers encounter a stop signal in their major natural target, layer IV, arborize, and make functional synaptic contacts with cortical neurons (Bolz et al., 1992; Yamamoto et al., 1989; Blakemore and Molnar, 1990; Molnar and Blakemore, 1991; Lotto and Price, 1995). This ingrowth is specific as regards the vertical dimension of the cortex, but unspecific in the tangential dimension. Outgrowing fibers from a posterior thalamic explant will invade an adjacent explant taken from any area of the neocortex, or even from the hippocampus—but not one from the cerebellum (Blakemore and Molnar, 1990). The *efferent* axons of neurons growing out from a neocortical explant display the layer-specific target preferences typical of normal neocortex *in vivo* (Novak and Bolz, 1993; Yamamoto et al., 1992).

Efferent axons of cortical neurons are attracted to their targets over

Secondary Events in Cortical Histogenesis

the final short range by target-generated diffusible factors. Efferent axons of layer V pyramidal cells in the rat project initially to the spinal cord, bypassing one of their subcortical targets in the basal pons. Collaterals later emerge from those axons, not from growth cones, to innervate that pontine target. O'Leary et al. (1990) used *in vitro* co-culture experiments to show that explants of the pons attracted the descending axons and initiated the collateral branching from the sides of those axons. Time-lapse microscopy revealed that the frequency of branch formation was greatly increased and that some of those branches reached the pontine target and were stabilized; cortical co-cultures with nontarget structures did not elicit these events (Sato et al., 1994). The diffusible factor has not been identified. It is unlikely that single diffusible target-cue molecules exist that are unique for each system and each of its targets. The remarkable target accuracy of the developing brain is achieved by a regulation in time and space of many factors (Korsching, 1993). Although diffusible molecular attractants are necessary, they are not sufficient to account for the specific patterns of connectivity in the mature neocortex (Jones, 1990b).

The Role of Neurotrophins in the Maturation of the Synaptic Microstructure

A major idea in developmental neurobiology is that the number of neurons innervating a particular target is determined by a signal from that target itself. What that factor is was discovered in a series of experiments carried out by Bueker, Levi-Montalcini, Hamburger, and Cohen, then working at Washington University in St. Louis (Levi-Montalcini, 1987; Loughlin and Fallon, 1993; Korsching, 1993). They identified a neurotrophic agent, nerve growth factor (NGF), elaborated by target cells innervated by sympathetic efferent neurons. NGF exerts a powerful sustaining effect in regulating the survival of those preganglionic efferents during development and in mature life. Antisera to NGF destroy all para- and prevertebral sympathetic neurons, producing an "immunosympathectomy." NGF also sustains these neurons in dissociated cell cultures. A general neurotrophic hypothesis evolved from this work and much that followed it, that the number of neurons in the nervous system and their continuing capacity to innervate their targets is determined by trophic factors produced by target tissues, which support the viability of innervating neurons and for which those neurons compete. Those winning survive; those losing die. NGF also promotes the outgrowth of axons and dendrites and the initiation of transmitter synthesis, actions not commonly regarded as neurotrophic. The original neurotrophic idea has come to include neurotropic effects as well.

NGF-sensitive neurons are limited in the mature brain to the derivatives of the neural crest, the autonomic efferents and the dorsal root ganglion cells, and to one set of central neurons, the cholinergic cells of the basal forebrain that project upon the cortex. During ontogenesis NGF is expressed in many cortical neurons, including those of the cortex, and its receptor is localized to neurons of the subplate (Allendoerfer et al., 1990). Five neurotrophic proteins have been identified in the brain, together with their relevant postsynaptic receptors (Anderson et al., 1995): NGF, brain-derived neurotrophin factor (BDNF) (Hohn et al., 1990), neurotrophins-3, -4/5, and -6 (NT-3, NT-4/5, and NT-6). These five are short basic proteins (110 amino acid residues) with about 50 percent sequence identity between them. They are among the most strictly conserved proteins in mammalian evolution, for those from rat, pig, and human are identical. The receptors for the neurotrophins are the *trk* family of protein kinases, *trk*A for NGF, *trk*B for BDNF, and *trk*C for NT-3. Receptor activation initiates second-messenger events that lead to an increase in intracellular Ca^{2+} and to gene expression. Receptors *trk*B and *trk*C are widely distributed throughout the brain and are thought to be expressed on the majority of CNS neurons. The equally widespread distribution of their ligands predicts an almost universal action of neurotrophins in the CNS. The production of BDNF depends upon neuronal activity, being increased by non-NMDA receptor activation and decreased by GABA action. NT-3 is expressed in central neurons that project to muscle and in afferents from muscle; its CNS distribution is limited to the hippocampus and the cerebellum.

It is not clear how neurotrophins act to promote and maintain the detailed synaptic patterns in cortical networks. Several recent observations suggest that when axons approach a candidate neuronal target they open a short time window of neurotrophin release, during which they must make synaptic contacts or die (Davies, 1994). This fits with the observation that the selective axonal pruning described in a following section is neurotrophin-dependent.

McAllister et al. (1995) measured dendritic growth in different layers of short-term organotypic slice cultures of developing ferret visual cortex and exposed each culture to a neurotrophin for 36 hours. Many neuron dendritic trees were then visualized, reconstructed, and compared with untreated controls. The results indicated that the basal dendrites in each cortical layer responded most strongly with elaboration of their arbors to a single neurotrophin; e.g., basilar dendritic trees were elicited in layer IV to BDNF, those in layers V and VI to NT-4. Apical dendrites, by contrast, appeared to respond indiscriminately to more than one neurotrophin. These findings suggest a differential distribution of different neurotrophin receptors in different parts of the dendritic tree. It is obvious that experiments of this sort mark the beginning of a surge of knowledge of what role neurotrophins—and perhaps other proteins as well—play in synapse formation and stabilization in the neocortex.

Local Synaptogenesis and the Role of Activity in Refining the Synaptic Microstructure

After sets of axons afferent to the cortex are guided correctly in pathway and target selection, they face the major problems of local synaptogenesis upon the appropriate zones of the correct target neurons; the stabilization of those connections; and the refinement of what are in many cases initially divergent distributions of terminal branches. The stability of these initial synaptic contacts and their refinement depends in part upon activity-dependent competition between axons aimed at common postsynaptic neurons. It appears likely that it is the phase relation between pre- and postsynaptic input that is important, rather than the level of activity per se. Initial synaptic contacts are strengthened when pre- and postsynaptic elements are active concurrently, weakened when they are not. This selection and stabilization of synapses at cortical neurons by phase-related pre- and postsynaptic activity is achieved by the mechanisms responsible for the activity-dependent changes in synaptic transmission, long-term potentiation and depression, described in Chapter 6. These NMDA-mediated changes are also thought to be the basis of the plasticity at cortical synapses during the early, critical period of cortical development. This plasticity—the capacity for change in the local microstructure of the cortex—persists in the mature cortex.

The segregation of geniculate axons into eye-specific ocular-dominance columns in the visual cortex is an example of activity-dependent competition between sets of axons for neuronal target space

(Stryker et al., 1990). Cabelli et al. (1995) have shown that the infusion of BDNF or NT-4/5 into the visual cortex prevents the formation of ocular-dominance columns in the infused area. The excess of neurotrophins is thought to remove the competitive basis upon which the formation of the columns depends. It is important to emphasize, however, that the extreme dependence upon afferent activity in maintaining intra-area specializations, like the ocular-dominance columns, may be unique to the visual system. Henderson et al. (1992) have shown that the specialized intra-areal structures in the trigeminal component of the somatic sensory cortex in the rat develop unperturbed when afferent activity in the system is silenced from the day of birth. Moreover, Chiaia et al. (1992) found that postnatal blockage of cortical activity with tetrodotoxin did not alter the development of intra-areal specializations in the cat's somatic sensory cortex related to the pattern of representation of the vibrissae.

The problem includes both the stabilization of single pre- to postsynaptic synapses and the mechanism operating during competition between adjacent presynaptic axons synapsing upon the same cell. Stent (1973) postulated on theoretical grounds that when a presynaptic axon (A) continually fails to excite a postsynaptic cell that is discharging under the presynaptic input from another axon or axons (the competitors of A), changes occur that render the effect of impulses in A less and less effective—A is the loser in the competition for synaptic space on the postsynaptic cell. Evidence has accumulated for the neuromuscular junction that what occurs is a loss of receptor molecules beneath the synaptic site of A (Lichtmann and Balice-Gordon, 1990). Whether this same mechanism is operative between competing presynaptic axons in the cerebral cortex is unknown.

This idea is almost universally, and I believe in part erroneously, attributed to the psychologist Donald Hebb, who elaborated it in his monograph of 1949 (Hebb, 1949). The requirement for near-synchronous activity in pre- and postsynaptic elements was the major idea behind decades of work by comparative neuroanatomists who sought to understand how synapsing neural elements are linked in ontogeny and how they move toward one another in an evolutionary series. The idea is described in detail by Ariens-Kappers in his monograph with Huber and Crosby of 1936 (Ariens-Kappers, Huber, and Crosby, 1936, pp. 73–94). Ariens-Kappers's central idea was that the relationships which determine connections are "synchronic or immediately successive functional activities," that synapses may form *de novo* as the result of selective association, and that changes in transmission result from the use or disuse of preexisting synapses.

The fundamental law of neurobiotaxis is that the temporal correlation of activity plays an essential role in establishing synaptic contacts during brain development. This differs qualitatively from the neurotrophic idea originated by Cajal. Cajal believed that the connections between neural elements are determined by the secretion of attractant and repellent substances and by the sensitivity of nerve cells to such substances. As it turned out, both Cajal and Ariens-Kappers were right!

Even though synchronous activity is necessary for the final maturation of synapses, it is not sufficient. Activity undoubtedly initiates a series of molecular events that complete the ultrastructural entities we recognize as synapses. These must include gene expression and protein synthesis to complete the membrane specializations of synapses, the formation of postsynaptic spines, the intramembranous movement and/or local synthesis of postsynaptic receptor channels, and the concentration of other large molecules in the subsynaptic regions.

At least in some systems this last series of events in synaptic stabilization is signaled by the expression of large proteoglycan molecules in the extracellular matrix (Hockfield et al., 1990; McKay and Hockfield, 1982). A monoclonal antibody, Cat-301, recognizes an antigen that appears on the surfaces of neurons at the last stage of the critical period. It is largely, but not completely, restricted to the motion components of the visual pathway, from the lateral geniculate to the prestriate visual areas (DeYoe et al., 1990; Hendry et al., 1984b; Hockfield and Sur, 1990; Hockfield et al., 1983). This large molecule is part of the extracellular matrix and appears on neuronal cell surfaces, but it does not contain a transmembrane spanning domain. It is thought to contribute to the final synaptic stabilization, but direct evidence that this is so is not available. It appears just at the end of the critical period, as plasticity is declining, and is regulated by neuronal activity. The inference is that in other systems equally specific extracellular matrix molecules may play similar roles in the final stabilization of synapses.

A great deal has been learned about these processes of selection and stabilization at peripheral synapses by studies of the neuromuscular junction (Changeux and Danchin, 1976), which serves as a model for study of synapse formation in the cerebral cortex. As presynaptic growth cones of motoneurons approach myotubes, they synthesize the transmitter-releasing machinery before contact is made, and transmitter is released both spontaneously and by nerve impulses (Haydon and Drapeau, 1995). Contact of a growth cone with the surface of the muscle cell initiates within seconds clustering of AChRs at the contact point, by intramembranous migration of receptor molecules and, perhaps on a longer time scale, an increase in receptor synthesis at the subsynaptic site and a decrease in extrasynaptic regions. A number of regulatory proteins play roles in synaptogenesis at the neuromuscular junction, including calcitonin-gene-related peptide, fibroblast growth factor, ARIA (Fischbach and Rosen, 1997), and agrin (McMahon, 1990; Bowe and Fallon, 1995). Agrin is synthesized in the motoneurons and transported via their axons to muscle cells, where it binds together synaptic basic lamina and appears to mediate the nerve-induced aggregations of large molecules that compose the postsynaptic apparatus, particularly the aggregation of ACh receptors. Agrin is expressed in many regions of the brain, but whether it or other proteins play a similar role in cortical synaptogenesis is unknown.

Projection and intrinsic cortical neurons develop more or less in tandem through the steps from proliferation, migration, and initial differentiation. The sequence proceeds as the layers of the cortex are formed, from layer VI to layer II. However, the pyramidal cells appear in many cases to differentiate more rapidly than do the intrinsic neurons, leading in the generation of neurites and achieving synaptic effectiveness through mechanisms described above. It is observed in slice experiments, e.g., that EPSPs can be recorded in developing cortex at a time when no IPSPs can be evoked, evidence that the intracortical inhibitory interneurons have not at that time achieved synaptic stabilization.

Subplate Neurons and Neocortical Innervation

A transient structure of the telencephalon, the subplate, is important for the guidance of axon systems to and from the neocortex, and it is thought that a subplate mechanism assures the areal specificity of the corticipetal projections. The neurons of the subplate are generated, simultaneously with those of the marginal layer, from the primitive plexiform layer, and they are among the first postmitotic neurons to appear in the incipient cerebral cortex. The subplate of the neonatal human cortex varies in thickness from 4 mm beneath the postcentral somatic sensory cortex to 1 mm beneath the visual cortex, everywhere separated by a thin line from the overlying cortical plate, and later from layer VI. Contrary to earlier belief, cell death in the subplate is no greater than elsewhere in the cortex (Valverde et al., 1995). The surviving subplate neurons are interstitial cells in the white matter beneath the mature neocortex (Chun and Shatz, 1989; Kostovic and Rakic, 1980). Subplate cells differentiate rapidly to achieve the ultrastructural characteristics and biochemical markers of mature nerve cells, enabling them to receive mature, asymmetrical synaptic contacts. Early in subplate history, many of these synaptic endings are monoaminergic and derive from the central core systems (Molliver, 1987); however, among the earliest afferents to reach the subplate are specific thalamocortical afferents (DeCarlos and O'Leary, 1992). Electrophysiological studies in slices of immediately postnatal rodent brains reveal that subplate neurons respond to afferent volleys with local EPSPs; no IPSPs were observed (Shatz, 1990; Friauf et al., 1990; Friauf and Shatz, 1991), although GABAergic neurons are plentiful in the subplate at this time.

It was suggested by Shatz that subplate neurons may function as "pioneers," marking out by their trajectories pathways followed later by the axons of thalamic and neocortical cells (Calloway and Katz, 1992; Ghosh and Shatz, 1992; Shatz and Luskin, 1986; McConnell et al., 1989; for reviews, see Shatz et al., 1988, and Allendoerfer and Shatz, 1994). Axons of the lateral geniculate neurons, for example, grow into and innervate synaptically neurons of the subplate before migration of neurons to the overlying visual cortex is complete, and only later (after a "waiting period") resume growth into the visual cortex, following a pathway established between subplate neurons and layer IV (Ghosh et al., 1990). Other subplate axons project through the internal capsule to the dorsal thalamus, but not to other subcortical structures or to the contralateral hemisphere. It has been proposed that these descending subplate axons function as guidance pathways over which the reciprocal sets of fibers linking thalamus and cortex project (Shatz et al., 1988, 1990; Kim et al., 1991; DeCarlos and O'Leary, 1992). However, a study by Birknese et al. (1994) indicates that early efferent and afferent axons leaving or approaching the developing cortex follow paths adjacent to but distinctly separate from each other and from the subplate efferents. The afferent pathway is enriched by chondroitin sulfate proteoglycans in the extracellular matrix, that of the efferent is not.

It is an attractive hypothesis that position-specified molecular cues are present in the subplate and control the accurate, area-specific projections of dorsal thalamic nuclei upon the cerebral cortex. If the region of subplate beneath a particular cortical area is lesioned, thalamocortical axons make their way toward the correct tangential position, but may pass it by. They do not invade their natural target, the intact cortical area above the lesioned subplate (Ghosh et al., 1990). The presence of area-specific marker cues in the subplate infers that subplate cells maintain their neighbor relations in the x-y dimension throughout development. Moreover, if the hypothesis that different molecular markers are specific for local regions of the subplate is correct, it suggests that local subplate regions are specified in relation to specific cortical areas early in neurogenesis within the neuroepithelium, independently of any afferent influence. This fits with Rakic's hypothesis that a protomap of the cortex exists in the neuroepithelium and is transmitted to the developing cortical plate via the subplate. The identities of the relevant molecular markers are unknown, although a number are under study, including chondroitin sulfate proteoglycans, extracellular matrix proteoglycans, etc. (O'Leary et al., 1994). Following a lesion of the subplate, the maturation of the overlying cortex is arrested. Nothing is known of this more general sustaining function.

Progressive and Regressive Phenomena in Cortical Development

It is a general and widely confirmed observation that a large proportion of the neurons produced in a developing nervous system do not survive to maturity. Overproduction of both neurons and synapses has been observed in many areas of the mammalian brain, including the neocortex (Cowan et al., 1985; Ferrer et al., 1992; Oppenheim, 1991; Hamburger and Oppenheim, 1982). Cell loss usually occurs when a population of neurons begins to make connections to its target field, or to receive afferents from its sources. The percentage loss appears to be somewhat less (15–30 prcent) in the neocortex than in other structures, and it is not known whether cell death is selective for neuron phenotype, cortical layer, or area. The question is further complicated by the recent observation that about 50 percent of cells in the ventricular zone die, as do a similar ratio in the upper cortical layers (Blaschke et al., 1996). This new discovery raises some doubts concerning the validity of lineage studies that have yet to be resolved. Some evidence has been presented to support the idea of a regional difference in the degree of cell death in the hamster neocortex (Finlay, 1992), and the matter must be left for further study.

There are two phases or modes of neuronal death. The first and smaller pattern is of cells that die soon after they are produced by asymmetric division and before they emit axons or dendrites. These cells appear to be destined for death by a genetic program regardless of other factors; this form of cell death is called apoptosis. Nothing is known of the function of these cells during their short lives. The second, and much larger, phase of cell death extends through the "critical" period of cortical development, a period of maximal susceptibility of the cortex to plastic change, largely through a competitive interaction between axons for synaptic space on target cells. The usual explanation is that target cells produce only a limited amount of sustaining neurotrophins, and that axons failing to make adequate connections die for lack of those substances. The production of neurotrophins is thought to be under the control of afferent neuronal activity, and some recent evidence suggests that presynaptic as well as postsynaptic factors may be important in determining survival or death (Linden, 1994).

Rakic and his colleagues counted the number of synapses per unit area of neuropil in electronmicrographs, in the motor, somatic sensory, visual, and frontal homotypical cortex (area 46) in monkeys' brains that varied in age from E80 to old age, about 20 years in the macaque (Bourgeois et al., 1994; Bourgeois and Rakic, 1993; Zecevic et al., 1989; Zecevic and Rakic, 1991). Synaptogenesis begins during migration, rises exponentially at about the time of birth, and declines to 60–70 percent of that maximum at the time of puberty—3 years in the macaque. A slower decline then persists throughout life, and may amount in the end to a further significant loss. The time course of synaptogenesis is virtually the same in the four areas studied. The loss of synapses is much greater in the supra- than in the infragranular layers, and much greater for the asymmetric synapses on dendritic spines (80 percent of those lost) than for synapses on dendritic shafts or cell somata. Synapses made on shafts appear to accumulate slowly until a steady state is reached that is maintained throughout life.

The cycle of overproduction of cells and synapses and their subsequent decline provides a degree of variability in the formation of the microstructure of the neocortex. As a result, the precise pattern of synaptic relations, at least for that on pyramidal cells, is open to modification by afferent input and perhaps by other factors not yet identified, such as hormonal levels. Moreover, this susceptibility to modification by afferent input continues throughout life, though to a lesser degree than in the critical period, and is a necessary postulate for present ideas of the action of distributed systems and the role they are thought to play in the higher functions of the brain.

There is thus an activity-dependent regulation of neuron number and interneuronal connectivity in the developing cortex. This opens the possibility that this variability is operated upon in a selective way, and may be important for evolutionary changes in the cortex—providing a mechanism for adaptation to genetic mutations that produce change in the genesis of the cortex itself or in the afferent systems that play upon it.

The Specification of Axonal Projections by Selective Collateral Elimination

Studies of the callosal and spinal axonal projections of cortical neurons reveal that a significant reorganization of those patterns occurs early in the neonatal period. Initially exuberant and frequently widespread projections of axonal collaterals in the rat are narrowed to the pattern of the mature brain by pruning of inappropriate collaterals. This discovery was made by Innocenti and his colleagues (Innocenti et al., 1977; Innocenti and Caminiti, 1980; Caminiti and Innocenti, 1981), and has since been studied by O'Leary, Stanfield, and others (for review, see O'Leary and Koester, 1993; O'Leary et al., 1990). In these experiments, cortical neurons are labeled early in the neonatal period by the retrograde axoplasmic transport of fluorescent dyes injected into regions of axon terminations. The dyes persist for many weeks in the cell bodies. Cortical neurons labeled by injections into their transient neonatal projection targets do not possess those projections when tested again later in development by injection of a second dye into the same target zone. The loss of collaterals is not due, or not due wholly, to cell death, for many neurons containing the first dye persist in the mature cortex and sustain other projections to appropriate targets.

The exuberant distribution of axonal collaterals by cortical projection neurons is not randomly distributed in the brain space. Cortical neurons with descending connections, for example, generate many more collaterals to subcortical targets than they will retain, including those that persist to the appropriate structure, but they generate none to the contralateral hemisphere. Likewise, the transcallosal systems undergo radical pruning of their original projections but send no collaterals to the spinal cord. The two sets of targets to which these two sets of efferent axons project initially are separate, but they include for each what will eventually be the appropriate targets.

The neurons of origin of the callosal fibers in the somatic sensory cortex of the monkey are initially uniformly distributed in the *x-y* dimension of the area, but are reorganized during development by axonal pruning to the disjunctive pattern of the mature cortex, in which the areas where the face and apices of the limbs are represented are relatively free of contralateral projections (Chalupa and Killacky, 1989).

Pruning is not universal in all cortical axonal projections. Thalamocortical projections to the barrel cortex of rodents, for example, are precise and topographic from the start. Vertical interlaminar connections within the cortex are generally precise in their mature form from the initial outgrowth of their axons (Burkhalter et al., 1989; Callaway and Katz, 1992; Katz and Callaway, 1992; Lund et al., 1977). Both inhibitory and excitatory interneurons emit their axonal trees in mature form and do not depend upon a later pruning for refinement. This is true also for the intrinsic vertically directed collaterals of the pyramidal cells, whose main stem axons leave the cortex for distant targets, make diffuse distributions there, and are subject to collateral pruning. The intrinsic projections of these same neurons that link cells in different layers are specific from the start; an example is the projection of layer II/III pyramidal cells to layer V. These same pyramidal cells also emit horizontally directed collaterals that project within the cortex. This set of collaterals reaches its mature form of a carefully structured, intermittently patchy distribution only after a long period of axonal pruning. It appears that the cortical neurons may emit some sets of axonal collaterals that are specific and mature from the start, others that are refined by pruning.

How inappropriate axonal projections are eliminated is unknown. Analogy with projection phenomena in segmental structures and in submammalian forms suggests that the target structures synthesize and release attractant and sustaining molecules for which the appropriate axonal growth cones possess membrane receptors. Such a

mechanism has been demonstrated for the cortico-pontine projection, although the attractant/sustaining molecules have not yet been
identified (Heffner et al., 1990; Sato et al., 1994). It is important to
emphasize that axonal exuberance and later pruning is a much more
subdued phenomenon in the development of the primate brain than
it is in that of the rodent.

Koester and O'Leary (1993) have used the phenomenon of axonal
pruning in a study of phenotype specification. In rodents, though
not in primates, layer V contains two sets of projection neurons,
corticospinal and transcallosal. These authors demonstrated the absolute separation of these two classes; neither ever emits even transient axonal projections into the domain of the other, although
within its domain each emits processes later eliminated, as well as the
appropriate ones to the correct target. The two sets of neurons are
generated virtually simultaneously within the neuroepithelium, as
predicted by their common laminar destination. The conclusion
drawn is that the two types of projection neurons are phenotypes
with distinct lineages set by cell-autonomous mechanisms within the
neuroepithelium. Phenotype distinctions are made before migration,
independently of the influence of corticipetal afferents or of any activity-dependent mechanism.

It is obvious that much has yet to be learned about how sets of
axons find their correct pathways and general target regions in the
brain, although there is little doubt that guidance depends upon the
recognition and selection of specific sets of molecular cues. A major
problem is how these axons, having reached the target region, make
correct and detailed synaptic impingements upon target neurons,
connections that are in many cases remarkably specific as regards
both the neuronal phenotype selected and the region of the neuron
upon which synaptic contacts are made.

Do Gap Junctions Play a Role in Specifying Local Cortical Circuits?

Gap junctions are ubiquitous channels of communication between
cells in many tissues, including the nervous systems of invertebrates
(Bennett et al., 1991). Attempts to demonstrate these junctions in
the adult mammalian neocortex by electron microscopy produced
equivocal results; when seen at all they were very small. Gutnick and
Prince (1981) demonstrated such couplings between neocortical neu-

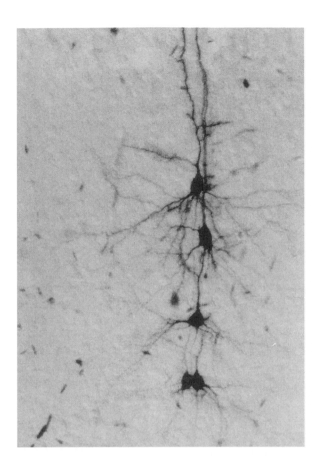

Fig. 9-1 A small group of neurons in the upper layers of rat neocortex are shown to be coupled through gap junctions by injection of neurobiotin into one cell, postnatal day P12. There is strong coupling between neurons in the vertical direction, little tangentially. This type of coupling is not seen in the adult cortex. Such assemblies of coupled neurons, which may be members of the ontogenetic unit of Rakic, are presumed to function together in the adult cortex. (From Peinado et al., 1993a.)

rons in the slice preparation by the intracellular iontophoresis of the fluorescent dye, lucifer yellow. Gap junctions are common in the immature rodent neocortex, as shown by intracellular iontophoresis of smaller tracer molecules such as neurobiotin. These preparations (Figs. 9-1 and 9-2) document the fact that early in development any single pyramidal cell is coupled with many others (Peinado et al., 1993a,b; Connors et al., 1983). Several important observations were made in these experiments: (1) gap junctions occur between dendrites; (2) pyramidal cells appear to couple only with other pyramidal cells, nonpyramidal with nonpyramidal; (3) couplings occur preferentially between neurons located in vertical arrays extending across the cortical laminae; (4) the couplings were common during the early postnatal period, days 5–12, but were not observed in these experiments after day 17.

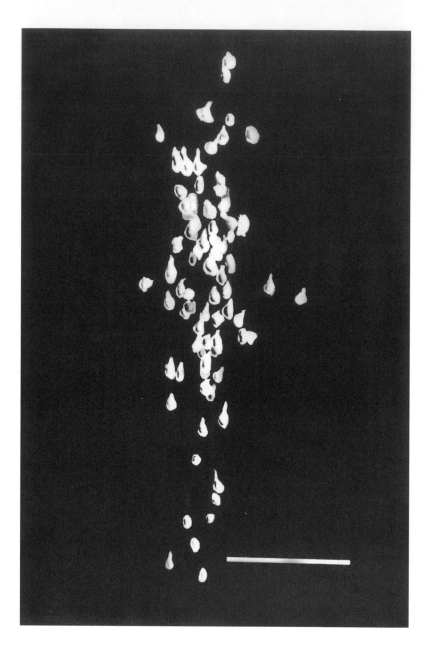

Fig. 9-2   A reconstruction of a set of cortical neurons shown to be coupled through gap junctions by intracellular injection of neurobiotin into one cell in the rat neocortex, postnatal day P5. There is a strong preferential distribution of the labeled cells in the vertical dimensions. (From Peinado et al., 1993a.)

What role gap-junction coupling plays in the neocortex during its early development is not known, nor whether such couplings promote the linking of neurons into local, vertically oriented circuits. Peinado et al. (1993a) suggested that when axons capture a single neuron they may, through coupling, capture a cluster. Gap junctions between neurons in the developing cortex allow direct diffusion of second-messenger molecules between cells. Thus, although much uncertainty remains, it appears likely that gap junctions serve as one means of signaling between neurons during development, and that they may contribute to the vertical linking of neurons across the layers in the mature cortex.

The Specification of Areas of the Neocortex

There is no more spectacular transition in cerebral ontogenesis than the chain of overlapping events that leads from a uniform expanse of virtually identical ontogenetic units to the mature neocortex composed of cytoarchitecturally specified areas. A general consensus has arisen that what is to be defined as a cortical area depends upon the combination of a unique cytoarchitecture with a set of dynamic functional properties of the neurons of the area, with a specific and often unique pattern of extrinsic connections, with a spectrum of biochemical markers, and with a set of characteristic and often localizing behavioral abnormalities after lesion. A cortical area can rarely be specified exactly by only one of these; almost always a precise definition depends upon the convergence of several. Given this complexity, it is no surprise that the specification of a cortical area in development depends upon a balanced cadence between interactions in time of genetic and "epigenetic" influences, or that the sequence of events varies the weighing of these two influences. This is particularly clear between the altricial and precocial status of cortical maturation at the time of birth—e.g., between rodents and primates. Certain more general aspects of the neocortex are relevant to the present discussion.

One major idea is that neurons produced in different zones of the neuroepithelium are specified to occupy certain areas of the neocortex and not others; i.e., that a predictive map of the neocortex exists within the neuroepithelium before migration begins. Areal specification and border definitions made in the mature neocortex are also influenced in a major way by events during and after the migratory phase, particularly by the ingrowth of cortical afferents. This is the *protomap hypothesis* of Rakic, discussed above, for which he has recently produced new evidence from experiments in primates (Rakic, 1995a,b). Other investigators propose that the neuroblasts of the neuroepithelium are not marked for a particular area, and that neocortical areas are specified only by a sequence of events imposed after the migratory period (O'Leary, 1989). Evidence adduced to support this idea is drawn almost exclusively from study of markedly altricial mammals, particularly rodents.

An Overlapping Sequence of "Intrinsic" and "Extrinsic" Factors Specify Cortical Areas

Since all cells in a given organism have the same genomic capacity, the problem of development is to discover the temporal sequence in which different genes are expressed and the mechanisms that control those expressions. It is obvious that early in development the timetable may be controlled by factors intrinsic to the cell, and it is just as obvious that there may then follow a gradual, overlapping transition during further development from the purely intrinsic to a stage of mixed control, and perhaps finally to one in which gene expression is dominated by extracellular events, such as afferent innervation and the patterns of impulse activity in those afferents to the cortex. These general ideas are developed fully in important reviews by Kennedy and DeHay (1993a,b, 1997), who define as *intrinsic* those constraints on gene expression a cell inherits stepwise from its ancestors, which constraints at that earlier time may themselves have been extrinsic, and *extrinsic* as the pattern of gene expression in a cell determined by signals from its environment. These authors emphasize that the separation between intrinsic and extrinsic refers to the time in the course of ontogenesis that the environmental stimulus to gene expression occurs. This temporal sequence varies greatly among mammals, and particularly between the two most commonly used in developmental studies, the precocial monkey and the altricial rodent.

Areal Specification within the Neuroepithelium

Kennedy, DeHay, and their colleagues (DeHay et al., 1993) have used pulse injections of ^{3}H-thymidine to show that the rate of neuron production in the zone of the neuroepithelium producing area 17 is more than twice that in the adjacent zone producing area 18. This difference produces a clear gradient, but not a sharp boundary between the two germinal zones, suggesting that the sharp boundary between 17 and 18 in the mature cortex is produced by extrinsic factors. Such a high rate of neurogenesis in area 17's germinal zone is achieved by a shortening of the cell cycle, particularly of its G-1 phase, a process greatly accelerated toward the end of neurogenesis. Moreover, the precursors of the area 17 zone of the neuroepithelium taken from the monkey at embryonic days E74–E80 and maintained in isolated cell culture continue to show higher rates of proliferation than do cells taken from the area 18 zone (Kennedy et al., 1995). The inference is clear: a regional specialization in the germinal epithelium specifies to a considerable degree a discrete cytoarchitectural area of the mature cortex (DeHay et al., 1991, 1993).

Molecular Specifications in the Germinal Epithelium

Convincing proof of the protomap hypothesis would be the discovery of discrete molecular markers outlining zones of the neuroepithelium, one for each of the topographically related cortical areas generated by each zone. That evidence is not available, but several neuroepithelial molecular markers have been described that label selectively regions rather than single areas of the cortex. Limbic areas are marked throughout by a membrane-associated protein (LAMP) (Levitt, 1984; Barbe and Levitt, 1991; Horton and Levitt, 1988), but this molecule does not label single areas of limbic cortex differentially. A comparable example for the neocortex is the discovery of Arimatsu et al. (1992) that a monoclonal antibody labels a group of primary and secondary sensory areas in the lateral neocortex of the rat. The antigen was not expressed until P6, but it was shown to recognize cells in tissue culture prepared from the lateral neocortex at E12. A molecular specification occurred within the neuroepithelium well before the invasion of the developing cortex by thalamocortical fibers. The specification is regional, of a group rather than of a single cytoarchitectural area (for a review, see Levitt et al., 1997).

More restricted labeling has been revealed by the transgene experiment of Cohen-Tannaoudji et al. (1994). They used the reporter gene *lacZ* to show that the transgene expression was confined to the representation of the body form in the somatic sensory cortex of the rat.

Grafts from visual to somatic sensory cortex did not show the transgene expression, illustrating that a molecular specification can be limited to a single cortical area.

I have described in an earlier section the hypothesis that molecular markers specific for local regions of the subplate are specified in relation to the local region of the developing cortical plate just above, and that they function as attractants for ingrowing thalamocortical fibers. This hypothesis awaits further direct evidence.

Finally, a number of studies indicate that the expression of putatively regulatory genes occurs in restricted regions of the forebrain. These are treated in the context of a neuromeric or prosomeric model of forebrain segmentation, but until now there is no direct evidence that the neuromeric model can be extended to include the neocortex (Puelles and Rubenstein, 1993; Bulfone et al., 1993; Rubenstein et al., 1994).

Afferent Control of the Sizes of Cortical Areas

It has been known for more than a century that in the brains of humans born without retinae there is a marked reduction in the sizes of both the lateral geniculate nucleus and the striate cortex. The reduced striate cortex is of normal thickness and vertical cell count and shows a normal laminar and cytoarchitectural organization. Haberland and Perou (1969) have studied such brains more recently and observed these reductions, as well as a novel transitional cortex at the border of the reduced area 17. Somewhat comparable experiments have been made in monkeys in the laboratories of Rakic and Kennedy, by bilateral enucleation at various times during gestation (Rakic, 1988a; Rakic et al., 1991; Williams et al., 1987; DeHay et al., 1991, 1989, 1996; for reviews see Rakic, 1991; Kennedy and DeHay, 1993a,b, 1997). Results comparable to those in humans were obtained if the enucleations were made at E70 or earlier in neurogenesis, before layer IV is formed. Early enucleations produced no change in the overall dimensions of the neocortex, but the geniculate and striate cortex were reduced in size by more than 50 percent. In the monkey, as in the human, the laminar and cytoarchitectural organization of the reduced area 17 appeared to be normal. A transitional cortex was identified at the anterior border of area 17, and sometimes also in isolated islands within the confines of the reduced area 17. This intervening cortex has a cellular organization different from that of either area 17 behind or area 18 in front, but it does not fully compensate for the decreased size of area 17. How this influence from the retina regulates the number of neurons within and the size of area 17 is still uncertain.

These results indicate that afferents from the retina exert a powerful control upon the overall size of their cortical target, area 17, but cytoarchitectural maturation of the cortex proceeds in apparently normal fashion in the absence of specific input over the relevant pathway. However, it should be recalled that the retinal are not the only afferents to the lateral geniculate nucleus, and the possibility that the central core systems play a role should be investigated.

The Rodent Model and the Peripheral Blueprint

There is little doubt that thalamic afferents exert a powerful regulatory influence upon cortical development; this is particularly obvious in the markedly altricial rodent. On the basis of studies in this animal, O'Leary and his colleagues presented the hypothesis that the neuroepithelium generates uniform lineages across its full extent, without any areal specification, and that specification of cytoarchitecturally defined areas after completion of migration is determined by subsequent events, particularly by the invasion of the cortex by thalamocortical afferents (O'Leary, 1989; O'Leary et al., 1992, 1994). This hypothesis includes the idea that many features forming the basis of areal differentiations emerge in a "protocortex," long after the conclusion of neurogenesis and migration, through such extrinsic processes as the invasion of this *tabula rasa* cortex by thalamocortical afferents.

This hypothesis has been tested in a series of cortical transplantation experiments in rodents. The usual protocol is to transplant a small piece of cortex (about 1×1 mm) from an E17 rodent embryo into a small cavity made in a recipient, host zone in a neonatal rodent; a transplant may be made, e.g., from the area of the future visual cortex to that of the future somatic sensory cortex, or vice versa. The results obtained have established two facts with certainty. First, the surviving transplant emits corticospinal and callosal efferents and receives thalamocortical afferents in patterns characteristic of the host, not the donor, area of cortex. Second, invasion of a transplant from the visual area to the somatic sensory area by the ventrobasal thalamocortical afferents induces the appearance of the intra-areal specializations—the barrels—characteristic of normal somatic sensory cortex (Schlaggar and O'Leary, 1991, 1994). These observations have been interpreted as evidence that cortical areas are *not* specified to any significant extent by cell-autonomous factors in the neuroepithelium, but are reliably specified by secondary histogenetic events, exclusively.

Several other observations bear upon these formulations (Porter et al., 1987; Barth and Stanfield, 1994). First, specializations that appear in the transplant to the somatic sensory cortex are intra-areal, and their appearance does not bear directly upon the question at hand, inter-areal specification. Second, the transplanted cortex with its induced barrels *is not capable of sustaining a placing reaction,* a simple, reliable, and classical test of the functional integrity of a somatic sensory cortex. Third, focal electrical stimulation within the transplant does not evoke a movement, even though the transplant has emitted some corticospinal axons into the pyramidal tract. This is readily understood in view of the observation that these particular corticospinal axons, originating in the transplanted cortex, do not arborize when they reach their presumed target zones in the spinal cord.

My own conclusion is that at E17 the visual cortex of the rodent has evolved intrinsic processing properties that are essentially visual; and that upon transplantation—even with emission of axons and the induction of barrels—*it does not possess the intrinsic operating capacity to function as a somatic sensory cortex.*

The hypothesis that after migration the cortex is essentially a *tabula rasa* upon which secondary events in histogenesis play to produce areal specifications remains, for the rodent, only partially supported by the available evidence. The results of these experiments do fit with the generally accepted proposition that the thalamocortical input is an important influence in the specification of cortical areas. The remarkable heterochrony of primate corticogenesis differs so greatly from the temporally compressed corticogenesis in the rodent that the rodent model is not a reliable predictor of the sequence or timing of events in primate corticogenesis.

Summary

I give here a summary of the chain of events referred to above. It is partly speculative, for concepts in this evolving field change continuously in the light of new evidence produced in many laboratories by the intense application of new methods.

1. The precursors of the subplate are defined by area-specific biochemical markers while still in the stage of neurogenesis in the neuroepithelium. The molecular identity of these markers and the mechanism of their production is unknown.

2. The precursors of the subplate migrate from the neuroepithelium to form the intermediate layer of the preplate, with the primordial plexiform layer (latter layer I) above. The migrating subplate neurons retain their area-specific markers. Alternatively, those markers might be expressed at any phase of neurogenesis, migration, and preplate-split; on this point there is no evidence.

3. After split of the preplate into the future layer I above and the subplate below, the neurons of the subplate retain area-specific markers; the overlying cortical plate is *not* specified by area.

4. Thalamocortical axons from specific thalamic nuclei grow into the internal capsule and then into a strongly labeled pathway leading through the subplate. Efferents emitted from the cortical plate avoid this pathway in their projection into the internal capsule. Sets of thalamocortical afferents invade their appropriate zones of the subplate and no others, and make effective synaptic contacts with subplate neurons. There is no evidence that the overlying cortical plate is biochemically marked by area at this time.

5. After the "waiting period," during which the migratory formation of the cortical plate proceeds, a biochemical gradient appears in the subplate leading upward, toward the overlying local zone of the cortical plate. Subplate neurons emit axon collaterals that invade that particular zone of the cortical plate and no other. These are the pioneer axons that made functional synaptic contacts with neurons of the cortical plate.

6. Invasion of the cortical plate by renewed growth of thalamocortical axons follows the biochemical gradient and/or the

pioneer subplate axons into the cortical plate at or just after the formation of layer IV.

7. Invasion of the cortical plate by the thalamocortical axons sets in motion a chain of events that produces:

   a. The specification of areas by cytoarchitecture, and the boundaries of those areas.

   b. Specification of intra-areal variations—e.g., loss of layer IV in area 4; fusion of II/III/IV in area 3b; ocular-dominance columns in V1; barrels in the rodent somatosensory cortex. The mechanisms of this interaction between afferent thalamocortical axons and the cortical neuronal population is largely unknown.

There is strong, though not yet completely convincing, evidence that, before any influence of thalamocortical afferents, neurons of the germinal epithelium are instructed of their future areal location. This stage is quickly overlapped by ingrowth of those afferents that contribute a major influence to the maturation of the immature cortex, leading to adult, area-specific features. These include intra-areal specializations, the sizes of cortical areas, the sharpening of areal boundaries, and the regulation of neuropeptide, transmitter, receptor, and second-messenger protein expression (Jones, 1990a; Huntley and Jones, 1991). However, there is some evidence that laminar and cytoarchitectural maturation may proceed in the absence of thalamocortical input. It is important to note that primates and rodents differ greatly; they are not part of any phylogenetic series. They are contrasted by the precocial nature of primate development and the altricial properties of that of the rodent. It appears very unlikely that any adequate model developed to account for the experimental findings in one will fit those obtained from the other, except in broad outlines.

The evidence available favors the dual proposition that a fate map of neocortical areas does exist in the germinal epithelium of the ventricular zone; and, in addition, that further specification of cortical areas depends upon the ingrowth of corticipetal afferents, particularly those from the dorsal thalamus.

Virtually all of the research done on cortical development has been made on the primary sensory areas of the cortex. Yet, it is well known, particularly in the primate, that the rate of maturation differs greatly between those heterotypical areas and the vast expanse of homotypical cortex, which makes up more than 90 percent of the neocortex of the human. The question is whether general conclusions drawn from studies of the sensory cortex, and especially those from the virtually unique striate cortex, are generally applicable.

10 The Distributed and Hierarchical Organization of Neocortical Systems

Discoveries made in studies of the sensory systems have revealed that different features of distal stimuli are in many cases transduced and signaled in separate sets of primary afferent fibers. The neocortical activity evoked by impulses in those sets of afferents, projected through the same sensory system, is processed divergently in separate cortical areas. In some cases this divergent channelling occurs in the primary sensory areas, as in the distribution of functions of areas 17 and 3b of the visual and somesthetic systems. No common target has been identified to which the successive processing areas of any sensory system project convergently to create the neural image of a holistic perception. Indeed, the present evidence indicates that no such integrating area exists for any of the sensory-perceptual processing systems of the neocortex. One must conclude that these systems are not strictly hierarchical in organization, as traditional intuitive appreciations of them had long supposed. Two methods of objective analysis, however, have revealed that a certain degree of hierarchy does exist at the early area-to-area progressions of sensory systems into the cortex from their sites of entry. Several lines of evidence indicate that for the neocortex more generally considered areas are heavily and reciprocally interconnected to form distributed systems that depart from the hierarchical arrangement. A distributed system is defined as a set of linked but distinct processing nodes that are spatially separate and that communicate with each other by exchanging messages (Lamport, 1978). One requirement for such a system is that the internodal transmission time be some significant fraction of the intranodal processing time. The slow conduction velocity of corticocortical fibers is certainly a significant fraction of transcolumnar processing time. Neocortical distributed systems are parts of more widely distributed systems in the brain, created by the dense and reciprocal connections of many cortical areas with extracortical structures (Bressler, 1995).

Coupling between nodes of such systems is described as re-entry, defined as "a process of parallel and recursive signalling along ordered anatomical connections that achieve integration by giving rise to constructive properties within and between (neural) maps" (Tononi et al., 1992a; Sporns et al., 1989). What those constructive and correlative properties are and how they arise remain unclear. The concept of distributed systems suggests the hypothesis that the holistic image of a perception is contained within the dynamic ongoing activity in the linked populations of the system. No single neuron signals the total image, nor is any single neuron essential for it. The image resides in the temporal relations between the discharges of many neurons. This is called *population* or *ensemble coding,* and I shall use these terms interchangeably. The nature of the linking function between spatially separate nodes of an active distributed system is a subject of intense enquiry at the present time. I discuss it in Chapter 12. It is important to note that agreement on this formulation is far from universal. Barlow (1995), e.g., has recently presented an updated account of the "neuron doctrine for perception" and has marshaled the evidence he interprets to support the view that the activity of single neurons or of small groups of neurons *can* provide a sufficient basis for perception.

Operations within distributed systems thought necessary for discriminations and categorizations, e.g., are executed within a few hundred milliseconds of intracortical processing time. For that fleeting instant the neural activities in widely separated, but interconnected, areas of the neocortex and relevant extracortical structures are welded into a coordinated and dynamic whole, a distributed system in action. Neocortical distributed systems selectively active in one or another perceptual operation function simultaneously within the ongoing activity of the brain. How that selective activity is successful in evoking a sensation when it occurs in the midst of the ongoing, sometimes synchronous and sometimes oscillating, activity of very large and widely distributed populations of cortical neurons raises a major problem. The difficulty of reaching a solution is particularly acute, for the electrical activity of the brain varies greatly in time and place and over a range of brain states that do not often disrupt perceptual constancy. I discuss some aspects of this problem in Chapter 12.

A number of important discoveries concerning the structure and the connectivity of the neocortex have contributed to the present hypothesis of distributed systems. The first is that a large number of previously unknown cortical areas have been defined in terms of their cellular and biochemical architecture, extrinsic connections, and their functional specialization. These properties differ from one area to another and express the specialized and sometimes unique "function" of an area. They appear to be determined by the particular set of afferent connections of the area, and thus by the functional properties of neurons in those source structures. It remains to be determined whether the specific function of an area is also set in part by intrinsic local circuit operations unique to the area. More than 70 areas have been described in the cerebral cortex of the macaque monkey (72 at last count), the nonhuman primate most commonly used in neuroanatomical research. The homologues of these areas are rapidly being identified in the human cortex, where some investigators believe a considerably larger number of cortical areas exist. The areas in the macaque are illustrated in Figs. 10-1 and 10-2 in the manner used by Van Essen and his colleagues in an extended series of studies of the neocortex of the macaque (Van Essen and Maunsell, 1980; Maunsell and Van Essen, 1983; Felleman and Van Essen, 1991). The method has many advantages: for defining areal boundaries precisely, for lo-

---

Fig. 10-1 A two-dimensional map of the cerebral cortex of a macaque monkey, prepared by the method of Van Essen and Maunsell (1980). Fine solid lines represent the contours of layer IV from a series of 16 horizontal sections taken at 2 mm intervals through the cortex. Numbers along the margins of the map correspond to the different section levels indicated in the lateral *(upper left)* and medial *(lower left)* views of the hemisphere. Shading indicates cortex lying within sulci; the fundus of each sulcus is indicated by the heavy dashed lines. Solid lines along the perimeter of the map indicate regions in which artificial cuts have been made to reduce distortions. Dashed lines along the perimeter represent the margins of the cortex where it adjoins subcortical structures. *AMT,* anterior middle temporal sulcus; *AS,* arcuate sulcus; *CaS,* calcarine sulcus; *CeS,* central sulcus; *CiS,* cingulate sulcus; *HF,* hippocampal fissure; *IOS,* inferior occipital sulcus; *IPS,* intraparietal sulcus; *LS,* lunate sulcus; *OTS,* occipitotemporal sulcus; *POS,* parieto-occipital sulcus; *PS,* principal sulcus; *RF,* rhinal fissure; *SF,* sylvian fissure; *STS,* superior temporal sulcus. (From Fellerman and Van Essen, 1991.)

Distributed, Hierarchical Organization of Neocortical Systems

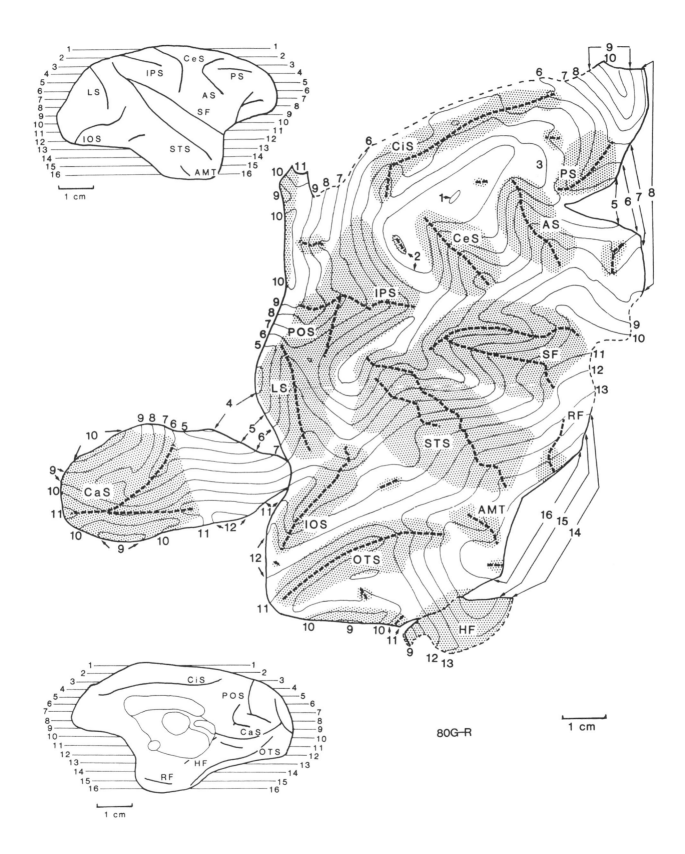

80G-R

1 cm

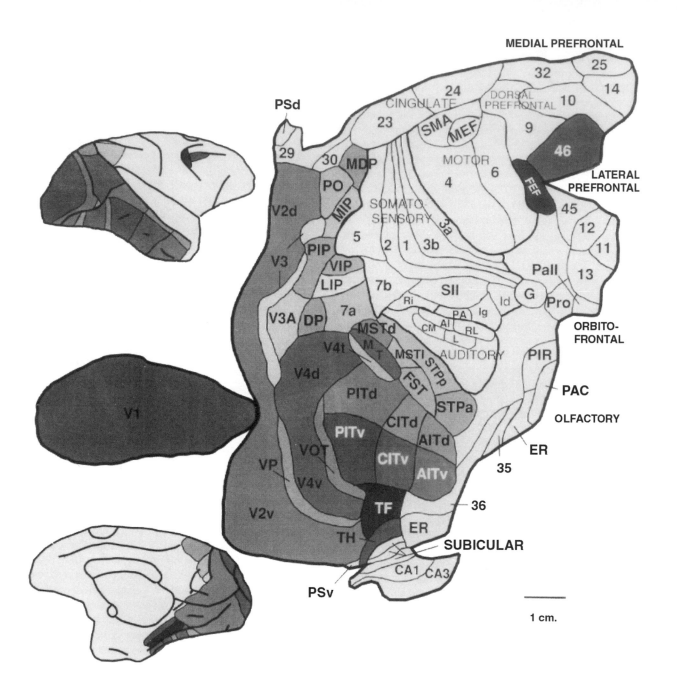

Distributed, Hierarchical Organization of Neocortical Systems

cating the sites of tracer injections and mapping the results, for measuring the surface areas of cortical regions, for mapping the distribution of labeled cells in immunocytochemical experiments, etc. This map should now be compared with that of Brodmann, prepared nearly 90 years ago (see Fig. 4-2). The map of Fig. 10-2 reveals the complicated terminology used to designate cortical areas. It is a mix-

---

Fig. 10-2   A map of the cerebral cortical areas of the macaque monkey, prepared by the method of Van Essen and Maunsell illustrated in Fig. 10-1. The presumptively visual areas are shown in different shades of gray. Arabic numerals are areal designations in the Brodmann system; alphabetic abbreviations are as follows:

AI	primary auditory area	PITv	posterior inferotemporal, ventral
AITd	anterior inferotemporal, dorsal		
AITv	anterior inferotemporal, ventral	PO	parieto-occipital
CA1\CA3	hippocampal fields	Pro	pro-isocortex
CITd	central inferotemporal, dorsal	PSd	prostriate, dorsal
CITv	central inferotemporal, ventral	PSv	prostriate, ventral
CM	caudomedial auditory	Ri	retroinsular
DP	dorsal prelunate	RL	rostrolateral auditory area
ER	entorhinal	SII	second somatic area
FEF	frontal eye fields	SMA	supplementary motor
G	gustatory cortex	STPa	superior temporal polysensory, anterior
HC	hippocampal cortex		
Id	insular, dysgranular	STPp	superior temporal polysensory, posterior
Ig	insular, granular		
L	lateral auditory	TF	area TF of the parahippocampal cortex
LIP	lateral intraparietal		
MDP	medial dorsal parietal	TH	area TH of the parahippocampal cortex
MEF	medial eye fields		
MIP	medial intraparietal	V1	striate cortex
MSTd	medial superior temporal, dorsal	V2	a prestriate visual area
		V2d	a prestriate visual area
MSTl	medial superior temporal, lateral	V3	a prestriate visual area
		V3a	a prestriate visual area
MT	medial temporal	V4d	a prestriate visual area
PA	postauditory	V4v	a prestriate visual area
PAC	periamygdaloid	VIP	ventral intraparietal
Pall	periallocortical	VOT	ventral occipitotemporal
PIP	posterior intraparietal	VP	ventral posterior visual
PIR	piriform		
PITd	posterior inferotemporal, dorsal		

ture of the original Brodmann numbers, of the V1–V5 system introduced by Zeki, and of many multi-lettered designations that indicate cerebral lobe, superior or inferior, dorsal or ventral (25 numbers and 16 letters are used in various permutations). A revision of terminology is badly needed. It may be doomed to failure, for the mixed terminologies of Fig. 10-2 are deeply embedded in the neurobiological community.

The second set of discoveries leading to the hypothesis of distributed systems is that a large number of connections exists between those areas. For example, 758 connections have been discovered to link the 72 presently known areas in the macaque monkey, and about 1100 have been formed in the cat, counting only those within the ipsilateral hemisphere and leaving aside connections with subcortical structures and with the opposite hemisphere. The increase in the numbers and the degree of specificity of the connections that exist between different structures in the brain, and particularly between different areas of the cerebral cortex, is so great as to constitute a new qualitative fact about the brain. It has come from use of neuroanatomical methods, such as Nauta's technique for tracing axon terminal degeneration after lesion and, more recently, methods that depend upon bi-directional axoplasmic flow. In the latter, chemicals injected extracellularly are transported into neurons and are moved throughout, allowing identification of both cell body sources and axon terminals of connecting elements. The actively transported substances used are, among many, radioactively labeled amino acids, horseradish peroxidase, and fluorescent dyes and microbeads. The connections between areas are often but not always reciprocal; 311 of the 758 connections in the macaque hemisphere are reciprocal pairs, 136 are one-way. The to-and-fro connections between areas are commonly not equivalent, for the source-target relations may differ between the members of reciprocal pairs. These irreciprocal laminar relations have been used as an indication of a hierarchical organization of the cerebral cortex, as described below. This type of organization is clear at the entry stages of the major sensory-perceptual processing systems in the cortex—e.g., for the somatic sensory and visual systems. With further traverse of systems into the homotypical areas of the neocortex, these hierarchical arrangements appear gradually to give way to the distributed nature of the overall networks.

The third set of discoveries is that cortical areas are organized in the modular format described in Chapter 7. Frequently one set of modules in an area entertains a certain subset but not all of the extrinsic connections of the area; other columnar groups, other subsets of connections. Several quasi-independent processing streams can be discerned embedded within the distributed systems of the neocortex.

These mixed hierarchical, distributed sensory-perceptual processing systems of the neocortex are parts of even more widely distributed systems within the brain. Cortical areas are densely and reciprocally connected with other brain structures, ranging from the opposite hemisphere, thalamus, basal ganglia, brainstem, and cerebellum to the spinal cord—the nervous system entire.

Analysis of the Patterns of Neocortical Connectivity

The number of cortical areas shown in Fig. 10-2 and the enormous number of fiber pathways now known to connect these areas with each other make it difficult by observation and intuition alone to reach other than informal and speculative conclusions about the functional organization of the system. A number of analytic studies have now been made, with the aim to uncover organizing principles from which testable hypotheses of functional properties could be generated. Among these are two I describe below. The first is based on a form of topological analysis, nonmetric multidimensional scaling; the second upon the irreciprocity of the laminar origins and targets of many corticocortical connections.

Topological Analysis by Nonmetric Multidimensional Scaling

This method is based upon the demonstration that if qualitative (i.e., nonmetric) information about the items in a data set—like similarity, proximity, or relative distance—are available in sufficient numbers, they can be used to generate a metric configuration of the set of points in Euclidian space (Shepard, 1980). The method has been used by Young and co-workers to analyze the connectivities between areas of the cerebral cortex. The available data are the presence or the absence of connections between cortical areas determined anatomically, for until now the number of axons composing area-to-area connections is unknown. In this analysis, each cell in the matrix relating each cortical area to all others in assigned a value: 2, if reciprocal connections exist between the two areas defining the cell; 1, if only a one-way connection exists; or 0, if no connections have been found, or if no study of that particular connection has been made neuro-anatomically. The connection matrix is then subjected to an optimization procedure and the result reduced from its high-dimensional state to a low-dimensional configuration by the method of nonmetric multidimensional scaling. The derived structure is one in which points are placed in an equilibrated tension such that they are as close as possible to the inverse of the rank order of the areal proximities defined by the presence or absence of connections, as defined above. For a full description of this program of research, see the monograph by Young et al. (1995a) and the original papers by Young (1992, 1993); Young et al. (1994a,b, 1995b); Scannell et al. (1995); Scannell and Young (1993). The two-dimensional image at this ordinal level of measurement is shown in Fig. 10-3 for the connectivity in the cortex of one hemisphere of the macaque monkey. It is as if these cortical areas have been rearranged so that those connected are close together in space; those not, separated. The result can be interpreted as a processing architecture that is independent of cortical geography.

The 758 connections between the 72 areas of the macaque monkey cortex shown in Fig. 10-3 account for only 15 percent of all connections that could exist between the areas (the maximum number is 5,112); undoubtedly others remain to be discovered. Each group, or "cluster," of areas of the major sensory systems is located at some distance from each of the others. The somatosensory and motor clusters overlap each other and are located at bottom right in the structure. Area 7b is drawn toward the center of the array by its many connections with other sensory systems. The combined somatic sensory-motor system appears to be partially inserted between the auditory and visual systems; the latter two are interconnected only minimally. The more "central" areas of each sensory cluster are connected with a group of areas in the limbic and prefrontal regions, shown at top left of the structure. These relations are shown more simply in the block diagram of Fig. 10-4.

Some hierarchical relations can be seen in the early stages of each sensory cluster; I shall discuss them further below. The more central (the "higher") an area in the somatic sensory or visual clusters, the more complex are the functional properties of its neurons. This undoubtedly reflects in part the convergence and elaboration of earlier stages of intracortical processing. In addition, some signs of partial separation of the parietal and temporal lobes' processing streams in the visual cluster can be seen to the left of the structure. In general, the curvature of the structure indicates its distributed, not its hierarchical, nature.

Hierarchical Analysis by Laminar Relations

An important discovery concerning corticocortical connections in the primate was made by Tigges, Spatz, and others in the early 1970s: that is, that pairs of linked cortical areas, like the 311 pairs in the macaque cortex referred to above, do not have similar laminar sources and targets (Spatz et al., 1970; Spatz, 1977; Tigges et al., 1973). Reciprocally linked pairs of cortical areas are frequently irreciprocal in the details of the sources and targets of the cells and axons that link the two. This observation was quickly confirmed and extended to include many areas in many primates, including both Old and New World monkeys (Wong-Riley, 1978; Rockland and Pandya, 1979; Tigges et al., 1981; Maunsell and Van Essen, 1983). Irreciprocity has now been described in a large number of studies in all major lobes of the neocortex—e.g., in the parietal cortex (Pandya and Seltzer, 1982; Seltzer and Pandya, 1980) and in the temporal lobe (Distler et al., 1993). It is particularly clear for the connections linking the initial and successive stages of progression of the major sensory systems into the cortex; or, in a different case, for the sequential invasion from the limbic cortex into the frontal lobe (Barbas, 1986; Barbas and Pandya, 1989).

Van Essen and his colleagues propose that these linking inter-areal connections fall into three classes, indicated in Fig. 10-5 (for review and summary, see Felleman and Van Essen, 1991):

Ascending or "feed-forward" connections, in which the neurons of origin are located most often only in the supragranular layers, less often in both supra- and infragranular layers. Their axons terminate in layer IV of the target area.

Descending or "feedback" connections, which originate mainly from neurons in the infragranular layers but in some cases from neurons in both supra- and infragranular layers and which terminate above and below but not within layer IV.

Lateral connections, which arise from neurons in both supra- and infragranular layers. Their axons terminate in a columnar manner, sending axonal branches to all cellular layers of the target areas. A second class of lateral connections will be described in a later section.

The axonal terminals of the "ascending" class of corticocortical connections converge in the target zone with the terminations of the specific thalamocortical projections, while those of the "descend-

---

Fig. 10-3 The topological organization of the macaque cortical areas in terms of their ipsilateral corticocortical connections, as known to 1993. A total of 758 connections between 72 cortical areas are shown; of these 136 are one-way. The connections shown are only 15 percent of the total possible connections. The structure is a best-fit representation of the topology of the system in two dimensions. The position of each area is specified as that which minimizes the distance from other areas with which it is connected, and maximizes the distances to areas with which it is not connected. Areas with similar patterns of inputs and outputs tend to be placed close together, those with dissimilar patterns far apart. The cortex is represented in a state of connectional tension, not in its true anatomical space. (From Young, 1993.) Arabic numerals are areal designations in the Brodmann system; alphabetic abbreviations are as follows:

AITd	anterior inferotemporal, dorsal	proA	auditory prokoniocortex
AITv	anterior inferotemporal, ventral	reit	auditory retroinsular temporal cortex
CITd	central inferotemporal, dorsal	Ri	retroinsular cortex
CITv	central inferotemporal, ventral	S2	second somatosensory cortex
DP	dorsal prelunate	SMA	supplementary motor cortex
ER	entorhinal cortex	STPa	superior temporal polysensory, anterior
FEF	area 8, frontal eye fields	STPp	superior temporal polysensory, posterior
FST	floor of superior temporal sulcus	TF	area TF of the parahippocampal cortex
G	gustatory cortex	TGd	temporal polar cortex, dorsal
HIPP	hippocampus	TGv	temporal polar cortex, ventral
Id	insular, dysgranular	TH	area TH of the parahippocampal cortex
Ig	insular, granular	Tpt	auditory area Tpt
KA	auditory koniocortical, primary	TS1	superior temporal auditory area 1
LIP	lateral intraparietal	TS2	superior temporal auditory area 2
MSTd	middle superior temporal area, dorsal	TS3	superior temporal auditory area 3
MSTl	middle superior temporal area, lateral/ventral	V1	primary visual cortex, area 17
MT	middle temporal area	V2	second visual area, part of area 18
PaA1	auditory parakoniocortical, lateral	V3	third visual area
PaAc	auditory parakoniocortical, caudal	V3A	visual area 3A
PaAr	auditory parakoniocortical, rostral	V4	fourth visual area
PaI	periallocortex	V4t	transitional zone of V4 abutting MT
PIP	posterior intraparietal	VIP	ventral intraparietal
PITd	posterior inferotemporal, dorsal	VOT	visual occipitotemporal area
PITv	posterior inferotemporal, ventral	VP	ventral posterior visual area
PO	parieto-occipital visual area		

Distributed, Hierarchical Organization of Neocortical Systems

ing" class converge with the layers of termination of the nonspecific, or generalized, thalamocortical projections. Both ascending and descending types of relations occur in one-way connections.

Van Essen and others have used these differences in the source-target relations between reciprocally linked pairs of cortical areas to form a generalizing hypothesis that cerebral cortical areas are organized into hierarchical systems (Felleman and Van Essen, 1991; Van Essen et al., 1990). Cortical areas were assigned by these investigators to different levels determined by the ascending-descending relations between reciprocal pairs. The areas shown geographically in Fig. 10-2 and topologically in Fig. 10-3 were placed in the hierarchical order of

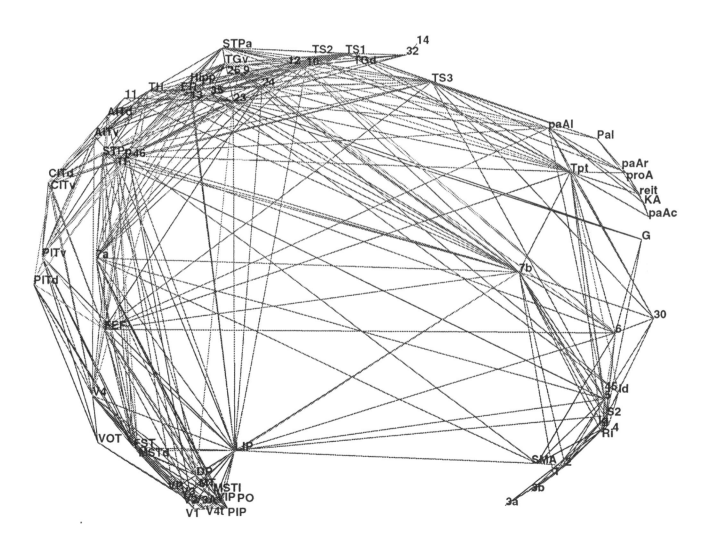

Fig. 10-4 The gross features of the connectional organization of the macaque cerebral cortex detailed in Fig. 10-3. The three major inflow sensory systems connect with a fourth complex, the fronto-limbic, which is topologically the most distant from the periphery. On this analysis, direct cross-talk between the three major inflow systems is limited; cross-talk is strongest through the fronto-limbic system. (From Young, 1993.)

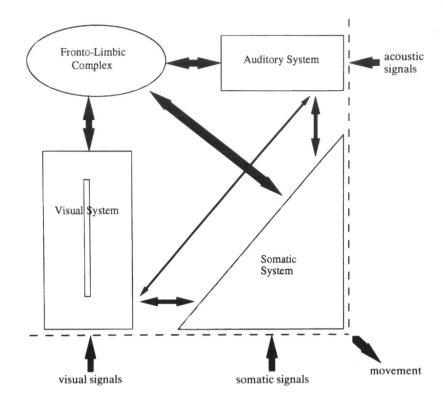

higher-lower levels, yielding the diagrams of Fig. 10-6 for the visual and somatosensory-motor systems. The concept of hierarchy is loosened to include aspects that are foreign to its traditional meaning, for the diagrams of Fig. 10-6 do not reveal a progression through a pyramidal shape to a supraordinate area; parallel channels can still be discerned in the hierarchy, with cross linkages. An area at any level may be reciprocally linked with areas at more than one step above, or even to those several levels "higher" or "lower" in the structure.

Several facts support the general idea of the hierarchical cascade of cortical areas, especially for those located early in the sequence leading from the primary heterotypical sensory areas into the homotypical cortex.

1. The ascending class of area-to-area projections engages a target at one of its major input portals, layer IV (and lower III). The descending projections specifically avoid layer IV to terminate above and below it. They project most strongly to

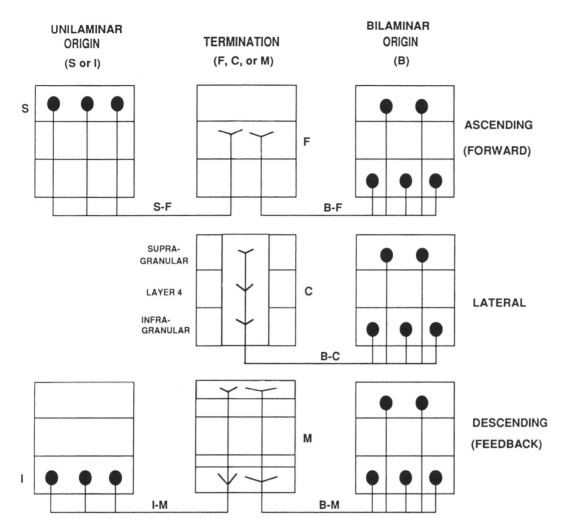

Fig. 10-5 Diagrams of the laminar patterns of origin and termination of corticocortical connections used by Felleman and Van Essen to assign hierarchical positions to cortical areas. The central column shows the characteristic patterns of terminations: the *F* pattern—with preferential termination in layer 4; the *C* pattern—the columnar pattern with equal density of terminations in all cortical layers; and the *M* pattern—a multilaminar pattern that specifically avoids layer 4. There are three characteristic patterns of the locations of the cells of origin of corticocortical connections: the bilaminar *(B)* pattern, with approximately equal numbers of cells of origin in superficial and deep layers; the *S* pattern, with origins predominately in the superficial layers; and the *I* pattern, with origins preferentially in the infragranular layers. The *B* pattern correlates with all three patterns of termination, the *S* pattern with *F*-type terminations in layer 4, the *I* pattern with *M*-type terminations. However, several variations on these general patterns have been observed. (From Felleman and Van Essen, 1991.)

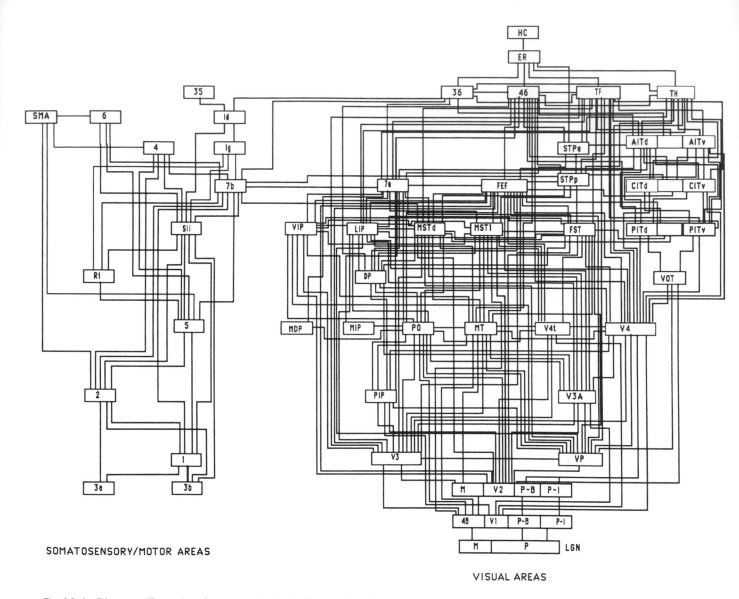

SOMATOSENSORY/MOTOR AREAS

VISUAL AREAS

Fig. 10-6 Diagrams illustrating the connectivities in the visual and somatic sensory distributed systems of the cerebral cortex of the macaque. There are 305 pathways linking areas termed visual, 62 pathways linking areas termed somatosensory, and a number of others, as noted at the tops of the diagrams, that link the two systems. (From Van Essen et al., 1990.)

layer I, whose intrinsic connections suggest a controlling rather than a driving function.

2. The functional properties of cortical neurons, determined by electrophysiological methods, become more complex in the transition from lower to higher stages of the putatively hierarchical array. These transitions include both increases in the sizes of peripheral receptive fields and a greater complexity of dynamic properties.

3. Removal of the first stage of such a cortical sensory system—its input funnel—leads to a profound sensory disorder. Removal of areas at higher levels of the hierarchy produces defects in one or another component of the sensation, not a global deficit.

4. The hierarchical arrangement at the input levels of cortical sensory-perceptual processing systems is revealed also by the method of nonmetric multidimensional scaling described above.

An equally formidable array of facts argues against the general applicability of the hierarchical concept.

1. There is nothing intrinsically directional (i.e., ascending–descending or feed-forward–feedback) about the reciprocal connections described, and there are some observations against the idea. For example, what are regarded as primary functional properties of neurons in lower areas depend in part upon projections from areas at higher levels in the hierarchy.

2. The sources and terminations of reciprocal pairs are frequently not spatially congruent. For example, Shipp and Zeki (1989) found that the return projection from V5 (MT) to V2 in the macaque is spatially more widespread than is the origin of the forward projection from V2 to V5. Thus this "reciprocal pair" is both reciprocal and in part one-way. This spatial mismatch has been observed in many "reciprocal" linkages classed as ascending-descending.

3. The data base from which the hierarchical generalization derives is restricted, for it includes only those corticocortical

connections intrinsic to a single hemisphere. All others are left out of the analysis, including the massive interhemispheric connections that are both areally homologous and heterologous; the heavy projections running both ways that link the cortex to subcortical structures, such as the thalamus, claustrum, basal ganglia, brainstem, and spinal cord; and the widely divergent innervation of the cortex that originates in the central core nuclei of the brainstem and in the basal forebrain. How the connection table would look were all these included is unknown, but it appears likely their addition would smear to a considerable extent the hierarchical relations described.

4. The hierarchical generalization ignores the many exceptions to the source-target relations between reciprocal pairs, on which it is based.

5. The generalization ignores the fact that certain subsets of the total array of modules within a cortical area entertain only certain subsets of the total pattern of the extrinsic connections of the area. Some of these may be in one relation to the areas with which they are connected, others in another relation. It is difficult to place such an area in a single hierarchical location.

6. Visual cortical areas previously regarded as purely hierarchical in their relation are activated virtually simultaneously by visual stimuli—e.g., V1 and V2 of the macaque (Bullier and Nowak, 1995; Nowak et al., 1995a; Raigeul et al., 1989). A lag of about 10 msec occurs between activation of V1 and V2, and the extended distributions of the latencies overlap almost completely, which indicates that processing is done simultaneously in the two areas.

Van Essen (Felleman and Van Essen, 1991) has emphasized that the concept of the hierarchical arrangements shown in Fig. 10-6 does not imply convergence to a peak, that it is adapted to the appearance of parallel processing pathways within the array, and that it accepts the many lateral connections between areas and the many exceptions to the strict ordering relations required by the hierarchical concept. Thus the general applicability of the hierarchical concept to the overall pattern of corticocortical connectivity is weakened, and when exceptions proliferate, parallel pathways are defined, and large classes of connections are excluded, it seems reasonable to conclude that the hierarchical concept is of limited heuristic value either for understanding cortical function or for planning experiments aimed at discovering it.

My own conclusion is this. There is a considerable variety in the source-target relations between reciprocal pairs of connected cortical areas, and among one-way connections as well. Where these connections link the primary sensory areas to the first several steps into the homotypical cortex, they do suggest a hierarchical arrangement, at least as regards the limited set of connections admitted to the analysis. However, these relations appear quite different when they link more "central" regions of the cortex, as I describe in the following section. At these levels the relations between areas resemble those marked "lateral" in Fig. 10-5, with added complications between the terminations of convergent projections to a single area. These reciprocal corticocortical circuits provide for parallel and re-entrant signaling, as do many between cortical and subcortical structures, particularly those that link different levels in afferent systems (Edelman, 1983; Tononi et al., 1992a).

I emphasize that although the neocortical system has the appearance of randomness when viewed *in toto, this is not the case.* The connections between nodes of even its largest and most widely distributed systems are highly specific and ordered. A case in point is the massively interconnected fronto-parietal system illustrated in Figs. 10-8 and 10-9. This system deals with space, with the orientation of the organism in that space and his operations within it, with spatial perceptions and memory. Moreover, in systems like the visual and somatic sensory, where hierarchy prevails at entry levels and where precise topography is present in the initial cortical representation of sensory sheets, that topography is preserved in terms of neighbor relations through many levels of the systems, although the mapping is less detailed and precise at more central than at entry levels.

Distributed Networks in the Neocortex

It has been known for two decades that the columnar mode of termination of the axonal projections between laterally interconnected cortical areas is intermittent. That is, the terminals are distributed across all cortical layers in the target area, most densely in the supragranular layers, in columns of 200–500 μm width, separated by columnar zones of equal width in which few terminals from that particular source can be seen. This discovery was made almost simultaneously in a number of laboratories (Goldman and Nauta, 1977; Grant et al., 1975; Jones et al., 1975; Kunzle, 1976, 1978; Jacobsen and Trojanowski, 1977). The cells of origin of such a projection are similarly arranged in intermittently distributed columns in the source area. An example of the columnar mode of termination taken from the work of Goldman and Nauta is shown in Fig. 10-7. In this experiment tritium-labeled amino acids were injected into the dorsal bank of the principal sulcus, a homotypical area of cortex of the monkey frontal lobe. After a delay to allow antegrade axoplasmic flow, labeled terminals were demonstrated by autoradiography in the cingular gyrus, one of the extrinsic targets of the peri-principal cortex. It can be seen in Fig. 10-7 that the labeled terminals occur in vertically oriented columns 200–400 μm wide that extend across all layers of the cortex. They alternate with columnar zones of equal width in which few labeled terminals occur. The widths of these columns are similar in macaque and squirrel monkey brains, which differ in size by a factor of 4.5 (Bugbee and Goldman-Rakic, 1983). This

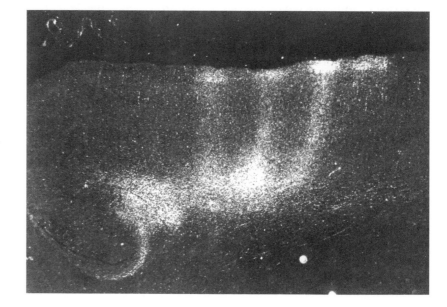

Fig. 10-7 A dark-field autoradiogram that illustrates columns of axons and terminals in the ipsilateral retrosplenial cortex labeled after a single injection of ³H-leucine and ³H-proline into the dorsal bank cortex of the principal sulcus in a 4-day-old monkey. The projection columns are on 500 μm centers. Three columns are seen here; the radioactive labeling is most dense in the plexiform layer I. (From Goldman and Nauta, 1977.)

Distributed, Hierarchical Organization of Neocortical Systems

interdigitated columnar pattern has been observed in many studies of connectivity in the neocortex, including connections between areas in a single hemisphere and between connections linking areas of the two hemispheres via the large commissures of the forebrain. The columns of terminals are frequently arranged in bands or stripes running in the tangential dimension of the cortex (Shanks et al., 1975; Jones et al., 1975), a pattern confirmed in many subsequent investigations. It is important to emphasize that bands or stripes are not functionally operative units. The static and dynamic properties of neurons vary intermittently along the axes of the stripes, in the columnar mode.

These observations raised the question of how the terminals that converge upon an area, or the cells of origin that generate separate sets of corticocortical axons leaving it, are arranged in space. The problem is formidable, for on average a cortical area generates or receives 10–20 sets of corticocortical connections, as well as many processes to and from subcortical structures. Goldman-Rakic and her colleagues have used the double-tracer method (tritiated amino acids and horseradish peroxidase) in a first approach to this problem, asking how the terminations of two convergent projections are distributed in target areas. They found that the interhemispheric and ipsilateral posterior parietal projections to the cortex of the principal sulcus of the frontal lobe terminate in sets of intermittently distributed columnar zones that are interdigitated with one another. One subset of columns of the frontal area is linked to one of the two sources, a second with the other (Goldman-Rakic and Schwartz, 1982; Schwartz and Goldman-Rakic, 1984).

These investigators then studied the patterns of termination of projections that originate in the posterior parietal and principal sulcus cortex and project convergently to other brain structures. These areas of homotypical cortex of the parietal and frontal lobes are themselves heavily interconnected (Fig. 10-8) and project convergently upon at least 15 other cortical areas (Fig. 10-9). The remarkable discovery was that the terminals of these two convergent projections are arranged in different patterns in different target areas. Those convergent upon the cingular cortex, e.g., are in intermittent columnar arrays interdigitated with one another. In other target areas, however, such as those of the temporal lobe cortex, the two sets of convergent projection terminals are interleaved in different layers of the target cortex. Fibers from the frontal cortex terminate in layers I, III, and V;

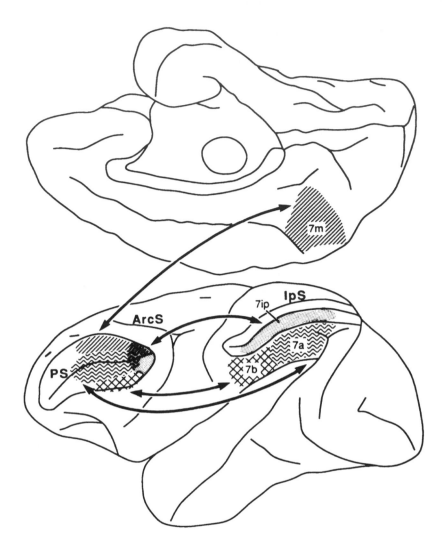

Fig. 10-8 A diagrammatic representation of the reciprocal, parallel neuronal circuits that link the posterior parietal cortex with the cortex of the frontal lobe in and near the caudal portion of the principal sulcus *(PS)*. Area 7ip of the posterior bank of the intraparietal sulcus *(IpS)* is linked with the cortex of the caudal end of the principal sulcus, area 7m with that of the fundus, and 7b with the cortex of the ventral rim of PS. (From Goldman-Rakic, 1988.)

those from the parietal cortex in layers IV and VI. Terminations of the last type were arranged over one another in a spatially congruent way, forming a column containing both (Selemon and Goldman-Rakic, 1988). Although these two patterns of termination were those most commonly observed, several variants occur in the 15 targets innervated convergently from the two source areas. Congruent projections from the two sources to subcortical structures like the basal ganglia also terminated in a segregated way, each preempting adja-

Distributed, Hierarchical Organization of Neocortical Systems

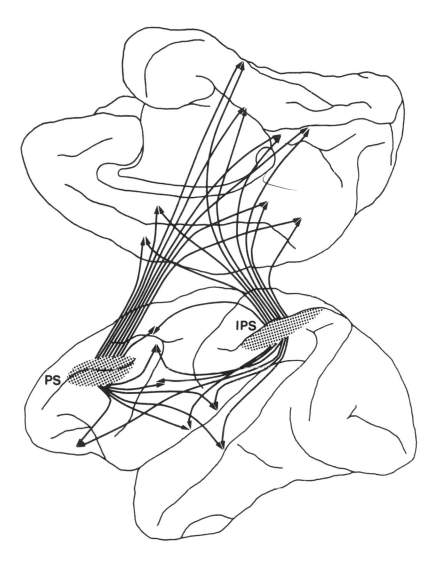

Fig. 10-9 Diagram of the mutually convergent projections of the posterior parietal and of the frontal cortex of the principal sulcus *(PS)*. Fifteen convergent projections are shown; there are five convergent subcortical projections as well, to the neostriatum, dorsal thalamus, claustrum, superior colliculus, and reticular formation. For some of the convergent cortical projections, terminals from the two sources are found in different layers of the same columns; in others, in adjacent columns in the target areas. (From Selemon and Goldman-Rakic, 1988.)

cent longitudinal bands (Selemon and Goldman-Rakic, 1985; for review, see Goldman-Rakic, 1988).

Distributive Properties of Neocortical Networks

How well do the patterns of corticocortical connections described fit the definition of a distributed system given above? The requirements are: (1) that the system be composed of a series of processing units that are spatially separate and that communicate with each other by exchanging messages; and (2) that the transmission delay be a significant fraction of the time between events in a single processing unit. A further inference is that the system possesses a real-time clock.

The first two statements could define the modularity of the cerebral cortex and the massive and distributed connections between its columns. This applies particularly to the homotypical neocortex, which makes up about 95 percent of the neocortex in the human brain. The input-output processing times in cortical columns are unknown. However, given that operations such as sensory discriminations can be executed with intracortical times in the range of 100–200 msec, and given that several iterations over the set of connections linking the columns active in a particular operation may be necessary, an estimate of 10–20 msec for the most rapid columnar processing time appears reasonable. The inter-columnar transmission time will be a "significant fraction" of the intra-columnar processing times, given the slow impulse conduction time in corticocortical axons, and especially in their small terminal branches. There is no evidence for or against the presence of a real-time brain clock operating in the dimension of msec, although slower cerebral clocks are well known.

Given the similarities between these definitions of a distributed system and the organization of the cerebral neocortex, it is of interest to consider certain properties of such a distributed system with reference to brain function.

1. Distributed systems are not hierarchical in their overall organization, although subsystems may possess hierarchical properties. This is exactly the result of the studies of cortical connectivity of the last two decades, summarized above.

2. Signal flow through such a system may follow a number of different paths, an obvious fit.

3. Action may be initiated at any of a number of loci within a distributed system. Recent studies by Galea and Darian-Smith (1994) provide a strong anatomical basis for this general statement. They have shown that separate populations of corticospinal neurons arise from widely distributed areas

of the cerebral cortex, in the frontal, parietal, and insular regions. Each of these sources of corticospinal systems has its own quite different sets of thalamic and cortical inputs. Each set has direct access to motoneuronal populations throughout the spinal cord.

4. Operations in a distributed system allow the "representation" in its dynamic activity of features by the combination of neural elements, where the specific feature is not contained within the activity of any single element, alone.

5. Local lesions within such a system may degrade its function but rarely eliminate function completely. This is the everyday experience of physicians dealing with brain lesions in humans, although a specific function may be lost completely if a brain lesion destroys an entry or exit funnel to the brain, such as a primary sensory area.

Some further implications of the idea of distributed systems as applied to the brain are the following.

Recovery of function of a distributed brain system after lesion results from a dynamic reorganization, is accelerated by training, and does not depend necessarily upon the formation of new connections. This is the common experience after cortical lesions in humans and in experimental animals—e.g., the partial recovery of motor function after lesions of motor cortical areas or after lesions of the cerebellar cortex.

The distributed system of the neocortex is a re-entrant system; its columnar nodes are open to both externally induced and internally generated activity. Phasic recycling of activity in the distributed system of the neocortex allows access first to primary and then to more general and abstract processing nodes. This allows for a continual updating of the central neural image of the world, and match or mismatch with the external state as sampled by afferent systems. This internal readout of stored information provides a mechanism for the awareness of brain events by the brain, a prominent aspect of consciousness.

A general hypothesis has evolved from the realization that the neocortex and its many interconnected structures together constitute a large number of mutually interdigitated distributed systems. High-order neuronal operations are embedded within the dynamic ongoing neuronal activity in those systems and are rarely localized in the traditional sense to single nodes of the systems. Each neuron in each of the nodes of a distributed system is connected with hundreds of other neurons in its own and in other nodes. What emerges is an interacting ensemble with dynamic properties not predictable from those of its individual members. Such interacting ensembles have emergent properties. This highlights the problem of how the results of operations upon the separated members of the set of stimulus features, carried out in separate but heavily linked nodes of such a system, are bound together into the dynamic activity of the system thought to constitute the central image of the perceptual whole. Presently the most intensely studied hypothesis is that this binding is accomplished by temporal correlation, a synchronization of the neural activity in even widely separated nodes that constitute parts of the whole. I consider the evidence concerning this hypothesis in Chapter 12.

I believe the concept of distributed systems is of some heuristic value, for newly developing methods allow recording the activity of many neurons in each of several nodes of such a distributed system simultaneously; already this can be done with numbers of microelectrodes implanted chronically in the neocortices of waking monkeys performing perceptual and/or motor tasks (Mountcastle and Steinmetz, unpublished studies, 1992). The combination in a single research effort of these methods with rapidly improving techniques for brain imagining, and with sophisticated methods of data analysis and large system modeling, promise a rapid advance in knowledge of brain function.

On the Conservation of Topology in Distributed Systems

The preservation of neighborhood relations between neurons within and between the nodes of distributed systems, and between nested distributed systems, is of central importance for orderly brain function. This conservation of neighborhood relations holds for both those systems which include a topographic map of some receptor sheet or its central transformation, and for those distributed systems in which the mapping is of some more abstract variable, as in what are called "computational maps."

What is the advantage of a conserved topology within and between nested distributed systems? First, it means that an exact point-to-point connectivity within the system is *not* required to retain accurate spatial signals or to make spatial discriminations. Second, a population of neurons carrying the distributed code will have near neighbors with only slightly different properties. This insures that the capacity for accurate signaling in the system will be virtually independent of randomly distributed local cell loss, of small processing errors, and of statistical variation in the spatial distribution of the active population.

This is one of the important results of the ubiquitous mapping functions in nervous systems and of the topological integrity of those maps through distributed systems. It endows brains with a built-in flexibility that allows them to compensate for the errors inherent in the operations of such a system.

Dynamic Operations in Neocortical Networks

I consider here the nature of the intrinsic operation of the neocortex, a major unsolved problem in cortical physiology. The central question is what transforms local microcircuits impose upon their inputs to produce their several outputs. Knowledge of the static connectivity within local microcircuits and of synaptic transmission between individual cortical neurons forms an essential base for further study. The properties of microcircuit operations are emergent, for they cannot be predicted from what is known of the action of single neurons. These network properties are likely to be highly dynamic, changing markedly and rapidly under the influence of modulatory inputs.

Direct electrophysiological studies of the neocortex *in vivo* and in isolated, surviving brain slices have yielded much of the knowledge of synaptic transmission in the neocortex detailed in earlier chapters. Use of these methods is beginning to reveal some aspects of microcircuit operation as well. Intracortical transforms have been studied indirectly in a wide variety of experiments in waking monkeys as they worked in sensory-perceptual or motor tasks. The electrical signs of impulse discharges of cortical neurons and the outcomes of behavioral tasks are recorded simultaneously in these experiments, and explanations sought in terms of the correlations observed. The hope has been that one might by retrospective inference identify the operations producing the transformations. Examples of these efforts abound: how the simple receptive fields and modality properties of the specific thalamocortical neurons that project into area 3b of the postcentral gyrus are transformed into the complex fields with directional preferences of the output cells of area 1; or, a more popular target, the continuing thirty-year effort to discover how the simple properties of geniculocortical axons are transformed in area V1 into the properties of orientation selectivity, directionality, etc., at the output levels of that cortex (Martin, 1988; Vidyasagar et al., 1996). Experiments in waking monkeys performing perceptual or motor tasks have revealed that remarkable transforms are executed between inputs and outputs in many areas of the homotypical neocortex. Although the results of the intracortical operations are clear in many cases, there are few instances in which the intracortical operations leading to the outputs have been discovered. The reasons are clear. The cortical microcircuits are embedded in the matrix of the brain and cannot be isolated for study. No method has yet been devised that allows direct observation of the neurons of such microcircuits as a transformation is executed. The developing methods of multiple microelectrode recording give some promise of a solution to this difficult technical problem.

Consequently, the functions of cortical areas are still defined—and cortical areas labeled—in terms of their extrinsic connections, as they have since the golden era of clinical neurology. The similarity of the lamination plan, neural phenotypes, and intrinsic connectivity, as well as afferent and efferent innervation patterns in different cortical areas, has led some to suggest that the internal operations in different areas may be similar. While there is little doubt that a vertically organized columnar arrangement exists in all neocortical areas, some anatomical studies suggest that imposed upon that basic plan are microcircuits that may differ between different areas—e.g., between the striate and homotypical frontal cortex in the macaque monkey (Kritzer and Goldman-Rakic, 1995; Lund et al., 1993). It seems likely that more or less identical intrinsic operations are used in different ways in different cortical circuits, and the dense projections into the neocortex of modulatory systems of subcortical origin suggest that intrinsic operations may be modified rapidly in a single microcircuit even with an unchanged anatomical connectivity. That is the inference derived from studies of small-numbered neural networks in invertebrate and simpler vertebrate brains, described in a following section. It is also consonant with some modeling studies of the neocortex (Aertsen et al., 1994).

Formulation of actions in distributed systems have not yet taken into account how system operations are sensitively determined by the local microcircuit operations in the nodes of the distributed system. It is in the nodes that the essential system operations are played out; internodal linkages carry but do not modify signals. Microcircuit operations are not revealed by the slow wave field potentials that sometimes accompany them. Therefore, *it is necessary to go beyond the characterization of single cortical neurons to determine the dynamics of their actions in microcircuits.* Local or intrinsic circuits of the neocortex are embedded within dense networks of extrinsic connections that link each neocortical area with some—usually many—other neocortical areas and with other brain structures; consequently, intrinsic networks cannot be isolated for study. What is termed intrinsic or extrinsic is arbitrary, for while the pyramidal cells are the sources of extrinsic cortical projections, they are also the most plentiful interneurons by virtue of their profuse axon collaterals. I give below a description of a microcircuit operation in an invertebrate ganglion that is understood at the levels of both single neurons and circuit operation, and using it as a model I draw inferences for the function of cortical microcircuits. I then turn directly to the cortical microcircuits themselves.

Neural Operations in Small-Numbered Neural Networks

The idea is to seek the simplest small-numbered neural circuit that can be isolated, establish the intrinsic properties of its neurons and the system properties of the network, and use it as a first-order model of the operation of a cortical microcircuit. A ubiquitous property of neural networks is a coherent periodicity of neuronal discharge and self-sustaining oscillations, properties displayed by invertebrate small-numbered networks as well as by the mammalian neocortex. Studies have been pursued in a number of invertebrates, nonmammalian vertebrates, and in reduced mammalian preparations. These small-numbered circuits display oscillatory activity reminiscent of that of the cerebral cortex, and hence they may serve as useful models of some intrinsic cortical operations.

Networks of this sort are accessible for experimentation, and their intra-network connectivities have been identified. Many generate rhythmic activities that control motoneurons: they are central pattern generators of the cyclic muscular activity necessary for many forms of behavior. Some neurons of these networks are very large and can be recognized in conspecifics, which means that the same cell

A

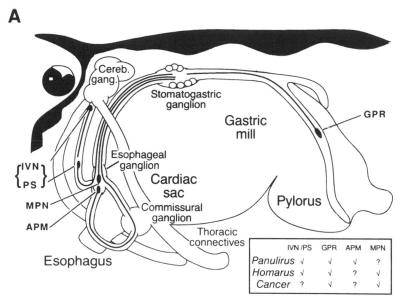

Fig. 11-1 (A) Anatomy of the crustacean foregut and the stomatogastric system, including the locations of the five types of modulatory neurons; the neurons were identified in different species (see chart to the right, in box) but are shown here in an idealized decapod. Only a single cell of each type is shown. The foregut is divided into three regions. Food enters the cardiac sac from the esophagus. Slow, irregular movements of the cardiac sac move food toward the gastric mill. The gastric mill consists of three internal teeth that macerate the food before it travels into the pylorus, where a series of fine filters allow fine particles to pass into the midgut. *APM,* anterior pyloric modulator; *Cereb. gang.,* cerebral ganglion; *GPR,* gastropyloric receptor; *IVN,* inferior ventricular nerve cell; *MPN,* modulatory proctolin-containing neuron; *PS,* pyloric suppressor. (B) Simplified synaptic connectivity diagrams for the pyloric and gastric mill central pattern generators in the stomatogastric ganglion of the spiny lobster, *P. interruptus.* Circles indicate inhibitory synapses; triangles, excitatory ones; resistors, electric coupling; diodes, rectifying electrical connections. Some electrically coupled cells have been combined; multiple cells are indicated by a number. Subsets of neurons are grouped in shaded boxes to indicate their function in control of the foregut. (From Katz and Harris-Warwick, 1990.)

B

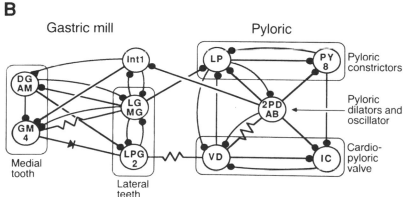

type can be studied repeatedly. Local circuits show persisting rhythmic activity after separation from extrinsic neural connections, so that the intrinsic operations can be observed in isolation. The results provide descriptions and synthesis of the circuit operations responsible for such rhythmic behaviors as locomotion and feeding (Fig. 11-1).

Oscillatory activity can be generated in small-numbered networks by endogenously bursting neurons that generate trains of action potentials separated by periods of silence, independently of extrinsic influence. Intermittent bursting is generated by the interplay of ionic

Fig. 11-2   (Above) Cable properties of the LP neuron of the stomatogastric ganglion (see Fig. 11-1). Simultaneous intracellular recording from the soma of LP and from one of its large neurites at 500 μm distance from the soma. Synaptic activation occurs in the neurite. The action potentials are greatly attenuated in passage to the soma; the EPSPs are not, illustrating the low-pass filter characteristic of the neurite to soma transit. Membrane potential about −50 mV. *(Below)* Simultaneous intracellular recordings from the LP cell of the ganglion and from one of its antagonists, the PD neuron (see Fig. 11-1). *(Left)* Reciprocal activity patterns of the two cells in normal saline. The trains of action potentials are abruptly terminated by the action of PL and other inhibitory interneurons. Picrotoxin blocks the inhibitory inputs and isolates LP, which now discharges in a nonoscillatory mode. (From Golowasch and Marder, 1992.)

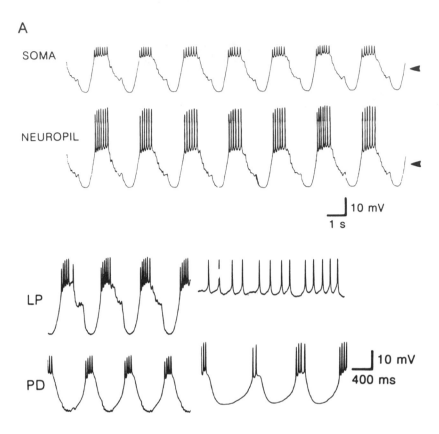

currents confined to the bursting cells. The membrane potentials of bursting neurons oscillate between hyperpolarization with no activity and strong depolarization with repetitive impulse discharge, spike frequency adaptation, postburst hyperpolarization, and postinhibitory rebound (Fig. 11-2, *top*). Oscillations can also be produced in such a network by the synaptic responses and the resulting conductance changes that produce slow changes in membrane potential, in the absence or inactivity of endogenously bursting cells.

Small-numbered oscillatory networks often contain smaller-numbered sets of neurons that drive the oscillatory activity. These "kernels" and their modes of operation are highly conserved, while the patterns of network connectivity are not. Network kernels produce oscillations by several neuronal interactions: recurrent excitations, recurrent or lateral inhibition, or parallel excitation and inhibition (Fig. 11-2, *bottom*). The final output is determined by the interaction

Dynamic Operations in Neocortical Networks

of synaptic and cellular properties and by the properties of the network itself. Many of these processes are inherently nonlinear.

The Stomatogastric Nervous System in Decapod Crustaceans

This small-numbered neural network generates patterns of rhythmic neural discharge that control the muscular activity of the digestive tract, in sequence the esophagus, cardiac sac, gastric mill, and pylorus (Fig. 11-1), each of which displays rhythmic muscular contractions (for reviews, see Cohen et al., 1988; Harris-Warwick et al., 1992; Jacklet, 1989; Selverston and Moulins, 1985). The ganglion contains about 30 neurons arranged in two overlapping, quasi-independent networks. The pyloric network controls the pumping and filtering action of the pylorus. The gastric network contains 10 motoneurons and one interneuron; it controls chewing movements of cartilaginous teeth within the gastric mill. The monosynaptic connections between the 11 neurons of the gastric network have been identified by paired intracellular recording. All the synapses are chemically operated, and several pairs of motoneurons are linked by gap junctions.

The gastric mill of the lobster is quiescent in the resting, unfed animal. Movements begin with feeding, recur at intervals of about 10 sec, and continue at slowing rates for many hours, even after food has passed into the pyloric chamber. The pattern of motoneuron discharge driving the repetitive motor activity disappears if the network is disconnected from extrinsic neural input, but it reappears if excitability is raised by suffusing the isolated network with a muscarinic agonist, revealing the presence of endogenous bursting cells within the network and modulatory cholinergic inputs.

Endogenous bursting is produced by the interplay of both sub- and suprathreshold ionic currents in combinations that vary greatly between species. At least six voltage-gated channels have been identified in neurons of the stomatogastric ganglion, three inward (I_h, $I_{Ca^{2+}}$, and I_{Na^+}) and three outward, all repolarizing K^+ currents (I_A, $I_{O-Ca^{2+}}$, and I_d) (Golowasch and Marder, 1992; Elson and Selverston, 1992).

The spike-initiation zone is located on a neurite several hundred microns from the cell body. Fig. 11-2 illustrates the low-pass filter property of the neurite; the action potentials are attenuated, the slow membrane potentials are not.

Stomatogastric neurons interact synaptically with each other and with the muscles they innervate by spike-evoked synaptic transmission. They are all excitatory to muscles by some axonal branches, inhibitory to other neurons by other branches. The same synaptic transmitter, glutamate, engages different receptors at different synaptic terminals (Cleland and Selverston, 1995). Many interneurons project into the stomatogastric neuropil, and 15 modulatory transmitters have been identified in their synaptic terminals: acetylcholine, GABA, dopamine, histamine, octopamine, serotonin, and nine neuropeptides. Synaptic transmission in this neuropil is complicated by the electrical coupling between neurons, by the graded release of transmitters from terminals without spike initiation, and by the multicomponent nature of synaptic responses.

What were previously thought to be rigidly operating central pattern generators (CPGs) can be modulated by factors that, without changing anatomical connectivity, cause the network to generate different patterns of output and thus different behaviors (Getting, 1989; Marder, 1994; Kaczmarek and Levitan, 1987; Harris-Warwick and Marder, 1991; Selverston, 1993). The oscillatory frequency is modified within a range set by the anatomical connectivity of the network, which through linking circuits with negative or positive feedback forms a generator producing many different patterns by altering synaptic potencies and neuronal excitability in network pathways (Bassler, 1986). The instantaneous distribution of activity in the network is a dependent variable and can be changed rapidly. For example, afferent input from chemoreceptors at the esophageal opening quickly silences the churning and chewing movements of the pylorus and gastric mill, and reorders the activity of all components to generate a sequential swallowing movement that transports food from the esophagus to the lower intestine. The independent activities of the pyloric and gastric circuits slowly return.

Two major inferences derive from these studies. First, local networks may display rhythmic patterns of activity by virtue of the presence of intrinsically bursting neurons; or, rhythmicities may be produced by the intrinsic network properties driven by extrinsic input, itself not rhythmic in nature. Second, the local circuit operations may be changed in a dynamic way by modulatory influences. Modulatory influences create *qualitatively* different patterns of activity in local circuits by influencing both voltage- and ligand-gated channels in circuit neurons, as well as direct and indirect synaptic transmission (Katz and Harris-Warwick, 1990). By analogy, one might predict

Dynamic Operations in Neocortical Networks

a variety of operating states for intrinsic cortical networks, for cortical neurons are equipped with many voltage- and ligand-gated channels and receive a dense synaptic input from the modulatory corticipetal systems of the brainstem core, the basilar forebrain, and from the generalized thalamocortical system. These systems operate with a variety of small-molecule transmitters, ACh and the monoamines, and a large number of peptide transmitters.

What Are the Intrinsic Functions of the Neocortex?

I define *function* in the present context as the intrinsic operation carried out by a local set of cortical microcircuits upon their inputs to produce their outputs. Cortical functions defined this way may have a general significance, and some of their characteristics may be similar in different neocortical areas. Such definitions give no hint of intrinsic operations. Given what Koch and Crick (1994) have called, rightly I think, the "pre-Copernican state of the field," one cannot define exactly the intrinsic function of the neocortex. I give here a list of candidate operations ("functions"); there are undoubtedly others I have neglected.

1. *Thresholding:* a nonlinear relation between the level of presynaptic input and cortical neuronal discharge; for many neurons a linear region is present between impulse threshold and saturation.

2. *Amplification* of inputs: e.g., a single impulse in a single myelinated fiber of a peripheral nerve in an attending human suffices to evoke a conscious perception. The amplification occurs in each synaptic station of the afferent pathway but is especially strong in the primary sensory areas of the cortex (e.g., area 3b).

3. The *derivative* function: cortical operations tend to accentuate and amplify transient inputs, adapt to constant ones.

4. *Feature convergence:* the creation of a neural representation of a complex feature or set of features by combining signals of two or more simpler ones.

5. The *distribution* function: some areas receive the neural signals of certain simpler features of sensory stimuli and distrib-

ute them separately to other cortical areas. Areas 3b and V1, in addition to having other functions, serve as distribution centers.

6. *Coincidence detection* by convergence of excitation, linking together two events that occur closely in time.

7. *Synchronization* and coherence of activity in the different nodes of distributed systems (see Chapter 12).

8. *Long-term storage and recall:* the mechanism is unknown (see Chapter 6).

9. *Pattern generation:* creation of spatial and temporal patterns in output signals that are not present in inputs (e.g., induced rhythms).

10. Specific *neuronal coding and decoding,* which allow precise detections and discriminations between different inputs.

Operations in Defined Neocortical Microcircuits

The classic outline of intracortical connectivity was first described in terms of layer of origin and termination during nearly a century of study with the Golgi method initiated by Cajal (for a collection of Cajal's publications and an informative survey of his work, see DeFelipe and Jones, 1988a). A general summary of intracortical connectivity patterns is shown by the diagram of Fig. 11-3. If the reader will imagine that diagram overlaid with the terminal pattern of even one of the modulatory systems that project from the brainstem to the neocortex (e.g., Fig. 3-12), I believe he will be impressed, as I am, by the apparently impenetrable complexity of the cerebral cortex. It is the conclusion of many that a productive approach to the problem is to define the connectivity and functional properties of microcircuits in the cortex *as circuits.* This is what a number of neuroscientists have worked almost incessantly to do, and they have made significant progress in defining the static connectivity in cortical microcircuits. The problem of intrinsic dynamic operations within those microcircuits has remained relatively intractable, but some progress has been made; more awaits new methods.

There are several complementary approaches. One is to study cortical neurons by intracellular recording in slice preparations, and to

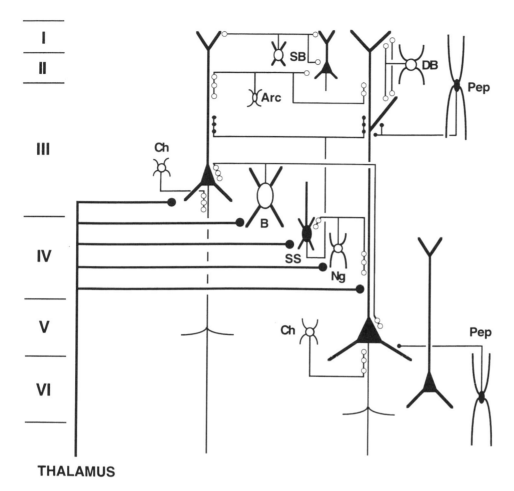

I

II

III

IV

V

VI

THALAMUS

Fig. 11-3 A schematic outline of cortical neurons and their interconnections, including the terminations of the specific thalamocortical afferents. Solid dots, excitatory terminals; open circles, inhibitory terminals; solid cells, excitatory; shaded cells, inhibitory. Cell designations are: *Arc,* arcade; *B,* large basket; *Ch,* chandelier; *DB,* double bouquet; *Ng,* neurogliaform; *Pep,* peptide cells; *SS,* spiny stellate, or spiny nonpyramidal; *SB,* small basket. (From Jones, 1991; modified by Yoshioka, 1997.)

combine this with methods for defining intrinsic cellular properties and connectivity. This has yielded a mass of new information, a part of which I describe below. Another approach is to record intracellularly from neurons in the intact brain, determine to the degree possible the functional properties of the cell impaled, inject it with marker, and reconstruct from sections prepared later the connectiv-

Table 11-1. General properties of neurons in the mammalian neocortex.

Cell type	Location (layer)	Transmitter[a]	Synaptic action[b]	Discharge pattern[c]	Intrinsic input[d]	Intrinsic output[d]
1. Spiny pyramidal	II/III	Glu	EX	RS-1	2–10	1, 2, 3–10, 30
2. Spiny pyramidal	V	Glu	EX	RS, IB	1, 5, 7, 8, 9, 10	1–10
3. Spiny pyramidal	VI	Glu	EX	RS-1, RS-2	1, 2, 5–10, 30	1, 2, 3–10, 30
4. Spiny nonpyramidal	III/IV	Glu	EX	RS-1, ?FS	4, 10	1–10
5. Large basket	III, V, VI	GABA	IN	FS	1–10	1, 2, 3
6. Small basket	II, III	GABA	IN	FS	1–10	1, 2
7. Double bouquet	II, III	GABA	IN	FS	1–10	1–3, 5–10
8. Chandelier	II, III, V, VI	GABA	IN	FS	1–10	1, 2, 3
9. "Peptide"	II, III	GABA	IN	FS	?	1, 10
10. Neurogliaform	II–VI	GABA	IN	FS	4	4, ?
11. Cajal-Retzius	I	Glu	EX	?	13, ?	1, 2, 3
12. Small (layer I)	I	GABA	IN	?	?	?
13. Martinotti	V, VI	GABA	IN	?	?	?
14. Interstitial	White matter	GABA	IN	FS	?	?
15. Inverted pyramidal	VI	?	?	?	?	?

a. Glu = glutamate; GABA = gamma-aminobutyric acid.
b. EX = excitatory; IN = inhibitory.
c. RS = regular spiking; IB = intrinsically bursting; FS = fast spiking (see Table 5-1).
d. Locations and cell types numbered as in table or as follows:
17. Acetylcholinergic cells of the forebrain and pons
18. Dopaminergic cells of the substantia nigra and pons

ity of the cell. Despite the laborious nature of this work, microcircuits slowly emerge, particularly from the research programs of Martin, Douglas, Whitteridge, and their colleagues (e.g., see Martin and Whitteridge, 1984; Martin, 1988; Douglas et al., 1989; Douglas and Martin, 1991; Ahmed et al., 1994), and of Gilbert and Wiesel (1979, 1983, 1989; Gilbert, 1983). Each of these groups has worked on the striate cortex of the cat. I describe some of the results obtained below. First, I shall describe in a general way prototypical intracortical microcircuits. These latter are processing chains of neurons linked together in specific connectivities; they are neither uniformly nor ran-

Table 11-1 (continued)

Cell type	Extrinsic inputs[d]	Extrinsic outputs[d]	Peptides	Calcium-binding proteins
1. Spiny pyramidal	17–21, 22, 23, 27, 28, 29	22, 23, 30	None	Calbindin
2. Spiny pyramidal	17–21, 27, 28	24–27, 30	None	Calbindin
3. Spiny pyramidal	17–21, 27, 28	28, 29, 30	None	Calbindin
4. Spiny nonpyramidal	17, 21, 28	None	None	Calbindin
5. Large basket	17–21, 27, 28	None	None	Parvalbumin
6. Small basket	17–21, 27, 28	None	?	?
7. Double bouquet	17–21, 27, 28	None	Substance P Somatostatin Tachykinin	Calretinin Calbindin
8. Chandelier	17–21	None	Corticotrophin releasing factor	Parvalbumin
9. "Peptide"	17–21	None	Cholecystokinin Vasoactive intestinal peptide Neuropeptide Y Somatostatin	?
10. Neurogliaform	17–21, 28	None	?	Calbindin
11. Cajal-Retzius	17–21, 27, 28	None	?	Calretinin
12. Small (layer I)	17–21, 27, 28	None	Neuropeptide Y	Calbindin
13. Martinotti	17–21	None	Substance P Somatostatin	?
14. Interstitial	17–21	None	Neuropeptide Y Substance P Somatostatin	?
15. Inverted pyramidal	17–21	None	?	?

d. (continued)
19. Noradrenergic cells of the locus ceruleus
20. Histaminergic cells of the hypothalamus
21. Serotonergic cells of the raphe nuclei
22. Ipsilateral cortical areas
23. Contralateral cortical areas
24. Spinal cord
25. Pons and medulla
26. Midbrain
27. Generalized thalamic nuclei
28. Principal (relay) thalamic nuclei
29. Claustrum
30. Horizontally distant patches

domly distributed or connected. The position of each neuron in such a processing chain is critical, and interchange of neuronal position or connection would radically change network operations. No neocortical microcircuit exists in isolation, for to variable degrees each is synaptically connected to others, and every neuron in every microcircuit receives direct synaptic inputs from the cortically projecting modulatory systems of brainstem and basilar forebrain origin.

A cortical microcircuit within a column contains a comparatively small number of neurons synaptically linked in a processing chain that leads from some particular input, intrinsic or extrinsic, to some particular targets that may or may not be cortical output channels. Some microcircuits appear to execute a particular operation (a "computation") upon their inputs to produce those outputs, but even the most canonical of microcircuits can be dynamically modified in its operation by modulatory control.

Many of the facts of cortical cell morphology, connectivity, and synaptic mechanisms are summarized in Table 11-1. Fig. 11-3 summarizes some of these facts in another way. Many exceptions and additions will be obvious to those interested in such specialized cortical areas as the primate striate area 17 (Lund et al., 1994). The facts gathered here come from the results of earlier studies made using the Golgi method (Peters and Jones, 1984; Peters and Rockland, 1994), and from the many new discoveries and clarifications of older uncertainties made with several new methods. This new knowledge of intracortical connectivity has led to speculative models designed to test which conjectured operations are feasible and which are not within the constraints of the known connectivity (Martin, 1988; Douglas and Martin, 1991; Worgotter and Koch, 1991; Somers et al., 1995); it has also motivated direct experimental study of microcircuits in the intact mammal.

The Prototypical Intracortical Circuits

I describe first the general pattern of microcircuit organization in a prototypical area of neocortex. It is not the detailed pattern for any particular area. The pervasive picture in cortical microcircuits is one of powerful excitatory drive coupled with a number of relatively short, superimposed inhibitory circuits—e.g., the basket cells to the somata and proximal dendrites of pyramidal cells; the chandelier cells to the initial axonal segments of pyramidal cells; the neuroglia-form cells to the excitatory interneurons; the double bouquet cells to the dendritic branches of the large majority of pyramidal cells. These local circuit connections have been determined by anatomical methods. We have no idea of the strength of those inhibitory loops in the active, waking cortex. Nor is it certain that the designated targets determined by these methods are the only ones engaged by the particular cells in question. What we do know is that even a mild suppression of GABA transmitter action leads quickly to a synchronized excitation of intracortical circuits by the intrinsically bursting cells of layer V (Chagnac-Amitai and Connors, 1989).

The most intensively studied neocortical microcircuits are those in primary sensory areas activated by afferent inputs from the related sensory thalamic nuclei: the auditory and visual cortices from the medial and lateral geniculate nuclei, respectively, the postcentral somatic sensory cortex from the ventrobasal complex. The advantages for experimental analysis are several. Brief stimuli delivered to the related peripheral sensory sheet elicit synchronous volleys of impulses relayed securely through the system and into the cortex. A sensory cortical area and its related thalamic nucleus can be isolated in a brain slice containing both for more detailed physiological study. Simultaneous observations can be made in the intact, waking monkey of sensory-perceptual performance and the discharge patterns of sensory cortical cells evoked by the same stimuli, and correlations sought between the two. Comparable studies made in motor cortical areas as monkeys execute motor tasks have been equally productive.

The thalamocortical afferents from a sensory thalamic nucleus, like those from the ventrobasal complex to postcentral area 3b, make monosynaptic contacts via collaterals of passage with the pyramidal cells of layers V and VI, and they synapse more densely with three classes of interneurons: the excitatory spiny nonpyramidal cells of layers III and IV, the inhibitory neurogliaform cells of IV, and the large basket cells of III and V (Fig. 11-3). Whether the direct inputs to the pyramidal cells of V and VI are sufficiently convergent to secure a monosynaptic rapid-action pathway through the cortex is unknown. The synaptic drive of the excitatory interneurons sustains very high frequency transmission, up to 200/sec in the unanesthetized monkey's postcentral gyrus (Mountcastle et al., 1969). These cells project to and receive synaptic input back from adjacent excitatory interneurons, creating a small microcircuit that provides powerful excitatory drive at the input level of the cortical column (Douglas et al., 1995). Its output is projected directly to the pyramidal cells of III and

II, as well as to inhibitory interneurons of the supragranular layers. The excitatory input to layer IV also drives the inhibitory neuroglia-form cells, which in turn project to the adjacent pyramidal cells. These fast-spiking inhibitory interneurons are driven at high frequencies when mechanical stimuli are delivered to the surround inhibitory receptive field of a postcentral pyramidal cell. The large basket cells are also thought to play a role in lateral inhibition, and perhaps also pericolumnar inhibition, by their horizontal projection to pyramidal cells located adjacent to the zone of action driven by the peripheral stimulus. The evidence from connectivity (Fig. 11-3) indicates that the pyramidal cells of II and III deliver a strong excitatory drive to the pyramidal cells of the infragranular layers via collaterals emitted from their axons as they leave the cortex. The pyramidal cells of those deeper layers innervate via their own axon collaterals virtually all cells in layers II, III, and IV, with some different distributions in different cortical areas. A proportion of the pyramidal cells of VI project, separately for separate populations, to the thalamic relay nucleus and to the claustrum, but many do not emit axons into the white matter, at least in some areas (Wiser and Callaway, 1996). The pyramidal cells of II/III receive and send monosynaptic links to cells of the same layers in other cortical areas, but whether these projections sustain monosynaptic input-output operations has not been established.

The operations of cortical microcircuits are carried out within the physical constraints of network connectivity, and at any given instant are determined by dynamic variations in synaptic excitability. Those variables are readily changed by action in the several modulatory systems that innervate the cortex; the range of activity states within a given microcircuit may therefore be considerable, as the example of the gastropod ganglion described above illustrates. It is obvious from the connectivity diagram of Fig. 11-3 that a number of other microcircuits exist and may be engaged sequentially and in parallel by afferent input over thalamocortical fibers. Included in these circuits are the double bouquet cells that, by innervating virtually all pyramidal cells and many classes of inhibitory interneurons, impose a strong columnar distribution of inhibition and disinhibition across the cortical layers; the recurrent collateral horizontal projections of pyramidal cells of layers III and V to local areas of cortex hundreds of micrometers away; and the chandelier cells' inhibitory clamp on the spike-initiation zone of pyramidal cells.

One can conjecture that activation of a cortical module over other afferent pathways, like those from other cortical areas projecting into layers III and II, will activate intracortical microcircuits in ways quite different from that described. It has not yet been possible to devise a direct experimental approach to investigate these problems. Inferences drawn from several indirect ones are described in that which follows.

Studies in Neocortical Slices

It was McIlwain who first showed that an excised slice of neocortex remains metabolically active for hours in an oxygenated, artificial cerebrospinal fluid. Later, with Li, he demonstrated that neurons in a slice maintain membrane potentials in the normal range (Li and McIlwain, 1957). (For general reviews, see Dingledine, 1984; Kerkut and Wheal, 1981; McIlwain, 1984.) Studies with this method have extended knowledge of cortical cell phenotypes derived originally from Golgi studies and provided a precise taxonomy of cortical neurons. The general conclusion is that there is a remarkable uniformity of cortical cell phenotypes both between different areas in a single mammalian neocortex and between different mammalian species. Research with the method has allowed definition of the biophysical properties of cortical neurons and how these change in development, and how response characteristics differ between different cell types, both to direct membrane polarizations and to synaptic excitation. It has also led to a description of voltage-dependent and synaptically evoked ionic conductances. The slice method is that most commonly used for study of long-term potentiation and depression at cortical synapses (Chapter 6) and of the mechanisms of cortical epileptogenesis.

The power of this method is increased by its combination with intracellular injection of markers, which permits definition of cell morphology and synaptic contacts (for examples, among many, see Mason and Larkman, 1990; Larkman and Mason, 1990), and now with pre-experimental injection into target areas of retrogradely transmitted markers to define both the cell and its extracortical target (Kaspar et al., 1994). In combination with scanning laser photostimulation for the photolysis of such caged molecules as glutamate or Ca^{2+}, it allows study of molecular events on a rapid time scale (Katz and Dalva, 1994; Yuste and Katz, 1991; Yuste et al., 1994, 1995) and of the transition from gap junction continuity to synaptic contiguity in the developing neocortex (Peinado et al., 1993a; Yuste et al., 1992).

Many groups of investigators have contributed to the astounding success of the slice method, notably among others David Prince and his colleagues (see, e.g., Connors et al., 1982; and *The Cortical Neuron,* edited by Gutnick and Mody, 1995). More than 2,000 papers have been published in the last two decades describing studies based on this method, with no end in sight.

Recently the use of double intracellular recording has provided information concerning microcircuit connectivity and synaptic transmission in rodent visual (Mason et al., 1991) and somatic sensory cortex (Thomson and Deuchars, 1994; Thomson et al., 1993a,b; Deuchars et al., 1994; Deuchars and Thomson, 1995). Action potentials are produced in one cell by electrical stimulation and postsynaptic responses recorded in the other, and the reverse, to determine whether a synaptic relation exists between the two and, if it does exist, its properties. Under these conditions the presynaptic input is confined to a single cell and its axonal tree, the only arrangement I know in which it is possible to study the cortical response to impulses in a single neuron. Iontophoresis of a cell marker allows definition of the cell types and morphological reconstruction of the synaptic targets of the stimulated cell. The results show that both the presynaptic and the postsynaptic neurons exhibit a wide range of synaptic properties. The results are summarized as follows.

PYRAMIDAL CELL TO PYRAMIDAL CELL

Synaptic transmissions from one pyramidal cell to another (P-P) in the same column are strongly excitatory. The postsynaptic response declines precipitously with distance between the two P cells. The axon terminals from one P cell occupy a restricted zone on the dendritic tree of the target P cell; these zones differ greatly between pairs. The synaptic connections between P cells activate both NMDA and non-NMDA receptors. P cells of the infragranular layers exhibit a strong paired pulse depression produced by presynaptic inhibition (Thomson et al., 1993a), perhaps by linking to non-NMDA receptors. By contrast, when P-P linkages to NMDA receptors are stimulated at a slow rate (1/sec), an enduring enhancement of the EPSP occurs. This mechanism will induce reverberating excitatory activity within a columnar pool of P cells (Fig. 11-4). Excitatory recruitment will be limited by the presynaptic inhibition described above.

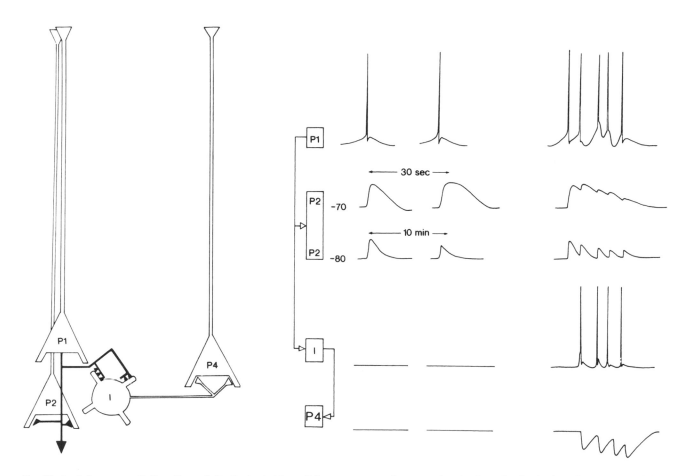

Fig. 11-4 Schema predicting the activity that might result from strong and repeated activation of a single deep-layer pyramidal neuron *(P1)*, summarizing the results of Thomson and her colleagues in double intracellular recording experiments in slice preparations of rodent brains. In these experiments one intracellular electrode remains in a single pyramidal cell and is used to stimulate that cell. The other electrode is used to penetrate and record from as many other neurons as possible. Thus the preparation allows study of activity evoked in cortical local circuits by activation of a single intracortical pyramidal cell. On the right the probable postsynaptic responses in P2, I (inhibitory interneuron), and P4 that would result from repeated 1/sec stimulation of P1 for 30 sec, are illustrated. Reverberating activity in intracortical excitatory circuits within columns recruit additional pyramidal neurons when a single one is repetitively activated. P1 excites P2, and the EPSPs increase in amplitude and duration, evoking an increasing number of action potentials in P2 as the stimulation of P1 continues. Eventually the input from P2 to P4 is sufficiently facilitated to bring P4 to threshold. P4 then excites P1 in turn, facilitating its activity. The burst firing in P1 activates the interneuron *(I)*, which then elicits trains of IPSPs in P4. (From Thomson and Deuchars, 1994.)

Dynamic Operations in Neocortical Networks

Transmission from a P cell to an interneuron (P-IN) is quite different, for these synapses exhibit strong paired pulse facilitation at non-NMDA receptors, a postsynaptic event. Interneurons insert non-NMDA receptors at P cell synapses in their membranes; pyramidal cells insert both NMDA and non-NMDA receptors. Thus the pattern of synaptic transmission is governed in part by postsynaptic mechanisms.

INTERNEURON TO PYRAMIDAL CELL

All the interneurons studied were inhibitory fast-spiking cells. Prolonged trains of presynaptic impulses produced IPSPs in P cells that declined only slowly in amplitude.

The Rodent Barrel Cortex as Model

I described in Chapter 7 the organization, the neuronal phenotypes, and the dynamic activation patterns within a barrel of the rodent trigeminal somatic sensory area. That information provides one of the strong supports for the general hypothesis of the modular organization of the neocortex. Here I return to this experimental model, for it is perhaps the best understood of local modules in terms of the patterns of activity evoked within it by a sensory stimulus. I first repeat here the basic description given in Chapter 7, without reference documentation—to save the reader page-turning.

The modular structures called barrels are most robust in the portion of the rodent somatic sensory cortex devoted to the representation of the contralateral mystacial vibrissae. A barrel is a column containing many minicolumns. There is a strong system-maintained synaptic relation between a single whisker and a corresponding single cortical barrel. Each barrel, limited to layer IV, consists of a cell-rich wall and a cell-poor interior. Neurons above and below each barrel of layer IV are aligned in the columnar manner. Neuronal phenotypes and the intrinsic synaptic connections resemble in general those described above for the prototypical mammalian neocortex.

Neurons of layers II, III, and IV of a rodent barrel are activated by movements of only a single contralateral whisker; 64 percent of infragranular neurons are activated by movements of more than one. The regular-spiking neurons are tuned to the direction of movement, the fast-spiking neurons are not (Simons, 1978). Armstrong-James et al.

(1987, 1991, 1992) took advantage of the fact that a brief deflection of a mystacial vibrissa evokes a synchronous volley of impulses in a few first-order fibers, and in the related neurons projecting through the system to the cortical barrel. Under conditions of light general anesthesia, activation latencies of cortical neurons can be measured and compared. The brief whisker deflection first activates the neurons of layers IV and Vb. Activity is then transferred upward from IV to III and II, just as the first activity reaches Va. Cortical activity evoked by a brief volley in thalamic afferents is first relayed vertically within the barrel, and only after 3–4 msec is there transcortical spread to adjacent columns (see Fig. 7-17). Invasion of a column by a specific thalamocortical afferent volley activates the inhibitory interneurons at shortest latency, accounting for in-field and surround inhibition, and is quickly followed by the pattern of excitatory transmissions described above.

Until now this work has dealt only with very brief cortical activations evoked by synchronous thalamocortical volleys. It has revealed little of what transformations might be imposed within these cortical circuits upon more extended neural activity. The whiskers of the rodent are used in whisking, from which he derives a spatially extended and temporally continuous image of his spatial surround. It is appropriate now to study, with multielectrode recording, the barrel transformations in a waking, whisking rodent.

Microcircuit Operations in the Visual Cortex

The studies of the striate visual cortex by Hubel and Wiesel (1962), Peter Bishop (Bishop et al., 1973; Henry et al., 1974), and Otto Creutzfeldt (Creutzfeldt et al., 1974), and by many who followed them, provided phenomenological descriptions of the representations of complex features of visual scenes in the activity patterns of striate cortical neurons. These features are for the most part not transduced at the first-order input of the visual system, but are constructed in the visual cortex. Binocularity is the most obvious of these, produced by the convergence upon cortical neurons of two sets of geniculocortical fibers, each driven from one of the two eyes (Barlow et al., 1967; Poggio and Fisher, 1977). Other transformations lead to spatial frequency and velocity tuning and to orientation and directional selectivity, etc.

Intracortical transformations have been subjects of intensive study

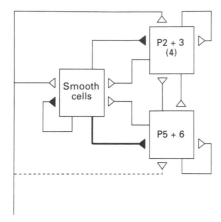

Thalamus

Fig. 11-5 Block diagram constructed by Douglas and Martin to model the intracellular responses recorded in the visual cortex of the cat, evoked by stimulation of thalamic afferent fibers. Three populations of cells are indicated: the inhibitory (closed synapses) nonspiny cells and the excitatory (open synapses) superficial *(P2+3)* and deep *(P5+6)* pyramidal cells. The layer 4 spiny stellate cells *(4)* are grouped with the superficial pyramidal cells. Some neurons in each of the three populations receive excitatory input from the thalamus; the thalamic drive to the superficial set of cells is stronger in the solid lines than in the dashed lines. The inhibitory cells activate both GABA$_A$ and GABA$_B$ receptors on pyramidal cells. The thick continuous line from the smooth cells indicates that the inhibitory input to the deep pyramidal cell population is relatively greater than that to the superficial population. (From Douglas and Martin, 1991.)

since their first descriptions, enabled greatly by definitions of cell-to-cell connectivity within cortical microcircuits—e.g., by the work of Gilbert and Wiesel (Gilbert, 1983, 1993) and of Douglas, Martin, and Whitteridge. The latter group has used the label-and-reconstruct method to define the initial microcircuit in the cat striate cortex engaged by geniculocortical afferents. Their diagram, as shown in Fig. 11-5, does not include the important discovery that a local excitatory microcircuit projects upon the first postsynaptic neurons to exert there a strong amplification (Martin, 1988; Douglas et al., 1989; Douglas and Martin, 1991). The majority of neurons of the striate (outside the puffs) and immediately prestriate cortical areas are orientation-selective, a feature regarded as a first step in the neural mechanisms of contour recognition. Orientation selectivity is a strong property of the simple cells in layer IV of the striate cortex. Simple cells subtend elongated ($2\times - 10\times$) receptive fields that consist of one or more pairs of on and off regions of roughly equal width, placed alongside. They are activated by visual stimuli, of appropriate sign in the appropriate subfield, that consist of elongated contrast steps, edges, or gratings placed over the long dimension of the subfield, and are acutely sensitive to stimulus orientation, with half-widths at half-heights of the tuning curves of about 20 degrees.

A question debated for some time is whether orientation selectivity is a projected feature that depends upon the convergence upon cortical neurons of sets of geniculate cells, that by virtue of either (a) a special arrangement of their own receptive fields along a line in space or (b) the projection of an orientation selectivity of retinal origin creates by that convergence the orientation selectivity of cortical neurons. Alternatively, much evidence suggests that while a weak orientation selectivity may indeed be a projected property, the florid selectivity of cortical neurons must depend upon a further, powerful elaboration of that feature by intracortical mechanisms. Several models have been proposed to account for orientation selectivity of striate neurons. Four are outlined schematically in Fig. 11-6 (Vidyasagar et al., 1996).

The simplest model has as its basis the origin of orientation selectivity in the elliptical receptive fields of (some) retinal ganglion cells, and projection of that property to cells of the lateral geniculate nucleus (LGN). Cat retinal ganglion cells respond in a weakly selective way to line-segment stimuli placed over the long axis of their receptive fields. The orientation bias of retinal ganglion cells is one-sixth

Dynamic Operations in Neocortical Networks

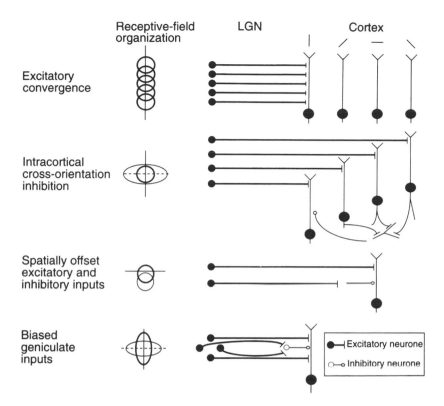

Excitatory
convergence

Intracortical
cross-orientation
inhibition

Spatially offset
excitatory and
inhibitory inputs

Biased
geniculate
inputs

Receptive-field
organization

LGN

Cortex

● ⊢ Excitatory neurone
○ ─● Inhibitory neurone

Fig. 11-6 Schemes that have been proposed to explain the orientation sensitivity of cells in the striate cortex. The receptive field organizations of various cortical cells are shown in terms of the relevant geniculate inputs; regions within thick lines mark excitatory input, those within thin lines inhibitory inputs. The straight line indicates the optimum orientation of the cortical cell responses, and the dashed line (where shown) represents the optimum orientation of inhibitory input to the cell. All direct geniculate inputs to the cortex are assumed to be excitatory; inhibitory inputs are routed through intracortical inhibitory interneurons. The four short lines above the cortical neurons represent the optimum orientation of different orientation columns. (From Vidyasagar et al., 1996.)

that of striate simple cells (Levick and Thibos, 1982). A similarly weak orientation bias is observed for LGN neurons in the cat, limited to certain spatial frequencies (Jones and Sillito, 1994; Schall et al., 1986; Shou and Levanthal, 1989; Soodak et al., 1987; Vidyasagar, 1984; Vidyasagar and Heide, 1984; Vidyasagar and Urbas, 1982; Thompson et al., 1994). This selectivity survives removal of the cortical projections to the LGN. The selectivity of LGN cells has not been observed in many other experiments, and few attribute the sharp orientation selectivity of visual cortical neurons to a simple projection property constructed at the LGN level.

The hypothesis proposed by Hubel and Wiesel to explain orientation selectivity puts a heavy requirement on developmental mechanisms. It requires that sets of geniculate neurons whose receptive fields are arranged along lines in space converge upon each single striate neuron to produce the latter's selectivity (Fig. 11-7A). Thus an *on* subregion of a simple cell receptive field is produced by the convergence of a set of *on* LGN neurons whose fields are arranged on a

Fig. 11-7 Receptive field mechanisms producing orientation specificity of simple cells of the visual cortex of the cat. (a) According to the original model of Hubel and Wiesel, afferent connections from LGN cells, whose receptive fields are aligned in a row to form an elongated line, project monosynaptically to the cortical neuron, thus producing its orientation. (b) The data obtained in a recent cross-correlation study by Reid and Alonso of the monosynaptic relations between LGN cells and cortical simple cells support the original hypothesis. The elliptical regions are the central (solid lines) and flanking (dashed lines) subregions of an idealized cortical simple cell. The circles represent the receptive field centers of X cells (23 of 74 cells studied with overlapping receptive fields) that were connected monosynaptically to a simple cell; solid line, same sign (on or off) as the strongest (central) simple-cell subregion; dashed line, same sign as the weaker, flanking subregions. The same-sign (solid) LGN cells tended to lie along the length of the central subregion, the opposite-sign (dashed) LGN cells tended to be over the more prominent flank. This result provides evidence for very precise connections between LGN and cortex and supports the original hypothesis of Hubel and Wiesel for the cat striate cortex. (From Reid and Alonso, 1966.)

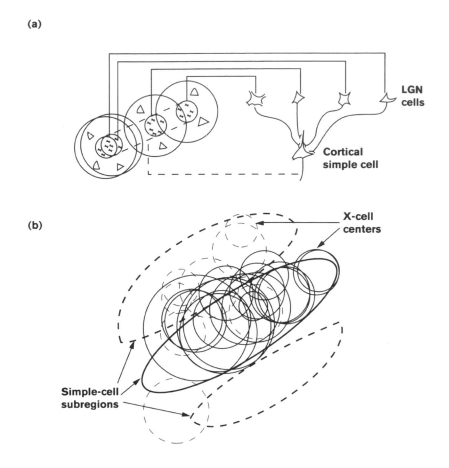

line in space, and a similar relation was posed for the projection of a line of *off* LGN cells to the *off* field of the simple cell.

On this model further intracortical processing to strengthen orientation selectivity is neither invoked nor denied. A number of experimental findings support this model. Chapman et al. (1991) eliminated with cytotoxins the activity of cells in the ferret striate cortex and recorded from the terminals of geniculocortical fibers in what was conjectured to be a single cortical orientation column. They observed that the receptive fields of the fibers were arranged in the linear spatial array required by the model. Ferster et al. (1996) cooled the striate cortex, to eliminate synaptic activity from intracortical sources, and recorded intracellularly the local postsynaptic responses of simple cells to visual stimulation. While cooling reduced the amplitudes of the evoked EPSPs by factors of 5 to 20, the remaining responses were orientation-selective. Reid and Alonso (1995, 1996) recorded simultaneously from LGN and striate cortex in cats and sought neurons in the two sets with overlapping receptive fields and a monosynaptic connection from thalamic to cortical cell. They then measured the cross-correlations between the two sets of impulse discharges (see also Toyama et al., 1981; Tanaka, 1983). The results shown in Fig. 11-7B indicate that when these conditions are met, the receptive fields of LGN cells do align along the long dimensions of the fields of simple striate cells. Nevertheless, it has seemed to many that some further intracortical process is necessary to account for the orientation selectivity of striate cells.

Considerable experimental evidence supports the eclectic model of the orientation mechanism schematized in Fig. 11-8. The model combines a weak selectivity in precortical elements with intracortical processes that accentuate that feature. Combinations of this sort are the centerpieces of several modeling studies (Worgotter and Koch, 1991; Somers et al., 1995; Vidyasagar et al., 1996). Each of these combines excitatory and inhibitory mechanisms in the local microcir-

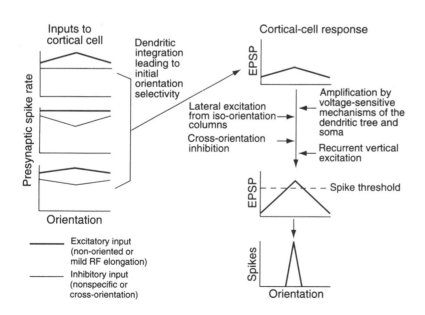

Fig. 11-8 A more eclectic model accounts for orientation selectivity of simple cells of the visual cortex. An initial mild orientation sensitivity can be produced in the postsynaptic potential (PSP) responses of a striate cortical cell by any one of three possible combinations of excitatory and inhibitory inputs shown in the left columns; any inhibitory input is assumed to be via cortical inhibitory interneurons. The biases of the thalamic inputs might reflect the biases seen in individual cells of the lateral geniculate nucleus *(LGN)* by some investigators; or, it might arise from a modest convergence of two or more LGN fields in a row. Such a mild orientation selectivity of the PSP response is amplified by a number of candidate cortical mechanisms, shown on the right. The contributions of each of these mechanisms may vary from cell to cell. *EPSP,* excitatory postsynaptic potential; *RF,* receptive field. (From Vidyasagar et al., 1996.)

cuits to account for the cortical operation. The relevant experimental observations are as follows.

EXCITATORY MECHANISMS

Douglas and Martin (1991) proposed that layer IV spiny neurons are connected with adjacent spiny neurons by tight excitatory loops that function to amplify synaptic transmission from the weakly oriented geniculocortical input to the layer IV simple cells. This was suggested by the observation that only 5–20 percent of the excitatory synaptic terminals (which are 85 percent of all synaptic terminals) on layer IV spiny stellate cells are derived from geniculocortical afferent fibers (Ahmed et al., 1994; Anderson et al., 1994a,b). Direct evidence for this strong excitatory loop—e.g., recording of the activity of the cell in the proposed microcircuit as animals make orientation detections and discriminations—is not yet available.

INHIBITORY MECHANISMS

The question is whether excitatory mechanisms can account fully for the sharpening of orientation selectivity produced by striate micro-circuits or whether inhibitory processes are also at work. Some of the earliest studies of orientation selectivity led to the suggestion that responses to orthogonally placed stimuli were inhibited by the actions of adjacent or distant neurons with orthogonal selectivities, and thus by a cross-inhibition contributing to selectivity (Henry et al., 1974; Creutzfeldt et al., 1974; Morrone et al., 1991). This left unexplained how orientation selectivity was created in the cross-inhibiting elements in the first place. Sillito et al. (1980) found that local iontophoresis of N-methyl bicuculline, which inhibits GABA interneuron, suppressed orientation selectivity for many striate cortical neurons and eliminated it completely for some. Local injection of the same inhibitor some distance away (5–600 μm) from a recorded striate cell suppressed its orientation selectivity (Crook and Eysel, 1992; Crook et al., 1991). It was a surprise, then, when some of the first intracellular recording experiments revealed that the strongest inhibition of a striate cell was produced by iso-oriented stimuli, and that hyperpolarizing PSPs were only rarely evoked by nonoriented stimuli; no shunting inhibition was observed (Douglas et al., 1988, 1991; Berman et al., 1991; Ferster and Jagadeesh, 1992). The relative unimportance of inhibition appears to be supported by the experiment of Nelson et al. (1994), who found that orientation selectivity survived

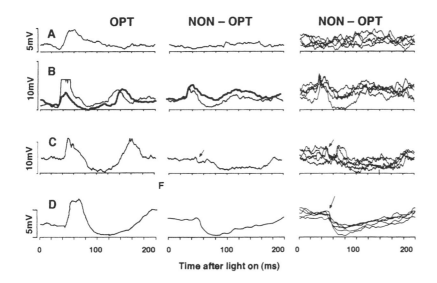

OPT   NON – OPT   NON – OPT

A

B

C

F

D

Time after light on (ms)

Fig. 11-9 Postsynaptic potentials of neurons in the visual cortex of anesthetized cats, recorded intracellularly from four different cells (A–D, thin lines) with the whole-cell *in vivo* technique. The responses were evoked by flashing bars on the receptive fields of the cells placed at different positions and orientations. The traces on the left, evoked by the optimally oriented bars, are averages of five responses each. The excitatory postsynaptic responses are obvious, but no clear inhibitory responses are present. The five individual traces on the right and their average, displayed in the middle, were evoked by nonoptimally oriented bars. Three of the four cells show clear inhibitory postsynaptic potentials. The thick lines in B are postsynaptic responses to stimuli delivered during passage of a hyperpolarizing current. X. Pei, T. R. Vidyasagar, and O. D. Creutzfeld, "Receptive field analysis and orientation selectivity of postsynaptic potentials of simple cells in cat visual cortex," *Journal of Neuroscience* 14(11): 7130–7140 (1994).

blockade of inhibitory action by intracellular injection of chloride channel blockers. However, the patch-clamp experiments of Pei et al. (1994) indicate that inhibition is indeed produced by nonoptimal stimuli (Fig. 11-9), although it may be small and in some neurons absent altogether. The model of Fig. 11-8 takes this into account. The discovery that orientation selectivity, as measured by PSPs, narrows in the first few tens of milliseconds after the onset of a visual stimulus is interpreted as further evidence that intrinsic cortical operations play an important role in orientation selectivity (Eysel and Shevelev, 1994).

The question is not settled whether orientation selectivity is produced by a simple projection/convergence mechanism, or whether such a convergence is combined with intracortical microcircuit operations that enhance this feature, or whether orientation selectivity is generated by intracortical processing alone. The weight of evidence appears to favor the latter, particularly in the primate. The respective roles and importance of excitation and inhibition in those intracortical operations remain uncertain. This model also accommodates the patterns of connectivity and dynamic operations in the macaque striate cortex, where neurons in the direct geniculo-recipient sublayers 4A, 4Cα, and 4Cβ have small, nonoriented, monocular receptive fields. Neurons in sublayer 4B, which does not receive direct geniculate input, are orientation-selective and frequently binocular (Hubel and Wiesel, 1968, 1977; Blasdel and Fitzpatrick, 1984). Studies of the dynamic operations producing orientation selectivity in monkey V1 show that tuning of neurons develops within 35–45 msec after stimulus onset and persists for 40–85 msec (Ringach et al., 1997). Cells of the geniculo-receptive layers have a single orientation selectivity that does not change and that may be sharpened in time with further intracortical processing. Cells of the output layers are more broadly tuned to orientations that may change with time and even reverse. The properties of these latter cells are best understood in terms of feedback in intracortical circuits. It appears likely that properties other than binocularity per se are produced by intracortical operations in striate and prestriate areas; a huge literature has accumulated describing their phenomenology, but little is known of the mechanisms producing them.

Transformations in the Homotypical Cortex of the Monkey

The phenomena of feature convergence and new feature construction reach an epitome in the homotypical frontal, temporal, and parietal cortex (for reviews of parietal studies, see Mountcastle, 1995). Feature convergence/construction is true for every neuron class identified in area 7a of the monkey parietal lobe. These combinations of sensory and motor features are integrated with the neural mechanisms of drive states. Parietal neurons display their full feature profiles only if the particulars of the behavioral tasks in which the monkey is engaged have meaning for him—i.e., only if he is interested in and attends them (Mountcastle et al., 1981, 1984). Reach and manipulation neurons are active only when those complex motor acts are directed at targets with similar meaning. Fixation neurons are active only during the interested, visual regard of such objects. Their responses are influenced by the angle of gaze, as are the receptive field distributions of visual neurons (Andersen and Mountcastle, 1983). Saccade neurons are active only during eye movements induced to targets of interest, and not during the spontaneous eye movements that occur in casual regards of the surround. These powerful effects of drive states have been observed routinely, but virtually nothing is known of the mechanisms by which they affect integrative action at the level of homotypical cortex.

The visual neurons of area 7a of the parietal lobe (PVNs) provide a striking example of feature construction. This area receives converging, relayed projections from several prestriate visual areas, as well as from the retina-collicular system via the pulvinar nucleus of the dorsal thalamus. The neurons of no single one of these sources display the full profile of PVN features. Many PVNs are activated from large, bilateral receptive fields that require interhemispheric projections for their composition (Mountcastle and Motter, 1981). PVNs are remarkably sensitive to motion and to the direction of motion of visual stimuli, as are the cells of several source areas projecting to area 7a. In 7a, however, the directionalities are arranged radially, either inward toward the fixation point, as illustrated in Fig. 11-10, or, for another set, outward toward the edges of the visual field (Motter et al., 1987). Moreover, these particular features depend in part upon the act of interested fixation and may not be evident without it, as shown in Fig. 11-11 (Steinmetz et al., 1987). Studies of area 7a revealed a few neurons with more limited properties, as if they might have contributed part features to the final sum, but the cells observed were too few in number to provide direct evidence of how the properties described are composed by intramodular processing. Further knowledge will require multiple microelectrode recording in waking, behaving monkeys.

Modulatory Control of Intrinsic Neocortical Operations

Of the many seemingly intractable problems that confront even the most dauntless experimental neuroscientist, a high place on the list must be given to the mode of action of the modulatory systems upon the intrinsic operations of the neocortex. I gave in Chapter 3 a description of the sources and distributions of these systems, which latter in some cases include much of the brain and spinal cord as well as the neocortex. Modulatory systems engage the cortex in a quasi-tangential way, and their axons run for long distances within the cortex itself, frequently ignoring columnar, areal, and sometimes even lobar divisions. They innervate by the terminals of collaterals, and by *boutons de passage,* thousands of cortical neurons, and perhaps in some cases blood vessels as well. Some may release transmitters directly into the extracellular space, which then reach their receptors in neural membranes by diffusion in volume conduction, although this possibility is much debated. A number of tracer and immunohistochemical experiments have shown that in the primate, if not in the rodent, there are differences in the terminal densities of the nor-

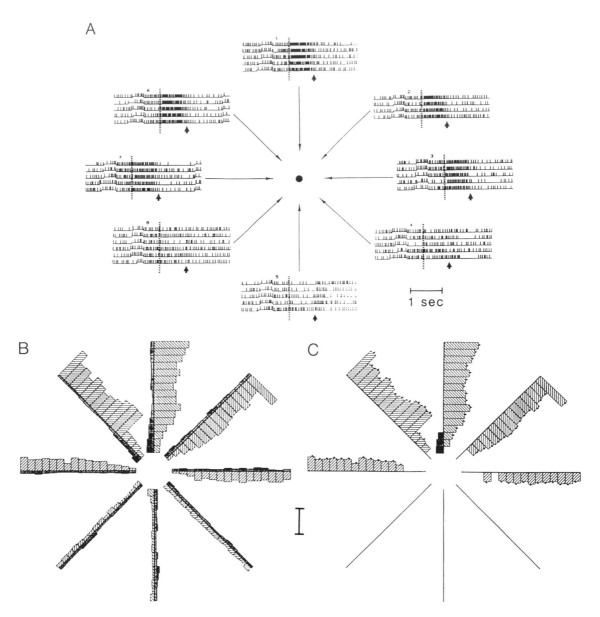

Fig. 11-10 An example of the transformation of visual input in the inferior parietal cortex of the monkey, area 7a. Recordings were made extracellularly from a parietal visual neuron as, in each trial, a waking monkey fixated a target light and detected its dimming for reward. The impulse replicas and radially oriented histograms shown in A display the responses evoked during repeated trials when a 10-degree square visual stimulus moved in each of eight radial directions through the visual field, crossing the fixation point (long arrows). Vertical dashed lines indicate stimulus onset and small arrows the instant the stimulus crossed the fixation point. The radially oriented histograms in B and their statistically significant residues in C show the frequencies of discharge as the stimuli moved inwardly (diagonal shading) and outwardly (solid shading) from the fixation point in each of the eight directions. This is an example of opponent vector organization of this large bilateral visual field, requiring interhemispheric convergence. Bin size, 50 msec; vertical bar = 100 impulses/sec; stimulus velocity, 60 degrees/sec. (From Mountcastle et al., 1984.)

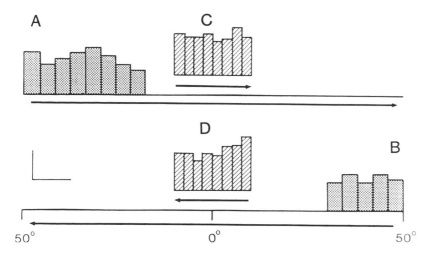

A   C   D   B

50°   0°   50°

Fig. 11-11   Evidence for a transformation of visual input that creates the properties of opponent vector organization and feed-forward inhibition in the posterior parietal cortex of the monkey, area 7a. There is a mismatch of the receptive fields when studied with short- and long-range moving stimuli. Histograms A and B show responses evoked by stimuli moving inwardly along a meridian at 90 degrees/sec. The receptive field extended to the edges of the 50-degree radius tested but spared a large central zone, much in the manner illustrated in Fig. 11-10. Inset histograms C and D show intense but nondirectional responses to identical stimuli moving along 20-degree segments of the same meridian, centered at the point of fixation within the central zone that was unresponsive to the full-field stimuli. This is an example of an intracortical dynamic transformation requiring interhemispheric convergence. (From Motter et al., 1987.)

epinephrine, dopamine, serotonin, and acetylcholine fibers in different cortical areas, between laminae, and between lobes (Wilson and Molliver, 1991a,b; Morrison and Hot, 1992; Morrison et al., 1982, 1992; Lewis et al., 1986, 1987; DeFelipe and Jones, 1988b; for reviews, see Fallon and Loughlin, 1987; Eckenstein and Baughman, 1987; Mesulam et al., 1984; and Saper, 1987). Nevertheless, although densities differ, there is scarcely a cortical area or indeed a cortical neuron devoid of modulatory projections. Complementary studies of the distributions of the receptors for the transmitters of modulatory systems have been made with autoradiographic methods. The results in general conform with the distributions of the terminal fibers of the systems, although in some cases spatial mismatches have been described. A very large literature has accumulated; for reviews see Rakic et al. (1988); Goldman-Rakic et al. (1990, 1992).

An earlier section of this chapter describes how modulatory systems can change in a radical way the output generated by a microcircuit in the gastric ganglion of the lobster, and do so on a rapid time scale without change in microcircuit connectivity. This is likely to be true also for the intrinsic neocortical microcircuits considered here, for each cortical neuron is innervated to some degree, from slight to heavy, by modulatory input. The arrangement in the neocortex resembles in one important way that in the gastropod ganglion, for the modulatory systems in each case deliver to the microcircuits the same array of small-molecule transmitters, as well as a large number of neuropeptides co-localized in the synaptic terminals of the modulatory axons.

Spectacular advances have been made in defining the effect of modulatory transmitters upon the excitability of single cortical neurons by a combination of intracellular recording in cortical slice preparations and local iontophoresis of putative transmitter agents; for general reviews see McCormick (1992); McCormick et al. (1993). The general result is that the responses of cortical neurons to the iontophoretic release of modulator transmitters (e.g., acetylcholine, norepinephrine, serotonin, dopamine, or adenosine) are mediated by the transmitters' effects upon K^+ channels, some of which lead to decreases, others to increases in neuronal excitability. The three principal effects are schematized in Fig. 11-12, which also illustrates the important generality that a coupling of a variety of transmitters, via their specific receptors, to a common second-messenger system leads to changes in channel conductance. The three major effects are these:

1. All the transmitters suppress the Ca^{2+}-activated K^+ current, called I_{AHP}, which normally suppresses the after-hypopolarization and thus slows the rate of discharge of spike frequency in regular-spiking cortical neurons, even during a sustained excitatory input. The suppression of the I_{AHP} current increases cell excitability and the sustained impulse discharge (Fig. 11-12, upper right).

2. Activation of some modulatory receptors shown in Fig. 11-12 (as those for serotonin, $GABA_B$, and adenosine) leads to hyperpolarization by increasing K^+ conductance, shown in Fig. 11-12 as I_{KG}. Increasing the conductance of this channel suppresses cell excitability.

3. Stimulation of serotonin and muscarinic acetylcholine receptors suppresses the I_M (for muscarinic) current. This voltage-dependent K^+ current is completely suppressed at resting membrane potentials more negative than about -75 mV, but it is activated by depolarization and tends to prevent cell discharge and to hyperpolarize the membrane (Fig. 11-12, lower right). Suppression of this current increases cell excitability.

This brief summary of what has been learned about the molecular and cellular mechanisms by which modulatory inputs affect the excitability of single cortical neurons reveals the difficulty in specifying

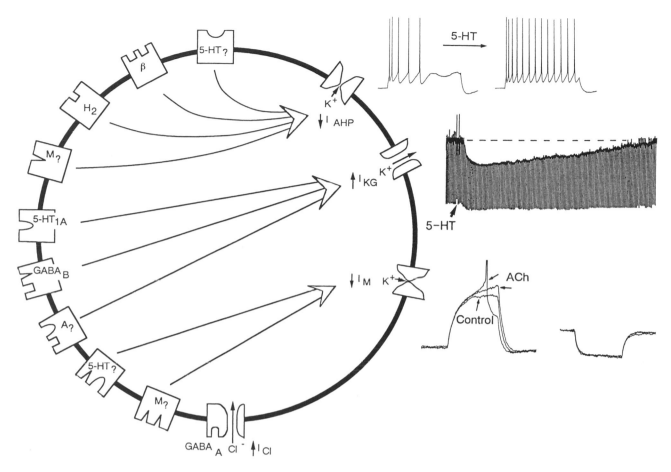

Fig. 11-12 This diagram by McCormick illustrates the postsynaptic action of acetylcholine, adenosine, GABA, histamine, norepinephrine, and serotonin in a schematized cerebral cortical pyramidal cell. Activation of muscarinic, histaminergic, β-adrenergic, and serotonergic receptors results in a suppression of the Ca^{2+}-activated K^+ current (I_{AHP}) and subsequently decreasing spike frequency adaptation, shown in the impulse records (top right). Activation of 5-HT$_{1A}$, GABA$_B$, and adenosine receptors results in a hyperpolarization and inhibition (middle trace, right) through an increase in a potassium current (I_{KG}) that is associated with a G-protein. Stimulation of serotonin *(5-HT)* and muscarinic receptors results in suppression of I_M. Suppression of I_M enhances the response of the cortical neuron to a depolarizing pulse so that after application of acetylcholine a previously subthreshold depolarizing pulse (control, lower right) becomes suprathreshold and generates an action potential (ACh, arrows). In contrast, the response to hyperpolarizing inputs remains unchanged due to the voltage dependence of the M current (bottom traces, right). Only the activation of GABA$_A$ receptors is found to increase membrane chloride conductance. Question marks indicate incomplete identification of receptor subtypes. (From McCormick, 1992. Used with permission of Lippincott-Raven Publishers.)

what effect a particular profile of modulatory inputs will have upon a microcircuit of interconnected neurons. Each of the neurons in the circuit will have a different concentration and distribution of receptors, and perhaps will respond differently to any particular modulatory input; the permutations are virtually endless. What is needed is an experimental arrangement that will allow one to control a particular input to a defined microcircuit, to record a particular output from that microcircuit, and to examine in this way the effect of modulatory influences upon the microcircuit transformations. A formidable experimental challenge!

Microcircuits Are Not "Cell Assemblies"

The use of the word *assembly* (or *collective*, or *aggregate*) to describe sets of neurons linked by connectivity in the neocortex leads to conceptual confusion. One definition of a "cell assembly" is that it is a group of neurons with strong and reciprocal internal connections, so that excitation of some neurons of an assembly leads to spreading activation in the network, and finally to ignition of the whole assembly. Equally misleading is the metaphor comparing the spread of activity in such an assembly to the waves produced in a still body of water by a dropped stone. I know of no population of neurons anywhere in the brain to which these statements apply. Neurons in any local region are arranged in microcircuits that are processing chains, not random distributions. The positions of neurons within such microcircuits are not interchangeable. Neocortical microcircuits have input channels and output channels that vary in number from several to many. Each input channel contributes qualitatively different signals to the processing network. The microcircuit imposes upon these inputs transformations that appear as its outputs. Even for such a small region as a minicolumn of the neocortex, it is likely that the transformation differs in different output channels. These are speculative statements, but they are grounded in knowledge of the connectivity within microcircuits and the properties of their constituent neurons. No cells within microcircuits are reciprocally and identically interconnected, and this is probably true also for the long-range connections between spatially separate modules of the neocortex.

Microcircuits are not cell assemblies; they are not indiscriminate collectives or aggregates. They are complex processing networks, and it is the operations within those network chains we need to know to understand the function of the neocortex.

The Layer V Hypothesis of Cortical Function

Connors and Amitai (Connors and Amitai, 1995; Amitai and Connors, 1996) propose that "the neural network within layer V is uniquely capable of ordering, controlling, coordinating, and synchronizing the activities of the neocortex." Layer V pyramidal cells projecting to subcortical structures are regarded on this hypothesis as the major output channels of the neocortex. All "outputs" to other cortical areas, to the dorsal thalamus, or to the opposite hemisphere are re-entrant to cortex, and are thus regarded as interneurons. They contribute through the distributed systems of which they are parts to the final "integrated" cortical output via the layer V pyramidal cells. This idea rests upon several facts concerning layer V pyramids (Kaspar et al., 1994). (1) Their exuberant, vertically directed recurrent collaterals and their dense horizontal collaterals impose powerful excitation upon large populations of cortical neurons of all classes. Excitation is especially strong in the local groups of neurons whose dendrites are arranged into ascending clusters (Peters and Setharcs, 1996). (2) Layer V contains pyramidal cells of the RS-1, RS-2 (regular spiking) and IB (intrinsically bursting) classes (see Table 5-1). The RS classes are callosally projecting cells; those of the IB class are the true efferents, for they project to extracortical structures. (3) The apical dendrites of layer V pyramidal cells can generate Na^+ action potentials. Excitatory inputs as far away as the dendritic tufts in layer I can have a powerful excitatory effect upon the spike-generating zone of the cell body. (4) Layer V pyramidal cells, especially those of the IB class, readily synchronize their activity, as when GABA inhibition is even slightly reduced. This ready escape from inhibition is of major functional significance for the action of layer V efferents in generating and propagating rhythmic activity in the cortical efferents. Synchronized coherence could have a major driving effect upon the downstream targets of the neocortex.

Koch and Crick (1994) have pursued the layer V hypothesis in an essay on the general subject of the neuronal basis of awareness, particularly of visual awareness. They emphasize that the output of layer V pyramidal cells must contain the results of intracortical computations, thought to be carried out mainly in the supragranular layers in activity that occurs at an unconscious level. The idea is that the layer V pyramidal cells, carrying the output of the intracortical operations, must contribute to conscious awareness. Koch and Crick put particular emphasis upon the intermittently bursting pyramids of layer V, which project to extracortical structures, and propose that the bursts will potentiate synaptic transmission from those axons to their target cells by loading synaptic terminals with excessive Ca^{2+}. This mechanism is proposed as a candidate form of short-term, nonassociative memory. How this idea will survive experimental tests remains to be seen.

It is an old idea that different cortical layers may in some way serve different functions. The early cytoarchitectonists had it just the other way, that the supragranular layers served "psychic" functions, the infragranular layers more workaday chores of brain function. None of these ideas, old or new, takes into account that the neurons of the supra- and infragranular layers are heavily linked in vertically oriented, translaminar processing chains. It seems unlikely that any layer can function independently of any other.

Summary

It is obvious from the above that our knowledge of the intrinsic operations of the cortex is still very limited; what we believe is derived as much from inference as from direct observation. I summarize in the following statements the properties of cortical operation I believe to be true.

1. There are no isolated channels through a cortical module, and no single "canonical" cortical circuit. Although no single afferent channel dominates any single output channel, there are several tight linkages; e.g., specific thalamocortical afferents drive directly the corticothalamic neurons of layer VI and the cells of origin of callosal fibers in layer II of area 3 of the somatic sensory cortex.

2. The neocortex is characterized by many short- and long-range re-current and re-entrant excitatory and inhibitory loops, with particularly strong excitatory drive linked to in-

hibitory control. The pervasive picture is one of a high level of excitation restrained by inhibition.

3. There is only one certainly known class of excitatory interneuron, but these are frequently linked together in powerful feed-forward circuits. There are seven classes of inhibitory interneurons in the cortex, give or take one or two depending upon different modes of classification. Pyramidal cells are both the major efferent channels and the largest class of interneurons in the cortex, by virtue of their exuberant axon collateral systems.

4. A more or less similar operation may occur in all neocortical areas; it is controlled and varied by the changing dynamic activity in many convergent afferent pathways, particularly by the modulatory systems originating in the central core of the brainstem, the basal forebrain, and the intralaminar thalamic nuclei. There is some evidence that microcircuit operations that differ in different areas are superimposed upon the basic pattern.

5. Yet the specificity of operations in cortical areas is maintained, at least over the intermediate time ranges, in the face of dynamically changing states. This must depend at least in part upon the specific nature of the thalamocortical inputs leading to specific patterns of activity in the distributed systems of which the cortical area is a part, for these patterns lead to detections and discriminations, etc., in spite of varying background activity. We retain superbly accurate perceptual functions over the wide range of central states from near-sleep to near-mania!

6. Output neurons "tap off" the internal operation at different stages for projection to different targets. The inference is that signals transmitted, e.g., by the cells of layer III to the contralateral hemisphere differ in some fundamental way from those transmitted via layer V to extracortical structures, or via layer VI to the dorsal thalamus.

7. No single neuron of any area of the neocortex is essential for any operation. The degree of convergence and divergence in

the system and the multiplicity of superimposed loops insures that patterns of activity within even a small population of neurons might continue virtually unchanged even after the randomly distributed loss of a considerable percentage of its members.

8. The modulatory systems set and control the general level of excitability in cortical local networks. Whether these systems can do so differentially for individual cortical areas is unknown.

9. Plasticity is a pervasive characteristic of cortical networks. It has at least three forms:

a. The first occurs almost instantaneously, as the modulatory systems change the "set of the center." The change may include up- or down-regulation of excitability in general, or more specific actions such as switching operations from one path to another.

b. Rapid plastic changes in synaptic patterns occur when afferent input to a neuron is removed. A cortical neuron is quickly captured by a change in the synaptic efficiency of fringe synapses previously below threshold (Chapter 6).

c. Longer-term changes are induced by changes in the pattern of afferent inputs to a neuron, leading to protein synthesis and ultrastructural changes at synapses. These are conjectured to play a role in learning and long-term memory.

Rhythmicity and Synchronization in Neocortical Networks

Oscillations characterize the activity of many living organisms in the plant and animal kingdoms. Much of the electrical activity of the brain, particularly that of the neocortex, is oscillatory in nature. Electroencephalographic (EEG) rhythms in the human cortex vary in frequency from 1 to about 100 Hz, and in amplitude from a few to a few hundred microvolts (μV), shifting readily over those ranges with changes in behavior or in central brain states. Rhythmic undulations in field potentials and the accompanying neuronal synchrony also vary in different areas of the brain. They are not homogeneous and may be produced by different mechanisms at different times and in different places.

The mechanisms producing the EEG include in varying proportions the corticipetal activity in certain thalamocortical systems, the intrinsic cellular properties of cortical neurons, and the system characteristics of local and distributed cortical networks. Following on the classical studies of Morrison, Bremer, Jasper, Moruzzi, and Magoun, a major advance of the last decade has been a substantial increase in knowledge of the cellular mechanisms that produce the EEG, particularly in the stages of and transitions between the sleep-wakefulness cycle. It has proven difficult to study the dynamic, emergent system properties of local neocortical circuits because they are embedded in dense intrinsic networks, and in the extrinsic connections that link each cortical area with other areas and with other brain structures. One approach to the problem is to use as a model a simple, small-numbered circuit that can be isolated, like the gastropod stomatogastric ganglion described in Chapter 11. Studies of that and of many other small-numbered networks have yielded useful inferences for understanding the operations of neocortical microcircuits. One is that the coherent periodicity and self-sustaining oscillations in such networks, properties displayed also by cortical networks, may be produced by either endogenously bursting neurons or by properties of the network itself, or both. Another is that the state of the network can be changed quickly and radically by modulatory inputs, in a circuit with unchanged connectivity.

Model Transition: Hierarchy to Distribution

Action levels in the neocortex extend from the molecular mechanisms involved in synaptic transmission through local cellular integrations to minicolumnar and modular network operations, to areal and system functions. Scholars working at these different levels often differ in the way they think about the brain, and in how they plan experiments and interpret the results obtained. Rather suddenly the intermediate levels between the actions of single central neurons and the global function of the brain in cognition have become major subjects for study, a change generated by new concepts and new methods. System-level studies revealed that the different features of distal stimuli are signaled in separate sets of primary afferent fibers, and that the resulting evoked neuronal activity is processed in spatially separate areas of the neocortex linked in large-scale distributed systems (see Chapter 10). Sets of neurons in these separate nodes from time to time display short periods of intense correlation, both when induced by sensory stimuli and during the brain activity accompanying cognitive states. These facts are essential parts of a number of theories of the integrative action of the brain—e.g., the theory of neuronal group selection, proposed by Gerald Edelman two decades ago (Edelman, 1978) and elaborated more fully since then (Edelman, 1987, 1993).

Studies of dynamic brain activity have led to a hypothesis quite different from the hierarchical model that prevailed hitherto: that is, that at higher levels, the "representation" of an evolving perception is contained in the activity in large-scale systems and is not localized to any single node of such a system (Mountcastle, 1978). Until now, few testable hypotheses have been presented about how the ongoing activity in the neurons of linked nodes of a distributed system can compose in a "representational mode" the central image of a complex stimulus.

The distributed-representation hypothesis requires a mechanism for linking the separate nodes of activity that allows identification of that activity as a coherent whole. It has been proposed that the linking mechanism is a transient (milliseconds in duration) synchronization of the activity of the neurons in the distributed population. Synchronization is regarded as a signature or label that identifies the synchronized set as a coherent whole, a representation. Techniques are now available for recording with many microelectrodes and for analyzing the results obtained so that this binding hypothesis can be tested directly.

The concept of temporal signal correlation as a binding mechanism between the evoked activity of sets of neurons in different locations in the neocortex recalls the principles of Gestalt psychology, in that the presence of synchronization may serve to bind local stimulus features into organized percepts (Rock and Palmer, 1990). While interest and experiment have centered on this problem in the visual sense, it is important also for other sensory modalities, and perhaps especially for those cerebral operations by which we construct holistic perceptions from afferent inputs arriving over two or more sensory systems. Many theorists have contributed further to the development of this idea. Reitboeck developed a theoretical and modeling background for the subject and devised methods both for recording simultaneously the activity of many neocortical neurons with multiple, independently movable microelectrodes and for analyzing the data collected (Reitboeck, 1983; Schneider et al., 1983; Reitboeck et al., 1987; Eckhorn and Reitboeck, 1988; Eckhorn, 1994). This idea has been formalized by Singer in the temporal-correlation hypothesis, for which he and Eckhorn have accumulated, independently, a body of evidence they interpret to support the hypothesis (Eckhorn, 1994; Singer, 1995; Singer and Gray, 1995). The general proposition has been reviewed by Bressler (1995). It is important to emphasize, as Singer has done (Singer et al., 1997), that the synchronization hypothesis is compatible with an earlier idea that for simple sensory events, the afferent relay and convergent projection of signals originating in tuned, feature-detector neurons may, after projection through the hierarchical structures at the entry levels of the neocortex, be sufficient for simple perceptions, such as a brief touch to the hand.

It is only in the last decades that the synchronization problem has been studied directly at the level of the mammalian neocortex. Two major fields have evolved. The first is the study of humans as they execute perceptual tasks, or engage in cognitive operations, with slow-wave phenomena recorded from the surface of the head as the measure of brain activity. Leaving aside the many important discoveries made with the methods of evoked and event-related potential recording, I shall describe coherent induced rhythms in the human brain, for they seem directly related to the present discussion. I introduce this subject with a review of the electroencephalogram, the record of the ubiquitous, rhythmic electrical activity of the mammalian brain.

The second general theme is the application of neurophysiological methods and analytic tools to the direct study of the neocortex in anesthetized and unanesthetized cats and monkeys, which leads us to tests of the temporal-correlation hypothesis. I discuss these findings in a following section.

The Electrical Activity of the Brain: The Human EEG

It has been known for more than a century that rhythmic oscillatory electrical activity can be recorded directly from the surface of the brain in mammals. The original discovery was made by Caton in 1874, demonstrated by him in Liverpool in 1875 and in London and Washington in 1877, and described in the *British Medical Journal* (Caton, 1875). Virtually identical discoveries were made independently at about the same time by Beck and Cybulski in Poland, by Danielewski in Russia, and by von Fleisch in Austria (for historical accounts, see Finger, 1994). Yet a period of 55 years elapsed between Caton's discovery and Berger's descriptions of the human electroencephalogram (the EEG), which appeared from 1929 through 1931. Berger's studies, however, had extended over many previous years, from his first attempts in 1902–1910 to record from the brains of dogs. From 1924 on, Berger succeeded in recording the electrical activity of the human brain, using string galvanometers without amplification (see Jung, 1963, 1965). Berger's observations were quickly confirmed by Tonnies (1933) and by Adrian (Adrian and Matthews, 1934; Adrian and Yamigawa, 1935). Berger discovered the alpha blocking in 1930 and attributed it to the onset of cognitive operations. From 1931 to 1938, then with amplification, he continued the intensive studies that established him as the pioneer of the human EEG. It was Berger who first proposed that explanatory correlations be sought between oscillatory wave patterns of the EEG, brain processes, and human behavioral states. He thus set with a single stroke the long-term research program of EEG, to relate the patterns of electrical activity recorded on the surface of the scalp to the brain processes that produce them. Berger's fourteen papers have been collected by Gloor (1969).

Over several decades, Berger's program was expanded by investigators who sought correlations between EEG patterns in humans and putatively related behavioral states, including psychotic states. Considerable success attended efforts to relate characteristic EEG patterns to the various stages of sleep and wakefulness (Steriade, 1991), as well as to such abnormal states as coma or anesthesia. Use of the EEG revolutionized the diagnosis and treatment of epilepsy, through the work of Herbert Jasper and many others, in conjunction with new methods in neurosurgery (Penfield and Jasper, 1954; Gloor, 1975). In general, however, the hope that the EEG could be used to specify the location and the dynamics of brain operations in relation to the behavior they control has been only partially successful. One reason is that the inverse analysis of the EEG pattern—the aim being to reveal underlying cortical operations—has no unique solution. The EEG field potentials are ambiguous reflections of neuronal activity. However, the use of new methods of recording and analysis is producing new discoveries of the relation between the function of the brain and its electrical activity.

General Properties of the EEG

Oscillations in electrical potential occur almost continuously between any two scalp or cortical surface electrodes; ordinarily, recordings are made from a large number of electrodes to allow detailed spatial analysis. The potential waves recorded vary in frequency over the range of 1 to 100 Hz, although higher frequencies are occasionally observed. When detected at the scalp surface, brain waves are 50–200 μV in amplitude and vary in frequency and amplitude from place to place on the head and in different states of awareness in any single individual. They persist in state-characteristic form during excitement, normal alertness, drowsiness, sleep, coma, and epileptic episodes, never ceasing short of cerebral catastrophe or impending

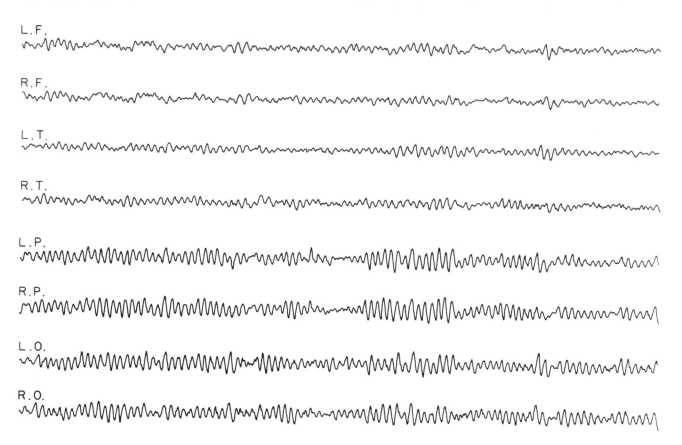

L.F.

R.F.

L.T.

R.T.

L.P.

R.P.

L.O.

R.O.

Fig. 12-1 Alpha rhythm recorded from the head of an adult male, age 42 years. Activity at 9.5/sec in all leads, maximal in parietal and occipital regions, from top down: left and right frontal leads, left and right temporal leads, left and right parietal leads, left and right occipital leads. Calibration: 7 mm = 50 μV. (From Gibbs and Gibbs, 1950.)

death. In a normal individual resting in a quiet room, with eyes closed, the dominant rhythm varies from 8 to 13 Hz and occurs at highest amplitudes over the occipital and posterior parietal regions; its amplitude may wax and wane. This is the alpha, or Berger, rhythm, shown in Fig. 12-1. Upon sensory stimulation or purposeful mental activity, alpha is quickly replaced, in most subjects, by faster frequencies of lower amplitudes (Fig. 12-2). This change was originally interpreted as a "blocking" or desynchronization of the alpha, but recent analyses have shown that it is a period of synchronization at higher frequencies, particularly including what I shall refer to as fast oscillations. These occur in the range of 20–80 Hz, with predominant power in the range of 30–40 Hz (Jasper, 1981; Steriade et al., 1996a,b; Steriade and Amzica, 1996). While the alpha frequency varies between individuals, it is remarkably constant in any one person (Fig. 12-3). Waves slower than alpha occur in normal individuals,

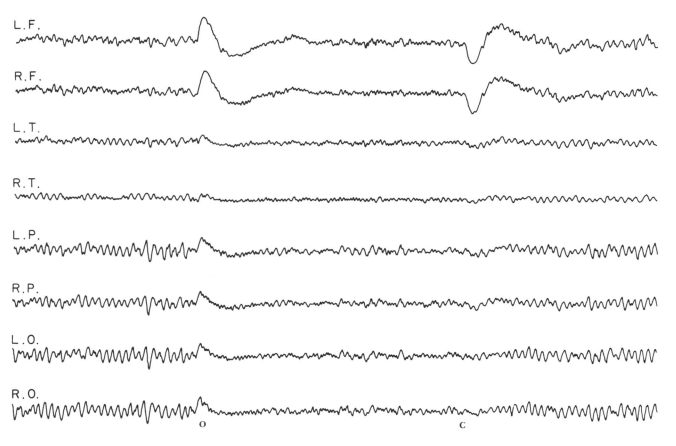

L.F.

R.F.

L.T.

R.T.

L.P.

R.P.

L.O.

R.O.

O   C

Fig. 12-2 EEG records made in a normal male, age 18 years. An alpha rhythm of 10/sec in all leads, maximal in parietal and occipital leads. At *O* the command "eyes open" was given. The 10/sec activity abruptly disappeared, to reappear when the eyes were closed *(C)*. This change was originally termed "desynchronization," but it is now known to be a synchronization at higher frequencies and lower amplitudes. Calibration and lead designations as for Fig. 12-1. (From Gibbs and Gibbs, 1950.)

particularly in the state of slow-wave sleep, but the appearance of waves in the range of 0.1–3.5 Hz in waking individuals is interpreted as a sign of brain pathology. The shift from alpha to fast oscillations, such as that evoked by sensory stimuli, can be made contingent upon preceding stimuli delivered over another pathway, stimuli to which the frequency shift can be "conditioned." Rhythms of 10–20 Hz are recorded in the rolandic region at rest (the *mu* rhythms); the 10 Hz rhythms predominate in the precentral region, the 20 Hz in the postcentral. They are modified during hand movement.

Associations between brain-wave patterns and pathological states were found to be so regular that the EEG rapidly became a valuable diagnostic and monitoring tool in the clinical neurological sciences. This purely phenomenological application led to the important clinical discipline of electroencephalography.

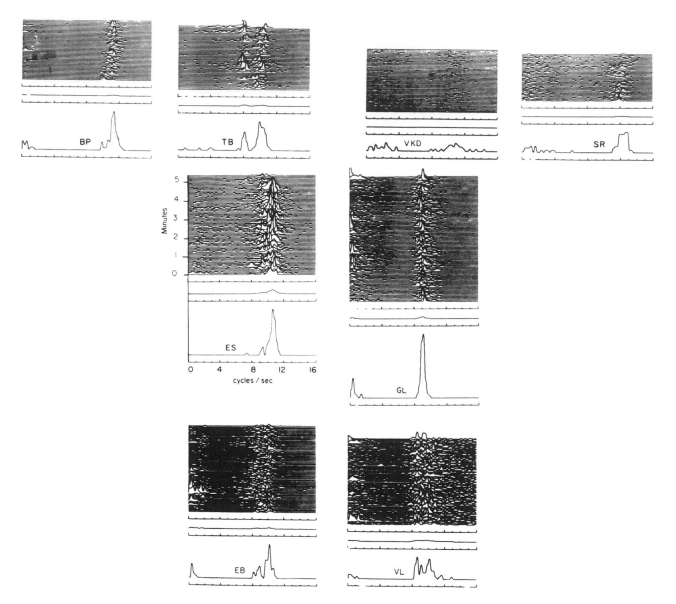

Fig. 12-3 Compressed spectral arrays, corresponding to 2–6 minutes of continuous alpha rhythm in 8 subjects. Each horizontal line for each subject is a plot of the power spectrum of a single 4 sec epoch of EEG recording. The recordings were bipolar between an occipital and a central lead. Note the flat spectrum for subject VKD, and that several subjects (TB, EB, VL) showed two or more peaks in their spectra, separated by 1–3 cycles. Most of the very slow activity is artifactual, produced by movements of the subjects. Each subject's spectral array is shown as upper plot, the average power spectrum in the middle, and the peak histogram below. (From Nunez, 1981.)

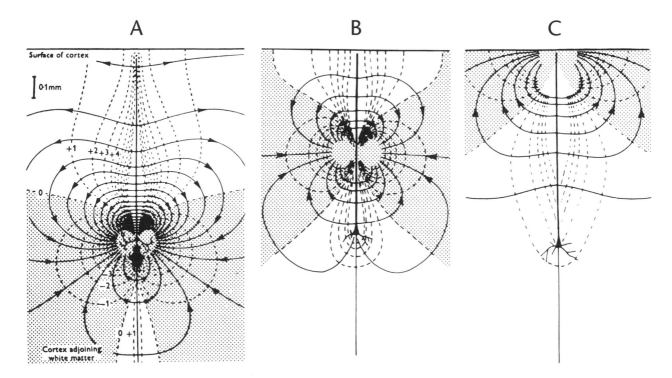

A   B   C

Fig. 12-4 Theoretical electrical fields produced by depolarizations at three different locations on a cortical pyramidal cell; from left to right, near the cell body, at the mid-dendrite level, and on the apical dendrite. Current flow is indicated by the solid lines with arrows; isopotential contours by dotted lines. Negativity indicated by the clear areas, positivity by the shaded ones. (From Creutzfeldt and Houchin, 1984.)

The Origin of the EEG

Electrical oscillations recorded from the surface of the head are generated within the cortex. On classical theory, they are thought to reflect the quasi-synchronous local postsynaptic responses of a set of geometrically ordered cells distributed in a layered array. These synaptically evoked local changes in membrane potential generate current flow through the extracellular spaces of the brain. Cortical tissue resistivity is no more than twice that of open solution of the same molarity, so the cortex is treated as a homogeneous medium, even though marked inhomogeneities occur on the micro-scale of space. Comparisons with the high resistivity of cell membranes indicate that more than 90 percent of imposed or induced currents will flow through the extracellular space. The elements of the layered "dipole" are the pyramidal cells in the gyral surfaces, where the longitudinal axes of the cells are more or less normal to the surface of the scalp. PSPs of either sign generate open fields of current flow in the surrounding medium (Fig. 12-4), including the skull and scalp. The net currents flowing into or out of the scalp are recorded across interelectrode resistances as the potentials of the EEG. If the pyramidal cells were distributed in a single layer, the shapes and signs of the EEG potentials could be analyzed directly in terms of volume conductor theory. However, the distribution of the pyramidal cells in several cortical layers and the convolutions of the cerebral cortex make the analysis uncertain. A major complexity is the variation in the angular orientation of the dipoles relative to the interelectrode axis of the recording pair (Fig. 12-5). The generators are not simple cellular dipoles; rather, they include a large number of subcellular elements, microgenerators such as synaptic terminals, axonal arbors, and perhaps the glial cells as well. Each of these when active may contribute to the net extracellular current flows. A simple model collapses all sources into a single equivalent dipole, for which all higher terms of a multipolar expansion are ignored because the distance between the dipole and the recording site is large relative to the assumed interpolar distance within the dipole. Attempts at spatial localization of current sources using this model often lead to large errors.

Fig. 12-5 Biophysical principles of recording potential changes on the surface of the head generated by dipoles in the cortical tissue. A potential P when recorded in monopolar fashion with reference to a distant electrode is proportional to the solid angle subtended by a dipole layer at the position of the recording electrode. The amplitude of P at any point around the dipole layer is determined by the equation at upper right, where e is the potential across the dipole layer, and Ω is the solid angle subtended at the recording electrode. (From Gloor, 1975.)

(A) The amplitudes of potentials P_1 and P_2 depend upon the solid angles Ω_1 and Ω_2 subtended at the two electrode positions by a hypothetical dipole layer with a circumference occupying the crown of a gyrus.

(B) Dipole layer occupying the crown and two sides of a gyrus. At P_1 the potential depends on the solid angle Ω_1^-, since the electrode "sees" only the portion of the negative side of the dipole. At P_2, two solid angles must be taken into account, Ω_2^+ and Ω_2^-, since the electrode at P_2 "sees" portions of both the positive and the negative sides of a folded dipole layer. The potential at P_2 is therefore proportional to the effective solid angle $\Omega_{2\text{eff}}$, which equals the difference between Ω_2^- and Ω_2^+, the sign of the larger angle determining the electrical sign at P_2.

(C) An illustration of the problem in obtaining a surface recording from a dipole layer occupying both walls of a sulcus. It is determined by the equation shown lower right.

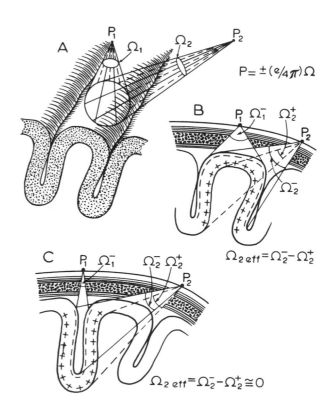

$$P = \pm (e/4\pi)\,\Omega$$

$$\Omega_{2\,\text{eff}} = \Omega_2^- - \Omega_2^+$$

$$\Omega_{2\,\text{eff}} = \Omega_2^- - \Omega_2^+ \cong 0$$

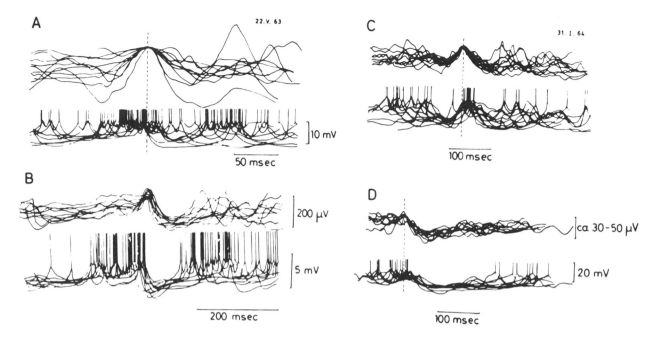

A   22.V.63

]10 mV

50 msec

B

200 µV

5 mV

200 msec

C   31. I. 64

100 msec

D

]ca 30–50 µV

]20 mV

100 msec

Fig. 12-6   Correlations between synaptic events recorded intracellullarly from cortical neurons and the EEG waves recorded directly above from the pial surface. The traces in panels A and C were recorded from the same cell; those in B and D from another. Superimposed line drawings of the EEG records and the intracellular records were collected and superimposed. Cell A–C: The surface waves were symmetrical and corresponded best with summated EPSPs, not with bursts of action potentials. Cell B–D: Negative-positive waves; the negative wave correlated best with synchronized EPSPs, the surface positive waves with synchronized IPSPs. Neither individual nor synchronized action potentials are reflected in the EEG. (From Creutzfeldt et al., 1966.)

Relations of the PSPs of pyramidal cells to EEG potentials have been studied by recording simultaneously the surface electrocorticogram and intracellularly from pyramidal cells just below. Results from the work of Otto Creutzfeldt (Fig. 12-6) show that the correlation between the two depends upon the types of EEG activity recorded (Creutzfeldt, 1995; Creutzfeldt and Houchin, 1984; Creutzfeldt et al., 1966). The correlation is tight for evoked potentials, but is less so for spontaneous EEG potentials. It remains uncertain whether the field potentials evoked in sensory cortical areas by appropriate peripheral stimuli are generated by a reordering (resetting) in time of cyclic components of the ongoing EEG (Basar, 1992), or whether they represent an impulsive addition with its own pattern of frequencies and amplitudes.

On the classic theory, rhythms of the EEG are generated in dorsal thalamic circuits and imposed upon the cortex in spatial patterns set by the relevant thalamocortical projections. Compelling evidence supports this idea in several special cases: e.g., the spindle waves that appear under special circumstances, or the cortical potentials evoked by sensory stimulation. The EEG depends in part upon afferent drive, for all except the very slow waves disappear when the cortex is disconnected from subcortical inputs. Nevertheless, the evidence that this hypothesis applies generally is not compelling, for many rhythmic activities of the EEG may depend upon a nonrhythmic afferent input that activates intracortical circuits that possess inherent rhythmic properties, a consequence of which is that the peaks of the frequency spectra of the waking EEG are characteristics of intracortical circuits. It is likely that each of these mechanisms plays a role in generating EEG rhythms of different types, at different times (Pedley and Traub, 1990).

The Thalamus as Neuronal Oscillator and the Generation of Thalamocortical Rhythms

It is remarkable that more is known about the cellular and network mechanisms of the brain rhythms in the various stages of sleep than in the waking brain. This is so because the rapid state transitions between the various stages of sleep—from waking to drowsiness to light sleep with spindling, to delta wave sleep, to deep sleep with very slow waves, to the robust frequency increments and reduced amplitude of the EEG of REM sleep—provide opportunities for direct correlations between behavioral and electrophysiological states. The electrophysiology of sleep is understood at the cellular and network levels, an increment in knowledge largely due to the studies of Steriade, Llinas, Hobson, and Jones. These investigators have expanded the knowledge base established by the classical researches of Bremer, Morrison, Jasper, Moruzzi, and Magoun, by demonstrating that the dorsal thalamus functions in two modes: first in its well-known relay function, and second, as a neuronal oscillator (Steriade and Deschenes, 1984; Steriade et al., 1994). Their accomplishment is one of the major contributions to understanding brain function of the last decades. Morrison's discovery that the rhythmic spindles of light sleep are generated in the dorsal thalamus was a major clue leading to the new discoveries. There were two key steps. The first was the application of intracellular recording, which revealed the two different modes of action of thalamic cells. The second was the discovery of the connectivity and direction of synaptic action of the cells of the reticular nucleus of the thalamus (RE).

Two modes of action of thalamic cells are illustrated in Figs. 12-7 and 12-8. Neurons are switched between the two by changes in membrane potential (Llinas and Jahnsen, 1982; Jahnsen and Llinas,

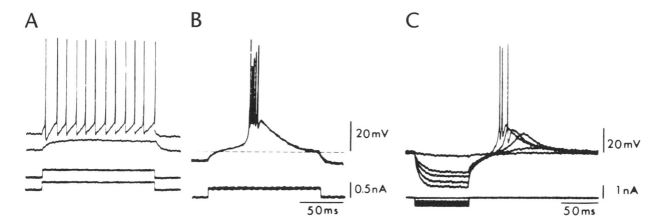

A   B   C

|20mV

|0.5nA

|50ms|

|20mV

|1nA

|50ms|

Fig. 12-7 Intracellular recordings from a neuron in a slice preparation of guinea pig thalamus. (A) Subthreshold current pulse (lowest trace) produced a subthreshold depolarization of the cell. The same stimulus, delivered after an imposed DC depolarization of the cell, produced repetitive impulse discharge (upper trace). (B) After hyperpolarization of the neuron, current pulse similar to that in A produced a single high-frequency burst of impulses. (C) Rebound burst responses are produced after hyperpolarization pulses of different amplitudes, followed by a slow return to baseline. (From Llinas, 1990.)

1984a,b). When depolarized from membrane potential levels of -60 mV or more by injected current or by afferent excitatory inflow, thalamic neurons in relay nuclei respond with a continuous barrage of action potentials that range in frequency from 10 to 165 impulses/sec; frequency is determined directly by the degree of membrane depolarization. This is the relay mode of action. If these same cells are depolarized from more hyperpolarized levels of membrane potential, they respond in a quite different pattern. First there is de-inactivation of a previously inactivated Ca^{2+} conductance, and a slow, low-threshold Ca^{2+} spike that leads at the height of its depolarization to a burst of Na^+ spikes. The slow return to a hyperpolarized level is produced by the sum of post-spike after-hyperpolarizations and the two K^+ currents shown in Fig. 12-8. The sequence then repeats itself at one of two preferred frequencies, 6 or 10 Hz, determined by the interplay of the conductances shown in Fig. 12-8. These oscillating burst discharges in thalamocortical neurons produce oscillating field potentials at the cortical surface.

As sleep supervenes, the high-frequency, low-amplitude rhythms of the waking EEG are replaced by low-frequency, high-amplitude waves characteristic of the several stages of sleep. Spindle waves have long been recognized as characterizing the onset of sleep and loss of consciousness (Fig. 12-9); they also occur at certain depths of barbiturate anesthesia. A spindle is a sequence of EEG and thalamic field potentials with intraspindle frequencies in the range of 7–12 Hz; the sequences recur at intervals of 3–10 sec. Cortical waves at first increment and then decrement within a single spindle. Spindles are generated by actions within a reverberatory, re-entrant network that includes the reticular and relay thalamic nuclei and the cerebral cortex (Fig. 12-10). (For reviews, see Steriade, 1991; Steriade et al., 1993, 1994, 1996c.)

The reticular nucleus (RE) is a thin, extended layer of cells that covers the lateral and dorsolateral surfaces of the dorsal thalamus. That portion adjacent to the lateral geniculate nucleus is called the perigeniculate nucleus; its cells and their functional characteristics are identical with those of RE (Von Krosigk et al., 1993). Reticular neurons are GABAergic (inhibitory) and innervate all thalamic relay nuclei except, in cats, the ventral anterior (VA) and ventromedial (VM), and the nuclei of the anterior group. Thalamocortical fibers from and corticothalamic fibers to dorsal thalamic relay nuclei pass through RE and innervate its neurons with axon collaterals, thus composing the re-entrant circuit shown in Fig. 12-10. With the drift into sleep and the associated decline in thalamic input from afferent systems, and from the central core activating systems, the RE cells slowly hyperpolarize. This initiates in RE cells much the same sequence shown for thalamocortical cells (TC) in Fig. 12-8. The burst of Na$^+$ spikes at the peak of RE cell depolarization produces a deep inhibition of TC cells. Their rebound burst of impulses evokes the spindle waves of the EEG and elicits the return discharge of the corticothalamic pyramidal cells of layer VI, and the reverberation contin-

Fig. 12-8 Diagram demonstrating the oscillatory properties of thalamic neurons, obtained by intracellular recording in a slice preparation of guinea pig thalamus. The fast Na$^+$ spike is followed by an after-hyperpolarization generated by a voltage-sensitive K$^+$ conductance (g_K) and a Ca^{2+}-dependent K$^+$ conductance ($g_{K(Ca)}$). The membrane potential is moved back to spike threshold by the slow, persistent Na$^+$ conductance $g_{Na(P)}$. In addition to the 10 Hz oscillations, slower oscillations at about 6 Hz can occur by the rebound excitation ($g_{Ca(inact)}$) following the hyperpolarization of the cell, $g_{K(Ca)}$, and inhibitory postsynaptic potentials (IPSPs). This hyperpolarization de-inactivates the low-threshold Ca^{2+} conductance and generates a rebound low-threshold spike, which triggers the entire process once again. (From Llinas, 1990.)

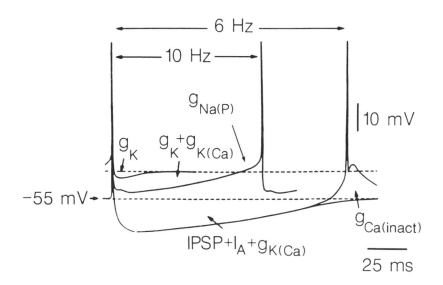

Rhythmicity and Synchronization in Neocortical Networks

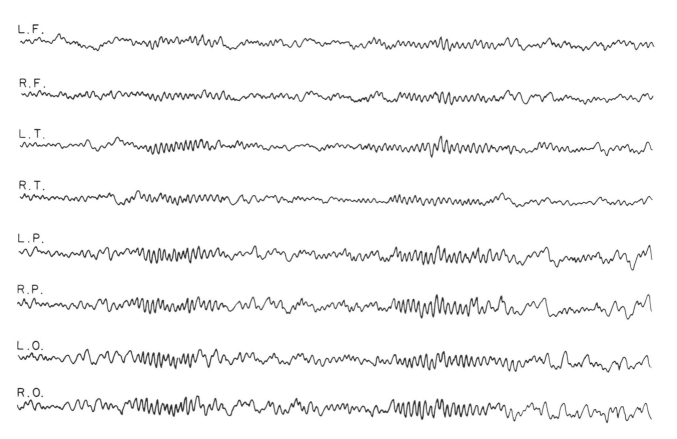

L.F.

R.F.

L.T.

R.T.

L.P.

R.P.

L.O.

R.O.

Fig. 12-9 Electroencephalographic records made during the spindle phase of sleep in a female, age 41 years. The spindles have an internal frequency of about 12/sec. Calibration and lead designations as for Fig 12-1. (From Gibbs and Gibbs, 1950.)

ues. Spindles continue to occur in an isolated RE nucleus, but not in thalamic relay nuclei after they are isolated, and not ever in those thalamic nuclei that receive no RE innervation. Although the reverberatory bursting activity is initiated in RE cells, it is sustained and strengthened by the reverberatory activity in the network. As sleep deepens, spindles decrease in amplitude and are gradually replaced by slower thalamocortical reverberations, the rhythms at 1–4/sec that characterize the delta phase of sleep. Waves at less than 1 Hz dominate the EEG record in very deep sleep. There is evidence that they are generated within the neocortex itself (Steriade et al., 1993; Steriade, Nunez, and Amzica, 1993a,b; Contreras and Steriade, 1995).

Transitions from sleep to waking may occur suddenly from any sleep stage, and they are accompanied by a surge-like increase in activity in systems located in the basal forebrain, posterior hypothalamus, and upper brainstem. Ascending modulatory systems in-

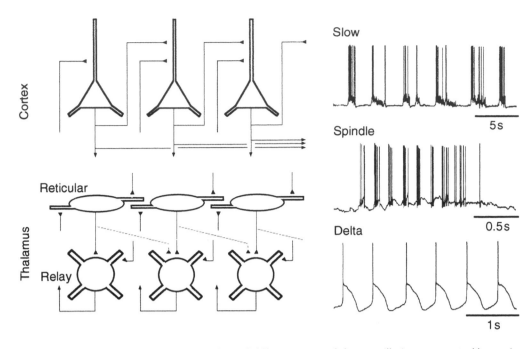

Fig. 12-10 The corticothalamic networks and different types of sleep oscillations generated by excitatory glutaminergic neocortical neurons (top row), inhibitory GABA reticular thalamic neurons (middle), and excitatory glutaminergic thalamocortical relay neurons (bottom). The direction of axonal conduction is indicated by arrows. Short- and long-scale intracortical pathways are illustrated. The divergent reticular thalamic axons are shown as broken lines. The different time calibrations in the intracellular traces show the cortical slow oscillation (c. 0.3 Hz), the reticular thalamic spindles (c. 7 Hz), and the intrinsic, clock-like, delta rhythm (c. 1.5 Hz) of thalamic neurons. These oscillations might be generated at each of these levels; they interact and their rhythms combine in complex wave sequences in the intact brain. M. Steriade et al., "Synchronization of fast (30–40) spontaneous oscillations in intrathalamic and thalamocortical networks," *Journal of Neuroscience* 16(8): 2788–2818 (1996).

nervate the dorsal thalamus and neocortex widely, as well as other structures of the forebrain. They release the modulatory transmitters norepinephrine (NE), serotonin (5-HT), histamine (HA), and acetylcholine (ACh), which evoke a strong depolarization of both RE and TC thalamic neurons and quickly abolish all sleep-related reverberatory activity (Steriade, 1993). Waking is accompanied by higher-frequency activity in the EEG, including the fast oscillations I discuss in a later section. Rapid eye movement sleep (REM) is a paradoxical state evoked mainly by the ACh ascending system. REM resembles waking in its EEG characteristics and is accompanied by a blockade of afferent input to the neocortex and of motor output to the spinal cord. REM sleep is often associated with dreaming.

I think it likely that more neuroscientists' years of effort have been spent in the study of sleep and its cerebral mechanisms than upon any other form of behavior controlled by the brain. The diagnosis and treatment of sleep disorders has become a medical specialty. We understand cerebral mechanisms of sleep as well as we do any other. Yet the paradox remains: although deprivation of non-REM sleep can be fatal in experimental animals, there are many documented cases of humans who do not sleep or sleep only rarely, without dire effects. How sleep serves the normal function of mammalian organisms remains largely a mystery. What we have learned from the study of sleep that has general significance is that, although exceptions occur, the ongoing electrical activity of the neocortex is frequently initiated and controlled by thalamo-cortico-thalamic reverberating networks. These networks are examples of the function of the thalamus as a neuronal oscillator (Steriade and Deschenes, 1984).

Fast Oscillations and Brain States

Steriade and his colleagues have defined the characteristics and the ubiquitous nature of the fast oscillations that appear in the EEG on the transition from the resting state with alpha rhythm to the alert state, shown in Fig. 12-2; for further analysis, see Fig 12-11 (Steriade and Amzica, 1996; Steriade et al., 1996a,b). Steriade's experiments were made in anesthetized and in waking cats prepared for chronic recording, using several electrophysiological methods. The results were that the fast oscillations include frequency components from 20 to 80 Hz, with dominant power within but not limited to the range of 30–40 Hz. Fast oscillations appear in the waking state, in slow-wave sleep during the depolarizing phases of cortical slow waves, during REM sleep, and during forebrain activation produced in anesthetized animals by stimulation of central core ascending cholinergic systems. They may also be evoked by sensory stimulation, which I describe in some following sections. Fast oscillations differ from evoked potentials, for they do not reverse as a recording electrode is moved down across the cortical layers, as slow waves do, and they do not appear in the white matter. They are produced by a series of local microsources and microsinks distributed through the depths of cortical columns, and their lateral coherency is restricted to closely neigh-

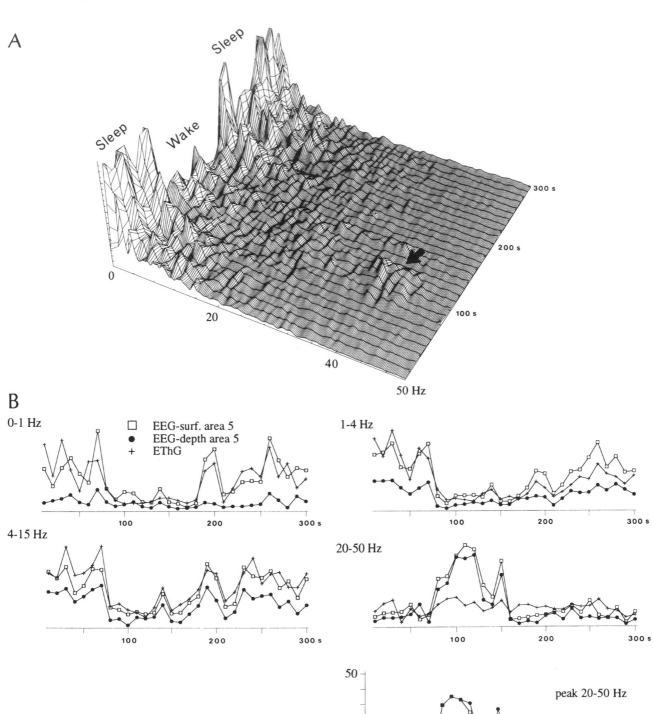

A

Sleep

Wake

Sleep

0

20

40

50 Hz

100 s

200 s

300 s

B

0-1 Hz

□ EEG-surf. area 5
● EEG-depth area 5
+ EThG

100   200   300 s

1-4 Hz

100   200   300 s

4-15 Hz

100   200   300 s

20-50 Hz

100   200   300 s

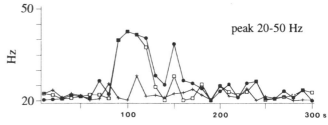

50

Hz

20

peak 20-50 Hz

100   200   300 s

boring columns. Fast oscillations are frequently coherent in reverberating thalamocortical circuits. Within the cortex, they appear in phase with the depolarization and impulse discharge of cortical neurons.

Steriade has emphasized that fast oscillations with dominant power in the 30–40 Hz range appear in a number of brain states, including anesthesia and deep sleep, but that this does not "preclude the possibility that the same intrinsic and network properties that underlie the fast oscillations during states of unconsciousness would operate to underlie perceptual integration by synchronization when relevant stimuli occur in wakefulness" (Steriade et al., 1996b). I discuss this hypothesis in relation to the binding problem in later sections.

Spatial Inhomogeneities and the Micro-EEG

Cortical tissue consists of a large number of densely packed neuronal elements of different sizes—e.g., synapses, dendrites, and axonal arbors. When active, these elements all contribute to extracellular current flow, but their specificities are lost in the smoothed sum of surface or large-volume recording. Intracortical sources are frequently small, sometimes oriented in different directions, and they change rapidly with time. Studies of the micro-EEG in humans with subdural

---

Fig. 12-11 Sequential spectral analysis of EEG waves recorded from the surface and the depth of cortical area 5 (in cat), and from the lateroposterior thalamus *(EThG),* during transitions from natural sleep to waking and back to sleep. Recordings were made through chronically implanted electrodes. (A) Three-dimensional surface is built up by successive fast Fourier transforms of sequential windows of 10 sec duration. Natural sleep is characterized by high peaks in the low-frequency range of oscillations; arousal is accompanied by the appearance of an epoch of fast oscillations at about 40 Hz and by a decrease in the low-frequency components. The epoch of fast oscillations follows abruptly upon arousal, but does not persist throughout the period of waking. (B) Spectral ranges are split into different frequency bands from both the surface and depth recording, for the same 300 sec period as in A. Each point in the graphs corresponds to the area within the indicated spectra (symbols). Arousal occurred at time 70–75 sec on the abscissa and was associated in all leads with a tendency toward a decrease in power in the range of 0–15 Hz and a large increase in the power spectrum in the 20–50 Hz band in the cortical EEG; the thalamic waves lagged the cortical fast oscillations. The peak frequencies, plotted below, indicate a dominant oscillation reaching 40 Hz. (From Steriade et al., 1996b.)

and depth electrodes reveal (1) a precipitous decline in coherence with distance, on a scale of a few millimeters and (2) a marked variability of coherence between records made from closely placed adjacent electrodes, on a scale of fractions of seconds (Bullock et al., 1995a,b). One inference of these results is that the classical model of the EEG as composed of several independent rhythms is not valid, and that the detailed microstructure of the EEG may contain as yet undiscovered information about the relevant intracortical neuronal activity (Bullock, 1989; Bullock and McClune, 1989; Petsche et al., 1988).

Brain microstructure also contains a large number of astrocytes, the K^+ scavengers of the neocortex. Whether the K^+ transport functions of these cells, and the associated extracellular currents, contribute to the surface-recorded EEG is still uncertain (Galambos, 1989). However, the time constants of the K^+ transport process are long relative to the EEG frequencies, and it seems more likely that astrocyte activity may contribute to the prolonged potential shifts recorded under some conditions from the surface of the neocortex.

Spatial and Temporal Analysis of the EEG

Traditional methods of recording brain waves with pens writing on moving paper and analysis of records by visual inspection have been replaced in EEG research by new methods of recording and analysis (Nunez, 1995; JS Barlow, 1993; Regan, 1989). An increment in knowledge of the dynamically changing topographic distributions of cortical activity has followed, particularly knowledge of activity occurring during perceptions, during the preparation for and execution of movements, and during many forms of cognitive behavior (e.g., Gevins et al., 1996).

Major efforts have sharpened the spatial resolution of the EEG and the capacity to locate intracerebral sources, and more precise analyses in the time domain are now possible. The hope has been that deeper analyses would reveal subtle aspects of cerebral electrical activity not readily seen by inspection of EEG records. A seldom-stated hypothesis is that aspects of brain function may be expressed in some hitherto unrecognized form in the surface-recorded electrical activity of the brain (Basar, 1992). Little evidence available to date supports that idea.

High-density recording (124 electrodes) improves spatial resolution by reducing the interelectrode distance on the average human head to 2.5 cm, approximately the cortex-to-scalp point spread function. The electrodes are aligned in 3 dimensions with head models derived from magnetic resonant images (Gevins et al., 1994b, 1996). A number of analytic methods have been introduced to improve localization. The current source-density analysis involves calculation of the second spatial derivatives of the potential field differences between any given electrode and each of symmetrically placed surrounding electrodes (Nunez, 1981). This spline Laplacian (the second spatial derivative) was used by Perl and Casby (1954) in recording from the auditory cortex of the cat, and by MacKay (1984) in his study of the visual evoked potential in humans. The spline Laplacian analysis yields a measure of the current entering or leaving each point on the scalp (Nunez, 1989; Nunez and Pilgreen, 1991; Nunez et al., 1991, 1994; Law et al., 1993; Le et al., 1994); it eliminates reference electrode effects, is independent of common mode signals, and yields an estimate of the potential changes at local points on the brain surface itself, and thus a more precise localization of sources within the brain to about 1 cm. Its validity has been confirmed by comparison with records made directly at the cortical surface in humans through closely spaced grids of subdural electrodes (Gevins et al., 1994a).

Analysis of the EEG as a time series is accomplished after high-frequency digitalization of the record. Spectral analysis then reveals the frequency composition of the original record in terms of relative amplitudes and phases. Fig. 12-3, which presents the compressed spectral analyses of the alpha rhythms in a number of subjects (Nunez, 1981), illustrates the relative constancy of the dominant alpha frequencies in most human subjects. An occasional individual never displays an alpha rhythm (see subject VKD in Fig. 12-3). Further analyses include cross-power and cross-phase analyses between records taken from different electrodes, and measures of coherence between the two. Methods have now been developed to display the shift in amplitudes and frequencies in the spatial domain. As a result of these advances, the EEG has become a valuable method of neuro-imaging, the spatial registration of electrical events to brain structure (Nunez, 1995).

Electroencephalography is linked to those fields in which evoked and event-related potentials are recorded in studies of cognitive functions (Gevins, 1995; Gevins et al., 1996). This combination forms the evolving discipline of human neurophysiology; for a scholarly review, see David Regan's monograph of 1989. One advantage of the EEG method is that the equipment is portable, small, and relatively inexpensive. EEG records can be telemetered over vast distances and stored for future analysis. Recordings can be made under almost any condition of normal life, as well as when the subject performs stressful tasks or must live in hostile environments (Gevins et al., 1995).

Magnetoencephalography

Electroencephalography is complemented by methods for recording the magnetic fields generated about active populations of neurons, the magnetoencephalogram (MEG), recently with large numbers of sensors ($n = 122$, Hari and Samelin, 1997). The magnetic fields normal to the scalp surface are not attenuated, frequency filtered, or distorted by the properties of tissues between source and detector. Low frequencies can be recorded in undistorted form. The fields are in the main generated by populations of neurons that induce current flows oriented tangentially to the surface of the head (Nunez, 1986). The MEG records preferentially the activity of populations of neurons within the sulcal banks of the cortex, orthogonal to the locations best observed with the EEG. Ioannides et al. (1993, 1994) devised a distributed current model to analyze the results obtained in MEG recording. Magnetic field tomography (MFT) is noninvasive and has a spatial resolution that approaches 1 mm and a time resolution of about 1 msec. Both cortical and subcortical zones of increased neural activity can be identified and localized and followed with clear resolution and in real time, as they shift from one place to another during evolving movements or cognitive tasks (Ribary et al., 1991; Tagaris et al., 1997). MEG has one disadvantage EEG has not, for it requires immobility of the subject within a massive apparatus. A combination of MFT and EEG appears to have considerable promise.

Induced Rhythms in Humans

It has been known since the earliest days of electrophysiology that a brief stimulus may evoke a rhythmic oscillation in the electrical activity of neural structures, from invertebrate axons to the mammalian neocortex (for reviews, see Bullock, 1992; Basar and Bullock, 1992; Bullock and Abramowicz, 1994). They are induced rhythms, a heterogeneous class of oscillations caused or modulated by sensory stimuli that do not themselves drive directly the successive cycles of oscillations. Periods of brief oscillations also occur during the central states of cognitive operations. The time structure of induced rhythms is determined by the intrinsic properties of the relevant neural networks. Unlike evoked potentials, induced rhythms may be either tightly or loosely linked to the stimuli that evoke them, and in the latter case may have long and variable latencies. Transient oscillations appear in many central structures, including cerebral cortex, thalamus, and hippocampus. The oscillations compose a broad power spectrum, with frequently a peaked focus in the range of 25–65 Hz. At many locations, however, the power spectrum includes the EEG spectral bands.

Potentially the most informative of the several classes of induced rhythms are those set in motion in separate cortical areas by peripheral stimuli. They occur over the full frequency range of the EEG, and conspicuously in the fast oscillation range (35–65 Hz). It is proposed that the fast oscillations evoked in different cortical areas, when coherent, contribute to the synchronization of the neuronal activity evoked in those separate areas by different stimulus features. Synchrony is thought to be the critical factor binding together those separate sets of neuronal activity to form the neural basis of a perceptual whole.

Induced fast oscillations appear in the EEG during periods of focused attention and during cognitive operations (Sheer, 1989). These latter have included calculations, thinking, reading, language translation, listening to music, the voluntary initiation of movements, mental rotations of imagined 3-dimensional objects, etc. In all of these, the fast rhythms appear differentially as regards cerebral lateralization and intrahemispheric locations, and in temporal relation to the presumed patterns of the cognitive operations. Linkages are often inferred from these observations, but in none has the study of induced rhythms led to an increased understanding of the brain operations in cognition. They are of value in suggesting which brain regions are active during the sequential stages of cognitive operations: they provide answers to geographical questions. Like slow wave events in general, they are derived and indirect measures of neural events in the relevant neural populations. These are the neural events we need to know to understand brain function.

Other studies have been concentrated on more direct sensory-per-

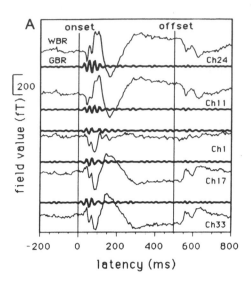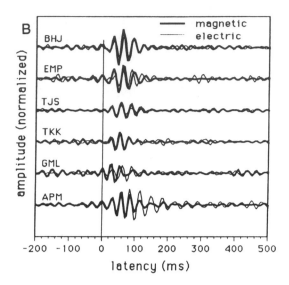

Fig. 12-12 A 40 Hz transient oscillatory response is evoked in humans by the onset of an auditory stimulus. The response consists of four or more cycles locked in phase with stimulus onset over the 20–120 msec poststimulus interval. The response is localized to the supratemporal auditory cortex. (A) Wide-band *(WBR)* and gamma-band *(GBR)* responses recorded from five electrodes located on the surface of the head over the temporal region. The initial WBR peaks are followed by a sustained field potential and an off response that contains no visible GBR. (B) Superimposition of simultaneous electrical and magnetic recording of GBRs from six human subjects. (From Pantev et al., 1991.)

ceptual tasks. Galambos and his colleagues recorded with EEG and MEG the transient responses evoked in the human cortex by brief auditory stimuli. They observed wide band responses with power peaks at about 10 Hz and about 40 Hz. The first was attributed to the primary auditory evoked potential. The latencies of the fast oscillations varied from 20 to 130 msec, and thus overlapped in time the slow-wave evoked potentials. Simultaneous EEG and MEG recordings were virtually identical (Fig. 12-12). The human subjects were alert in these experiments, but focused attention was not further controlled, and the auditory stimuli were not used in any behavioral task. Fast oscillatory responses were interpreted to reflect "the activity of a fundamental auditory perceptual mechanism," but no direct evidence supports this conjecture (Pantev et al., 1991; Galambos et al., 1981).

Llinas and his colleagues have used many-channel MEG recording to study the global distribution of the fast oscillations (c. 40 Hz) in

Rhythmicity and Synchronization in Neocortical Networks

both the waking and sleeping states (Joliot et al., 1994; Llinas et al., 1994). They propose that this activity is directly related to perceptual and cognitive neocortical operations. Widespread and intermittently coherent 40 Hz activity that occurs in the waking state is reset by a brief auditory stimulus. Parallel psychophysical and MEG recording experiments revealed an identity between the threshold interval at which human observers identified two stimuli as two, and not one, and the appearance of a linked 40 Hz response to the second of the two stimuli. The interval for both was 13–14 msec, close to a half-wave of the 40 Hz activity. Spontaneous 40 Hz activity appeared with a phase lag from the front to the back of the head of about 12 msec. It was proposed that the 40 Hz phenomenon—or what it represents—might serve as a scanning or global binding mechanism in the more global aspects of cognition. Forty Hz activity was greatly reduced in deep sleep, but strong and widespread in the REM stage of sleep with dreaming (Llinas and Ribary, 1993, 1994). An anterior-to-posterior phase lag was also observed in REM sleep, but in this state an auditory stimulus did not reset the rhythm; this was taken as further evidence for the disconnection of the brain from the periphery during REM sleep. The authors propose that the neural mechanisms of cognition in the waking state and in the state of dreaming in REM sleep have much in common, and depend at least in part upon similar cerebral mechanisms.

These important observations and ideas deserve further intensive study, for they bear upon the cerebral mechanisms in cognition at a level not previously explored so directly (Llinas and Pare, 1996). In a recent study made with multiple subdural electrodes in two epileptic patients, Menon et al. (1996) observed coherent 40 Hz activity on a spatial scale more limited than was observed by Llinas. The differences between the results of these two methodological quite different studies remain to be resolved.

Fast oscillations appear over the sensory-motor areas in humans during the preparation for and execution of self-paced movements, beginning about 2 sec before movement onset and continuing during the movement. Both the desynchronization of the low-frequency activity and the transient fast oscillations are localized close to the central sulcus (Pfurtscheller and Neuper, 1992). These observations resemble those of Sheer (1989) and of Rougeul et al. (1979), described in a later section, that increase in fast oscillations is correlated with focused attention rather than with movement preparation, *per se.*

Fig. 12-13 Evidence for a transient phase-locking between fast oscillations recorded over the frontal and parietal regions of the head in a human subject as he executed a somatic sensory task. The two locations are thought to be involved, respectively, in the cognitive and sensory processing aspects of the task. The subject was required to identify by toe movement when one finger designated the "target" was stimulated, in a sequence of stimuli delivered in random sequence to four fingers of the contralateral hand. Stimuli were twice the threshold for electrical stimuli delivered to the finger skin. Recordings were made at the locations indicated by the head figurines at a wide frequency band (1–500 Hz) and later filtered at the two bands indicated, 35–45 Hz and 28–35 Hz. (From Desmedt and Tomberg, 1994.) (A) Stimulation of the target finger was followed at about 150 msec by synchronized fast oscillations selectively for the 35–45 Hz band; they were at about 40 Hz. The latency varied from trial to trial; only a single trial is shown here, without averaging. The period of synchrony of the fast oscillations lasted about 125 msec, about 5 cycles, and ended long before the end of the reaction time at 490 msec, which was preceded by a P_{300} slow wave (record C). (B) No synchronization occurred over the hemisphere ipsilateral to the stimulated finger.

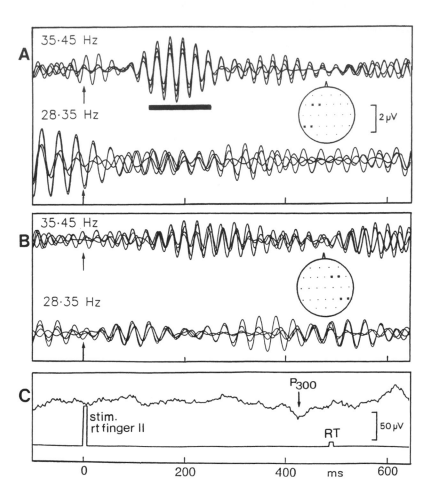

Experimental discrimination between these two interpretations is difficult, and the problem remains unsolved.

Fast oscillatory responses recorded in widely separated locations on the head are induced to phase synchronization by sensory stimuli delivered during a somesthetic discrimination task requiring close attention and choice of a correct motor response. Desmedt and Tomberg (1994) asked human subjects to identify by toe movement to a target which one of several fingers was stimulated with a weak electrical current. The records of Fig. 12-13 show a task-related, transient, phase locking of the gamma band responses in the contralateral parietal and prefrontal areas. These correlated oscillations began well after the direct sensory and early cognitive potentials recorded over the primary postcentral sensory cortex. The results are interpreted to represent the binding of the several cognitive features of the task in a widely distributed system of the neocortex thought relevant for conscious perception and sensory-motor linkage.

Temporal Correlation and Perceptual Integration

The Temporal Correlation Hypothesis

The proposal is that the neural activity defining the features of an object is labeled and bound in such a way that it can be differentiated from the activity defining the features of other objects. Discrimination between overlapping objects we view or the extraction of a melody from a varied auditory background are things our perceptual systems do almost instantaneously. This problem of linking or "binding" was posed for experimental study with the discovery that the neural activities evoked by the complex features of perceptual targets are processed in separate neocortical areas. The question is how the activities within and between those separate processing areas are unified in momentary association to form a coherent representational state—the neural basis of a perception.

This idea differs from that of a sequential convergence of separate feature-detector systems upon targets consisting of only a few neurons—in the limit only one. Such a small set of neurons is on this hypothesis thought to signal an integration of the total stimulus feature set. What target these neurons engage to achieve the transition to conscious perception is unknown. The single (or several) neuron hypothesis was proposed by H. B. Barlow in 1972 and updated by him in 1995. Two general principles are emphasized by Barlow: first, that single neurons detect peripheral events with features that are of behavioral significance to the organism—the feature-detector idea; second, that objects might be represented in the brain by the fewest number of active neurons—the efficiency idea (K. A. Martin, 1994). It is possible that the central projection and convergence of activity generated in single peripheral feature-detector neurons could suffice for the perception of simple sensory events. It seems unlikely, however, that there is a sufficient number of feature detectors to account for the virtually infinite number of sensory stimuli we readily perceive, nor for solving the binding and relational problems in perceiving complex scenes.

A second idea defines sets of neurons (or modules) as projection targets, called equivalent recognition units (Bullock, 1986). These are thought to receive a total convergence, each set located in some restricted area of neocortex. Convergence sets may exist at different levels of a single sensory system or between different systems—e.g., between visual and somatic systems in the parietal lobe. Such a case has been described by Oram and Perritt (1996), who discovered sets of neurons in the anterior superior temporal polysensory area of the macaque monkey that possess a complex of feature sensitivities to both the form (faces, bodies) and motion of objects. These neurons receive convergent input from both the dorsal and ventral processing pathways of the prestriate cortical visual system. Form and motion neurons are intermingled in this cortical area with others sensitive only to form or motion, which suggests a convergent processing chain. Sets of form and motion neurons may be regarded as recognition units in the sense given by Bullock. Oram and Perritt's discovery suggests that recognition units are embedded within the nodes of distributed systems. The recognition-unit model is of heuristic value, but other cases are needed to give it general support.

The temporal correlation hypothesis is based upon different ideas: that total convergence targets do not exist; that each processing unit contributes its output to the dynamic ongoing activity in the nodes and internodal linkages of a distributed system; and that the neural image of the stimulus is signaled by the activity in relevant sets of neurons, whose members are distributed in different nodes of the system. Those different loci of the neocortex are selectively but widely interconnected (see Chapter 10). The central idea is that the members of each such linked set are labeled and thus made identifiable by a transient synchronization of their activity; for distantly located nodes, coherent oscillations of slow-wave events may be important for securing that synchronization. On this model several ensembles might exist at the same time in a single distributed system, or in a single topographic mapping, perhaps distinguishable by different synchronizing frequencies. The superimposition of temporal maps upon spatial ones increases the number of representations (functional states) that can be sustained within a single group of re-entrantly connected maps (Llinas et al., 1994). Further, it is assumed that the synaptic linkages between sets of neurons are relatively direct, allow rapid synchronization, and are modifiable quickly to allow formation of new ensembles driven by new combinations of stimulus features. Focal attention is thought to play a role in promoting synchronized ensembles related to the attended stimuli. The experimental tasks are to discover if synchronized periods of cortical neuronal activity relate directly to the relevant perceptual experiences evoked by the same stimuli and to determine what mechanism produces the synchronizations.

The linking problem is combinatorial in that different objects within a sensory display may evoke similar but not quite identical patterns of activity in overlapping but not quite identical populations of neurons. Combinatorial questions are general in perception: how can one synthesize tactile, pressure, pattern, and proprioceptive inputs from the hand that allow one to discriminate, without vision, between a new tennis ball fresh from the can and one that has endured three hard sets of tennis? Or, what mechanism is responsible for the "cocktail party effect" discussed by Von der Malsberg and Schneider (1986) in one of the first theoretical formulations of the problem (see also Von der Malsberg, 1995; Abeles, 1982; Milner, 1974)? Even more mysteriously, we make such identifications using only a few or even a single stimulus feature. It seems likely that the full contexts of stimuli that are evoked by single features are recalled and reconstructed from memory. Memory recall mechanisms are unknown.

Singer and Gray (1995) listed the predictions of the temporal correlation hypothesis, as follows:

1. Neurons in different nodes recorded simultaneously should be synchronized on a time scale of milliseconds, including cells within a single column, in separate columns in the same cortical area, between different areas in the same distributed system, and between homologous areas in the two hemispheres.

2. Cell ensembles can be formed and dissolved in milliseconds. Transitions from one ensemble to another may match the serial orders of selective attention to and perception of successive events. Individual neurons should be free rapidly to change from one synchronized ensemble to another.

3. Neurons of an ensemble within a distributed system should show synchronous episodes during stimulus-evoked responses, but they should show no such relations with neurons simultaneously active in other ensembles within the

same distributed system. Thus more than one but not many ensembles may be active simultaneously within the same system.

4. The node-to-node connections over which synchronizations are effected should be specific, and their synapses modifiable by experience.

5. The episodes of synchronous activity in ensembles within a distributed sensory-perceptual system should relate specifically and directly to appropriate sensory-perceptual experiences of detections, discriminations, categorizations, etc.

Experimental Observations

Neurophysiological study of this problem was accelerated by new methods for recording simultaneously the activity of many cortical neurons with either acutely or chronically inserted microelectrodes. Analysis of the data obtained in such experiments is facilitated by the concepts and methods developed by George Gerstein and his colleagues (for reviews, see Aertsen et al., 1994; Gerstein et al., 1985, 1989; Gerstein and Aertsen, 1985; Palm et al., 1988). Neurophysiological experiments relevant for the temporal correlation hypothesis have been made in the visual cortical areas of anesthetized and waking cats (Eckhorn et al., 1988; Gray and Singer, 1989; Nelson et al., 1992; Konig et al., 1995) and in the visual areas of anesthetized (Nowak et al., 1994; Shaw et al., 1993) and waking monkeys (Ahissar and Vaadia, 1990; Kreiter and Singer, 1992, 1996; Frien et al., 1994; Eckhorn et al., 1993; Bressler et al., 1993). Visual stimuli with features appropriate for the loci of recording in several visual cortical areas evoke oscillating bursting discharges of single cortical neurons (called single-unit activity, SUA) and the discharge of local cell groups within the electrical view of low-impedance microelectrodes (multi-unit activity, MUA). These are frequently accompanied by but do not depend upon oscillating field potentials (the local field potentials, LFPs). The interburst and LFP frequencies in cats vary in the range of 35–85 Hz; broad-band distributions are observed in monkeys. Similar experiments have been made in the somatic sensory (Ahissar and Vaadia, 1990), motor (Sanes and Donahue, 1993; Murthy and Fetz, 1992; Murthy et al., 1994), frontal (Abeles et al., 1993a,b; Aertsen et al., 1991; Vaadia et al., 1995), and temporal (Nakamura et al.,

1992) cortical areas in monkeys. Although studies of the visual cortical areas by different investigators have in some cases yielded results compatible with the temporal/correlation hypothesis, several have obtained quite different results in similar experiments. I summarize them in a later section.

Oscillatory Synchronizations within Single Columns in the Visual Cortex

Fig. 12-14A illustrates the responses of a single neuron in cat area 17 to a moving stimulus and its correlations with the negative phases of the LFPs evoked by the same stimulus. The long latency to the LFP is preceded by a nonrhythmic state with no correlation with the discharges of the single neuron. Fig. 12-14B shows the records of another neuron of cat area 17, on slow (C) and rapid (D) time scales. The bursting nature of the discharge is documented by the auto-correlogram in panel B. Fig. 12-15 gives the results of an analysis of several neurons of a single column of area 17, recorded together. It illustrates the strength of the oscillatory responses and indicates that the latencies, amplitudes, and temporal phases of those responses are not time-locked to the stimuli that evoke them, although they are determined by stimulus features. The bursts of action potentials occur mainly on the negative phases of the LFPs. Responses are evoked by optimally oriented bars or grids drifting slowly across the receptive fields of the cortical neurons (1–12 degrees/sec). Bursting responses are rarely evoked by similar stimuli flashed briefly, without movement (Eckhorn et al., 1992). Oscillating activity evoked by slowly moving stimuli is abruptly suppressed by rapid accelerations, which evoke stimulus-locked responses (Kruse and Eckhorn, 1996). LFPs and associated neuronal activities vary in latencies and burst frequencies from one response to the next in a slowly repeated stimulus train, in the degree of synchronization between the discharges of adjacent neurons, and in their long latencies (compared with those of the primary visual evoked responses). The synchrony between neurons recorded by single microelectrodes in the local intracolumnar populations is strong in the immediate locale and falls rapidly over the first 2 mm of electrode separation (Brosch et al., 1995), but occurs at up to 10–12 mm separations in the visual cortex. Synchronizations are quantified by auto- and cross-correlation analyses and derivation of power spectra. Those observed between the activities of neurons in different cortical locations occur with virtually zero phase

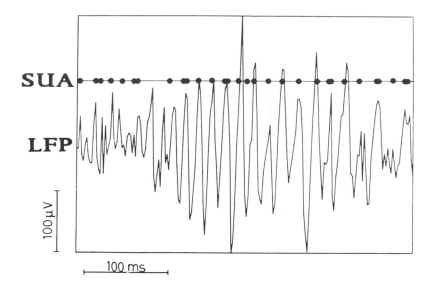

Fig. 12-14A Oscillatory activity evoked in the visual cortex of an anesthetized cat by a grating stimulus of 0.7 cycles/degree drifting across the visual field at 8 degrees/sec in the preferred direction and orientation for the neuron. Local field potentials *(LFP)* and single-unit activity *(SUA)* were recorded through the same intracortical microelectrode. Transition from a quasi-random state to an oscillatory state occurred at about 100 msec latency. On the SUA axis, each dot designates an action potential of the neuron; each is loosely synchronized with a peak of the slow waves. LFP frequency about 50–55 Hz. (From Eckhorn et al., 1988.)

shift. Modeling simulations show that sets of neurons with oscillatory firing patterns linked by long-range excitatory connections and local inhibitory interneurons can very quickly be brought into synchronization with zero phase shift (Konig and Schillen, 1991; Traub et al., 1996). The time constants of cortical neurons and the axonal conduction delays suggest that this oscillatory synchronization can vary from 30 to about 90 Hz. Synchronization may occur between nonperiodic patterns of neuronal activity.

Complex cells of the visual cortex commonly respond in the bursting mode (56 percent); simple and special complex cells do so less commonly (11 percent and 12 percent). Bursting cells are found in all layers of the visual cortex, with some differential concentrations in layers III and VI. Oscillations and synchronization between closely adjacent sets of neurons—within a single column—are almost always accompanied by LFPs, but not dependently so. Synchronization between more widely separated sets of neurons almost never occurs without the accompanying slow-wave oscillations (Konig et al., 1995).

Synchronization between Separate Columns in the Same and in Different Visual Areas

Optimal visual stimuli evoke virtually synchronous responses in visual cortical areas (Nowak et al., 1995a). A finding critical for the tem-

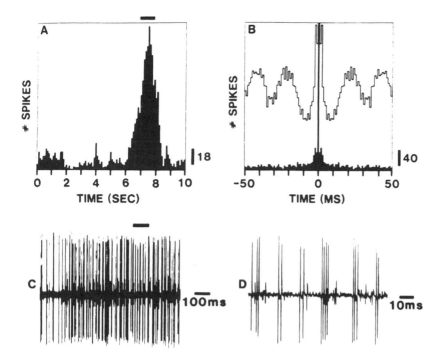

Fig. 12-14B Discharge pattern of an oscillating "standard-complex" neuron recorded in visual cortex of an anesthetized cat through an intracortical microelectrode (From Gray et al., 1990.)

(A) Post-stimulus time histogram summing activity evoked during 10 trials of stimulus movement in the second direction.

(B) Autocorrelogram, full and unfilled bars for the response evoked by the first and second directions of movement, respectively.

(C) Record of the impulse discharges of the neuron evoked during the second direction of movement.

(D) Part of the record of C at faster recording speed to show the oscillatory pattern of the single neuron activity.

poral-correlation hypothesis is that the co-activated responses are synchronized for brief periods during stimulus presentations. Synchronization occurs between the activities of single neurons, multi-neuron activities, and LFPs for sets of neurons in different columns of cat area 17, between columns of areas 17 and 18, and between homologous locations in the area 17s of the two hemispheres, in the cat (Eckhorn et al., 1990, 1992; Gray et al., 1989, 1992; Engel et al., 1990, 1991a,b; Freinwald et al., 1995). Sets of neurons in areas V1 and V2 and in separate columns in area MT of the monkey are synchronized by appropriately coherent stimuli (Frien et al., 1994; Kreiter and Singer, 1992, 1996)—e.g., by a match of the orientation of the stimulus with the orientation selectivity of the sets of neurons. Synchronization depends upon both common stimulus sensitivities of the two sets of neurons and, for locations separated by more than a few millimeters, upon the amplitudes of the accompanying oscillating field potentials. Oscillations in neural activity and LFPs occur at more or less the same frequencies. Slow-wave oscillations are not thought to carry specific information about the features of the visual stimuli.

Fig. 12-16 illustrates synchrony between two sets of neurons lo-

Fig. 12-15 Evidence that the latencies, frequencies, and amplitudes of oscillatory responses of visual cortical neurons are not time-locked to the onset of the stimuli that evoke them. Neuron discharges recorded through microelectrode in the visual cortex of anesthetized cat. Stimuli were moving light bars oriented at the cells' preferred orientations, moved back and forth across the cells' receptive fields. Multi-neuronal recording. (From Gray et al., 1990.)

(A) Post-stimulus time histogram of the neuronal responses to the preferred direction of stimulus movement.

(B) Autocorrelogram computed from the data of A; it shows oscillatory frequencies of about 50 Hz.

(C) Impulse trains for each of the 10 trials evoking the responses evoked for A, recorded during the second and third seconds of stimulus movement. The latencies vary.

(D) Autocorrelograms for each of the ten responses of C.

(E) Portions of the responses recorded at a faster time scale, for the period marked by the horizontal line in C.

(F) Recomputation of the autocorrelogram of B after shuffling trial sequences by one stimulus period.

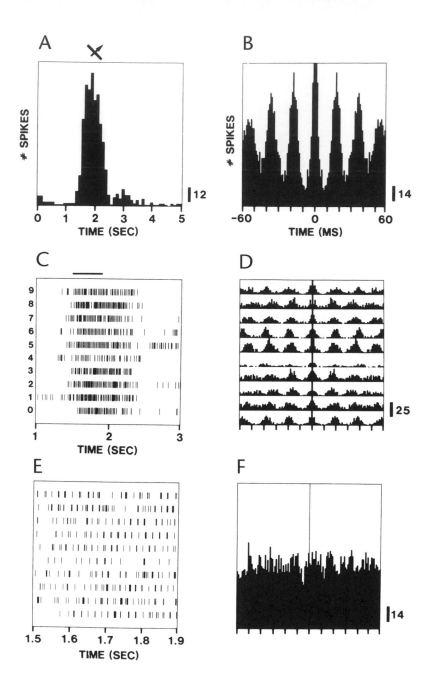

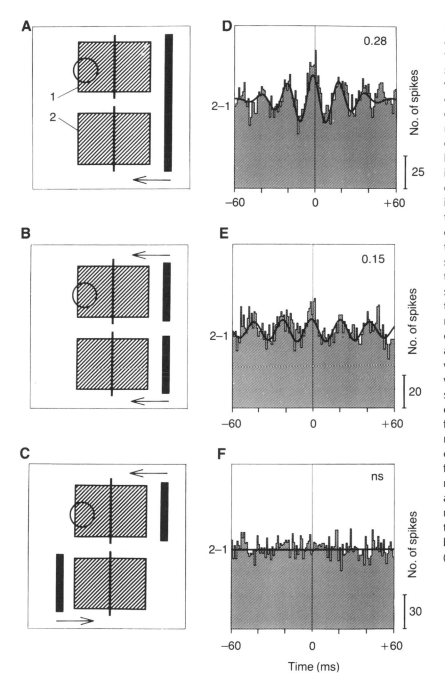

Fig. 12-16 The neuronal activity recorded at two locations 7 mm apart in the visual cortex of an anesthetized cat is synchronized by stimulus coherence. The two cell groups were selectively sensitive to stimuli with vertical orientations. Panels A, B, and C are plots of the receptive fields; their co-linear arrangement allowed the comparison of three different stimulus paradigms: a long continuous light bar moving across both fields (A), two independent light bars moving in the same direction (B), and the same two bars moving in opposite directions (C). The circle marks the center of the visual field; the thick line drawn across each receptive field indicates the selective orientation. Panels D, E, and F show the respective cross-correlograms between the data sets obtained using each stimulus paradigm. With the long light bar, the two oscillatory responses were synchronized, as shown by the modulation of the cross-correlogram with alternating peaks and troughs (D). The synchronization was weaker when the continuity of the stimulus was interrupted (E), and it disappeared if the stimulus motions were incoherent (F). The change in stimulus configuration did not affect the strength or oscillatory nature of the responses. The graph superimposed on each of the correlograms is a Gabor function fitted to the data; the numbers in the upper right corners indicate relative modulation amplitudes, determined by computing the ratio of the amplitude of the Gabor functions to their offsets. *ns* = not significant; scale bars indicate the number of nerve impulses. (From Engel et al., 1992.)

Fig. 12-17 Time courses of the coherent oscillations in the activity recorded at two corresponding positions in areas 17 and 18 of
an anesthetized cat; intracortical microelectrodes. Binocular stimulation with 0.7 cy-
cles/degree grating moving at 8 degrees/sec
in the optimal direction, with best orientation. Black bar and arrow indicates stimulus
movement. *(Left)* Data from area 17. *(Right)*
Data from area 18. (From Eckhorn et al.,
1990.)

(A) Single sweep recordings of local field
potentials (LFP). Oscillations occur during
stimulus movement, followed by more stochastic records after movement ceases.

(B) Amplitudes of the LFP frequency spectra, calculated for successive 256 msec epochs and averaged in the frequency domain
for 19 responses. The peaks at about 47 Hz
begin with stimulus movement and cease at
"stop." Numbers in the spectrograms indicate frequency of the maximum.

(C) Autocorrelation functions, calculated
by fast Fourier transformations of the data of
B; they show stimulus-evoked oscillations.

(D) Normalized cross-correlation functions calculated from the respective 256
msec epochs of LFP. Numbers at the peaks
are amplitudes.

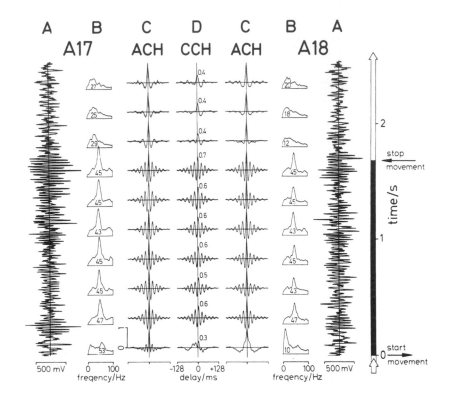

cated 7 mm apart in area 17 of the cat (Engel et al., 1992). The long
bar of panel A is virtually co-linear with the orientation selectivity of
both sets of neurons and covers the area of the visual field between
the two multineuronal receptive fields. This stimulus elicited oscillating and synchronized responses in the two sets of neurons (panel D).
Two short bars, each just covering one of the two receptive fields,
evoked a weaker synchronization (panel E). The two short bars moving in opposite directions across the receptive fields elicited oscillating and synchronous responses within the two populations (not
shown), but no synchronization between them. The two populations
are united in a synchronously discharging ensemble by the stimulus
conditions of A, less intensely so by the stimuli of B. For stimulus
condition C, the ensemble is dismantled, and the two sets of neurons
are presumed to be synchronized in other ensembles within the same
distributed system. Thus the two sets of neurons are switched between ensembles by change in stimulus configuration.

Fig. 12-17 illustrates the time course of the coherent oscillations of

LFPs recorded simultaneously in areas 17 and 18 of the cat by Eckhorn et al. (1990). The binocular visual stimulus was a 0.7 cycle/degree grating swept in the optimal direction at 8 degree/sec. The responses to a single stimulus traverse show the delay from stimulus onset to the transition from a stochastic state to coherent oscillation, at about 200 msec, and the reverse transition when the movement stopped. The auto- and cross-correlograms of columns C and D illustrate the synchronization of the oscillatory activity at each of the two recording locations. Fig. 12-18 presents the analysis of records made in cat visual cortex cortical areas with five microelectrodes (Eckhorn et al., 1992). The cross-correlograms show the strong coherence between stimulus-induced LFPs at gamma frequencies between recording locations in the same visual area, between two areas of the same hemisphere, and the much weaker interhemispheric correlations.

Linkage between sets of neurons in distant locations in single cortical areas is thought to be effected over the horizontally projecting axon collaterals of pyramidal cells (Chapter 3). These make excitatory connections with cells in all layers in target patches that average 400 μm in diameter, at interpatch intervals that differ between areas and species. The stimulus-feature sensitivities of neurons in the target

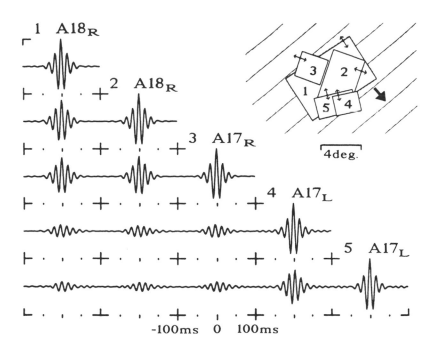

Fig. 12-18 Strong intrahemispheric and weaker but significant interhemispheric correlations between stimulus-induced gamma frequency spindles evoked simultaneously at 5 intracortical microelectrodes. Normalized auto- (at diagonals) and cross-correlograms (at off-diagonals) of the slow-wave oscillations evoked by 14 stimulus repetitions. Recording in areas 17 and 18 of the right *(R)* and left *(L)* hemispheres. The 5 receptive fields and the direction and orientation of the moving stimulus grating are shown upper right; grating of 0.25 cycles/degree, moving at 8.5 degrees/sec. (From Eckhorn et al.,1992.)

and source patches are usually similar. The maximum horizontal projection distances of these axons varies with cell type from 4 to 8 mm in cat area 17 (Galuske and Singer, 1996), comparable with the synchronization of cell groups in that area. The horizontal projection distances of these axons in monkey V1 are shorter (average = 0.61 mm, Chapter 3), which means that in the monkey distant synchronization, if effected by the horizontal system, must depend upon several transpatch activations. Synchronization of neuronal groups in different cortical areas and in different hemispheres is thought to be effected via corticocortical connections (Nowak et al., 1995b).

Mechanisms Producing Oscillations and Synchrony in Cortical Networks

Long-distance synchronizations are seldom observed without accompanying oscillations. This fact emphasizes the need to understand how oscillations arise in cortical circuits and how they contribute to synchronizations. One hypothesis is that oscillations are evoked in cortical networks by afferent input that is not oscillatory in nature, and that oscillations arise in sets of neurons reciprocally linked by excitatory connections, with local inhibitory interneuronal loops. An alternative explanation is that oscillations are induced and maintained by cortical neurons with endogenous oscillatory properties. Such cells respond to nonoscillatory, stimulus-induced thalamocortical input, with high-frequency burst discharges that recur at burst frequencies in the fast oscillatory frequency band (Jagadeesh et al., 1992). They are imagined quickly to entrain the cortical networks they inhabit to oscillating discharges at the same frequencies (for reviews, see Singer and Gray, 1995; Jeffreys et al., 1996; Singer et al., 1997). They do so because the intrinsic frequencies of the endogenous bursts fit within the frequency range determined by circuit parameters.

Gray and McCormick (1996) discovered a class of bursting cells with these properties in the supragranular layers of the cat striate cortex. These investigators recorded intracellularly, studied responses to injected depolarizing current and to visual stimuli, and determined cell phenotypes by dye injection and later histological recovery. They identified again the three classes of cortical neuronal discharge patterns described in Chapter 3 (and illustrated in Fig. 12-19A–C), and discovered a fourth, a class of bursting spiny pyramidal cells of layers II and III with expected pyramidal cell dendritic and axonal distribu-

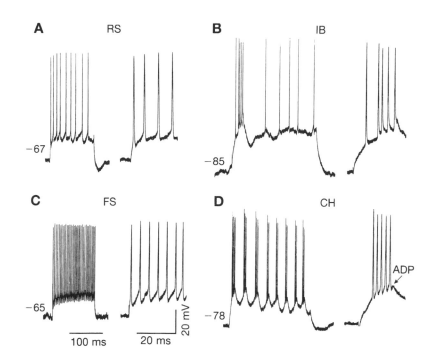

Fig. 12-19   Intracellular recordings from the visual cortex of anesthetized cats. Responses are shown for four classes of cells to intracellular depolarizing current injection. For each set, the initial phase of the response is shown by the record to the right of each pair. (A) Regular-spiking pyramidal cell in layer VI. (B) Intrinsically bursting cell of layer V. (C) Fast-spiking cell. (D) Chattering cell in layer III. Note that the intrinsically bursting cell switches from burst to tonic discharge with depolarization; note also the high-frequency train of impulses in the fast-spiking neuron and the repetitive bursts of discharge by the chattering cell. (From Gray and McCormick, 1996.)

tion patterns. These cells responded to depolarization and to visual stimuli with bursting discharges, with intraburst spike frequencies up to 800/sec, and interburst intervals from 15 to 50 msec, i.e., in the frequency band of 20–65 Hz. Both depolarizations and visual stimuli evoked oscillating membrane potentials at the burst frequencies, carrying the spike bursts on their negative phases (Fig. 12-19D). These responses were not tightly linked to visual stimuli but appeared with latencies and burst frequencies that differed from cell to cell. The oscillations and burst discharges never appeared spontaneously. It is likely that the coherent synchronization of large numbers of neurons in spatially separated areas requires both the presence of intrinsically bursting neurons and the oscillatory properties of neural networks.

An alternative or additional explanation for the oscillating activity in cortical networks is that they are driven by oscillating thalamocortical input. It has been known for a long time that oscillatory activity in the frequency range of 30–80 Hz occurs spontaneously in a significant population of cells in both the retina and the lateral geniculate. Visual stimuli evoke oscillating responses of retinal ganglion cells and lateral geniculate neurons of the cat (average frequency =

Rhythmicity and Synchronization in Neocortical Networks

88 Hz) (Neuenschwander and Singer, 1996). The retinal responses are correlated with those evoked in lateral geniculate neurons and accounted for the synchronization between the two lateral geniculate nuclei. They were also correlated with simultaneously evoked oscillating activity in visual cortical areas, commonly for neuron groups in area 18, rarely for those in area 17. While it appears that visually evoked synchronized activity in precortical levels of the visual system contributes to the synchronized patterns of neuronal activity in visual cortical areas, it is unlikely that this is the only mechanism producing those cortical rhythms.

The Relation of Synchronization to Perceptual and Sensory-Motor Performance

The results of many microelectrode recording experiments suggest the hypothesis that the synchronization of neuronal activity in the several nodes of a distributed system is a flexible mechanism for binding together the results of processing for different stimulus features in the nodes. Binding is assumed to delineate by recombination a neural image of the stimulus as a whole. Synchronized activity is linked to the stimuli that evoke it; only those activities evoked by stimuli with common stimulus features are bound together in a dynamically formed ensemble. A further test of this hypothesis is to discover whether a necessary and dependent relation exists between the synchronized activity and the perceptual or sensory-motor performance evoked by the same stimuli. Tests of this sort made in waking monkeys as they worked in such tasks have so far yielded equivocal results.

Murthy and Fetz (1992) studied the motor and premotor areas in waking monkeys working in simple motor retrieval tasks. They observed oscillatory activity in both the LFPs and single neuron discharges in the frequency band 25–35 Hz. These activities were on occasion synchronized between loci up to 14 mm apart, averaged 5 cycles in length, occurred in an irregular manner, were not related directly to movement parameters or to forearm muscle activity, and appeared most often in situations that required close attention to fine sensory-motor control. Sanes and Donoghue (1993) studied the motor and premotor areas in monkeys working in an instructed delay task. Synchronized oscillations appeared in widely dispersed loci in these motor areas during the delay period as the animal awaited a go signal and prepared for movement, but they were promptly suppressed by movement onset. These observations resemble those made by Rougeul and her colleagues, who recorded fast oscillating LFPs in the sensory-motor, premotor, and parietal areas of cats (at 35–45 Hz) and monkeys (at 15–18 Hz) during periods of motor inactivity but high levels of vigilance (Rougeul et al., 1979; Bouyer et al., 1981; Rougeul-Buser and Buser, 1994).The clearest behavioral correlate in all these experiments was attention to an expected event or object in the immediate environment. The rhythms were suppressed by bodily movement. No tests of synchronization were made.

The most direct links between synchronizations/oscillations and sensory-motor performance have been observed in multiple microelectrode recording experiments in the frontal cortex of monkeys working in spatial localization tasks (Abeles et al., 1993a,b, 1994; Aertsen et al. 1991, 1994; Vaadia et al., 1995). Recordings were made in the pre-arcuate and peri-principalis cortex, shown by lesion experiments to be essential for delayed tasks of this sort. Periods of correlation were observed between neurons widely distributed in these areas, frequently occurring during the delay period as the animal awaited a go signal for movement.

Abeles and his colleagues (Abeles et al., 1995; Seidmann et al., 1996) made analyses based upon a model of a hidden Markov process (Radons et al., 1994). They found that during the delay periods the activity of frontal cortical neurons occurs in successive discrete and identifiable states in which the activity is approximately stationary. These brief states occurred simultaneously in groups of neurons, and individual neurons shifted rapidly from one state to another. The states were reliably related to behavior; their analysis allowed prediction of 90 percent of trial outcomes.

The majority of visual cortical neurons in strabismic cats respond only to monocular stimulation (Konig et al., 1993; Roelfsema et al., 1994). Autocorrelation analysis of the responses showed that the proportion of cells responding with oscillating firing patterns is similar to that observed in normal cats. Cross-correlations between the responses evoked through different eyes revealed reduced synchronization between these sets of neurons, as compared with the proportion in normal cats. Fries et al. (1996) studied the visual cortex of waking cats with surgically induced squint with electrodes chronically implanted in areas 17 and 18. Visual images inducing binocular rivalry were delivered alternatively to the two eyes. Synchronized activity of neurons in areas 17 and 18 discharged at oscillating frequencies in the gamma range of 40–60 Hz. Synchronizations were enhanced between sets of neurons encoding the currently dominant stimulus, and suppressed for activity evoked by the nondominant stimuli, while the average discharge rates did not differ between the two sets.

Kreiter and Singer (1996) studied the middle temporal area (MT) in waking monkeys as they worked in a simple fixation task. They found that the responses of two separate sets of neurons could be synchronized only if they were activated by a "global" stimulus, in this case a long bar covering both receptive fields and oriented midway between the preferred directions of movement of the two sets. When two shorter bars were delivered, one to each receptive field and oriented to the preferred directions, vigorous responses were evoked, but they were not synchronized. These testing visual stimuli did not control behavior in these experiments—the fixation light did so—and thus no correlations could be made between synchronization and perceptual performance.

Modeling Experiments

The general subject has been explored in a number of theoretic and modeling studies (Hummel and Biederman, 1992; von der Malsberg and Schneider, 1992; Gerstner et al., 1993). Edelman and his colleagues have simulated aspects of integration within the cortical visual system in models based upon a sparse connectivity between excitatory elements, and between excitatory and inhibitory elements within local neuronal groups (Sporns et al., 1989, 1991, 1994). These aspects include *linking* re-entry between groups within a single feature domain and *binding* by re-entry between groups in different feature domains, i.e., within and between different cortical areas. Some of their results are the following:

1. Cortical integration occurs at several levels, locally within groups of a single area and between different cortical areas and systems. Distinctions between linking and binding are consonant with the distributions of neuronal connections within and between cortical areas.

2. Short-term correlations provide a way to achieve integration in one to a few hundred milliseconds, periods in which hu-

man observers achieve visual perceptions. The results suggest that changing patterns of temporal correlations may be just as effective in initiating and controlling behavior as are changes in neuronal frequencies. Correlations can change without changes in frequency.

3. Integration by re-entrant coupling can operate by correlation and by construction of new response properties.

Other Findings, Other Views

The experimental observations described provide some support for the temporal correlation hypothesis. Several others raise doubts about whether the phenomenon is a necessary neural concomitant of perception. The oscillations and synchronizations are highly variable in occurrence, latencies, durations, and internal frequencies. They vary widely in these parameters in a series of responses to a train of slowly repeated stimuli. The long latencies (frequently 200 msec or more) raise especial doubts, for the initial cortical processing of sensory input will have been completed before the onset of synchronization. More experiments are needed to determine whether in a waking monkey, working in a perceptual task, there is a direct and dependent relation between synchronizations and behavioral performance, tested on a trial-by-trial basis.

Several experiments designed to test the temporal correlation hypothesis have yielded results incompatible with it. Ghose and Freeman (1992) found the oscillations in area 17 of anesthetized cats to occur over a broad frequency spectrum, to be independent of stimulus parameters, and to be unstable in occurrence, duration, and internal frequency. They observed similar oscillations in a significant fraction of LGN cells and concluded that cortical oscillations are LGN-dependent and are unlikely to play a role in the cortical processing of visually evoked activity. They did not, however, examine the data for the synchronization of neural activity within or between cortical areas or between hemispheres. Singer has emphasized the role of synchronization, with or without oscillation, as the important parameter linking activity in distributed systems.

Young et al. (1992) studied areas V1, MT, and the inferotemporal cortex (IT) in anesthetized monkeys under conditions comparable to those used by Eckhorn and by Singer. They also studied area IT in waking monkeys working in a face-discrimination task. Oscillations independent of stimulus parameters were observed in the frequency range of 12–13 Hz at about 10 percent of the recording sites in area V1. No oscillations were recorded in area IT in anesthetized monkeys, and at only 2 of 50 recording sites in monkeys working in the discrimination task. Fast oscillations were observed at only 2 of 424 records made at 142 recording sites. No examinations were made for synchronizations either in or between cortical areas or between hemispheres.

Bair et al. (1994) made a power spectrum analysis of both bursting and nonbursting neurons in area MT of waking monkeys working in a directional discrimination task. They found 62 percent of cells with peaks in the power spectrum in the 20–60 Hz band, but only 10 percent of these peaks exceeded twice the control amplitude. The power spectrum did not change with changes in stimulus parameters, and it showed no significant relation to psychophysical measures of the animals' performances. No examinations were made for synchrony.

These three studies were interpreted to show that oscillations in neural activity, *per se,* are unlikely to play an important role in cortical processing. However, in none of the three were simultaneous recordings made from separated sites in areas or hemispheres to test for synchronizations. It is under these latter circumstances that oscillations have been reported to be important in securing synchronization, and it is synchronization that is emphasized as the essential linking parameter.

Summary

I have considered in this section what neuronal mechanisms achieve the transitions from the feature-detection functions of the peripheral, precortical, and primary sensory cortical areas of sensory systems to the population signals in distributed systems of the homotypical cortical areas thought to lead to the perception of complex scenes and objects. Activity in the homotypical cortical systems may be at preattentive levels, although many observations suggest it is influenced by attention. The hypothesis under study suggests that the synchronized neuronal activity within such a distributed system serves to label that particular neuronal set as evoked by a particular stimulus configuration. The synchronization dissects the ambiguities generated by the stimulus distributions in our sensory-perceptual environment. The frequency of the synchronized activity evoked by a single stimulus labels a linked ensemble as unique for a particular stimulus. More than one such ensemble may exist simultaneously within a distributed system. Different ensembles may be identifiable by frequency or phase differences in the oscillations, but direct evidence for this is not available. Such linked ensembles are transient associations, dissolving and re-forming on rapid time scales as the distal stimulus configurations change. Any single local neuronal group may from time to time participate in different linked ensembles.

It is obvious that more evidence is needed to establish these hypotheses as facts. Particularly, what is needed is strong evidence that the formation of a synchronized discharging ensemble is a necessary event for a successful execution of a perceptual task. This will require experiments in waking humans and nonhuman primates as they work in such tasks.

It is not yet clear how synchronization of the activity in distributed cortical systems could generate a holistic central "representation" of global stimulus features. The standard idea put forward is that synchronous activity in several nodes of a distributed system may converge on common targets and by virtue of its synchronization be more effective in transmitting to target neurons its own pattern of activity. But speaking of convergences and common targets raises for this hypothesis, as for the "single-neuron doctrine," the specter of an infinite regress.

13 Epilogue

A major research program in neuroscience is to determine the relations between the material order of the world around us and the sensory-perceptual order of our experience; and, to discover the central neural mechanisms of these transformations. Our perceptual experiences are generated by the integration of the central neural activity set in motion by sensory stimuli with the activation of the neural images of past experience and with those of the current central brain state. This combination I call a *construction,* as have many before me; the meaning of the term resembles the simpler part of what John Locke called *reflection* (see Locke, 1690, Book II, pp. 1–5). Whether the stored neural images of past experiences are themselves the result only of those past experiences, as I interpret Locke to have believed, or are determined in part by some innate properties of brain systems (innate ideas) generated a sustained controversy between empiricists and rationalists that engaged the attention of natural philosophers for generations, particularly in the age of the Enlightenment. These arguments have long since spent their force, and should now be set aside. Whether the doctrine of innate ideas has any basis in reality seems to me to be highly unlikely, but the evidence for and against it is uncertain.

The general problem of what brain mechanisms are involved in perception can now be studied directly. Indeed, it is an old idea that one might measure the performance of humans and nonhuman primates as they worked in perceptual tasks, and by some means record also the signs of the brain activity relevant for the tasks executed. What is new is that this *combined experiment* can now be executed with new methods for recording signs of the activity of large populations of central neurons and for correlating the two sets of observations. The methods range from indirect means of measuring changes in cerebral blood flow in local regions of the cortex in humans, or changes in the electrical activity of the human brain with large-numbered EEG recording, to the use of chronically implanted multiple microelectrodes in nonhuman primates. Causal explanations of sensory-perceptual experiences are then sought in terms of the neural activities that generate them. This is presently the most successful experimental paradigm used in perceptual neuroscience.

I have evaluated in preceding chapters several sources of knowledge relevant for understanding two of the many sets of unsolved problems in perceptual neuroscience. These are, first, the nature of the dynamic operations in neocortical microcircuits and, second, how neuronal operations are executed in widely distributed but heavily interconnected cerebral systems. I consider now in summary form several of those topics from earlier chapters and ask of each: what has this field of neuroscience research, valuable as it may be in its own venue, contributed to understanding of these two aspects of dynamic brain operations? The level of cortical function I address is the large in-between. Generally, we remain unaware of the complex integrated and spatially extended neuronal operations in distributed systems that follow an initial neural image (evoked by a sensory stimulus in a primary sensory area of the neocortex) or that precede a motor act (internally generated or reflexly evoked). The neuronal operations of construction, identification, categorization, discrimination, the interface with motor systems, and so on, are carried out within these widely interconnected systems. Only their final product flows across the threshold to conscious awareness, *fait accompli*. These intermediate mechanisms are the subjects of much of present-day research in perceptual neuroscience, endeavors sustained by the belief that until we have a better understanding of these intermediate processes, the workings of conscious awareness will remain obscure—absent some startling and presently unpredictable discovery.

What Have Phylogenetic and Comparative Studies Contributed to Knowledge of the Cerebral Cortex?

Perhaps there is no more startling event in evolutionary biology than the enlargement of the brain in hominids. Hominidae are thought to have emerged from stem Hominoidea during the Miocene-Pleisto-cene transition period, perhaps 5–7 million years ago, by a split from a common ancestor that produced australopithecines and pongids. A dramatic episode in our history followed: the early australopithe-cines assumed the upright stance and bipedal locomotion; perhaps they did so intermittently and perhaps they were not the first pri-mates to do so, but they initiated the chain of events leading to *Homo sapiens* (described in Chapter 2). They did so with brains no larger than those of modern pongids, but their new way of going must have required adaptations in the dynamic operations of central motor control systems that might not be evidenced by changes in brain size or external morphology. They did so using some postcranial skeletal adaptations for weight bearing in the upright mode, including lock-able knee joints unknown among pongids, but with no change in their pongid-like vestibular apparatus.

A tripling of brain size from 400 to about 1,300 grams marks hom-inid brain evolution—an enlargement that is associated with in-creased manipulative skill and in throwing with arm and hand. There followed the acquisition of a stone tool culture, family life, undoubt-edly gestural communication, and perhaps only much later a spoken language, the development of culture and civilization—and a tech-nology that could rescue *Apollo 13!* Some changes in brain structure accompanied its allometric enlargement: expansion of the posterior parietal and frontal cortices, the appearance of Broca's cap, increased bilateral asymmetry, etc.

A large effort has been made over the last century to understand neocortical evolution in hominids by study of the brains of living mammals. Even the most primitive mammals evolved cortices with 10–20 cortical areas, compared with about 100 in man, and the neo-cortex expanded in size in many lines. Comparative studies of the living hominoid descendants indicate that the general principles of brain organization resemble those in man, a strong example of con-vergent evolution. It is for this reason that the macaque monkey has become the essential experimental animal in perceptual neurosci-ence. None of these studies can inform us directly what the brain organization or synaptic patterns were in the extinct hominids but, to the extent that external morphology can be taken as an indicator, the general patterns of organization of the brains of the extinct homi-nids can be inferred with some confidence. Comparative studies have shown that the types of cortical neurons—their morphology, ultrastructure, and transmitter systems—appear to be quite similar over a very wide range of mammals, so that discoveries of cellular and molecular neurobiology made in living mammals appear directly applicable to the brain of man (see Chapter 3). We may infer from this that the major changes in hominid evolution were in size, numbers, systems organization, and patterns of connectivity, not in neuronal phenotypes and their proportions.

On the evidence from endocasts, the brain of *H. sapiens* has changed not a whit in size, form or external morphology since he appeared about fifty to a hundred thousand years ago. It is difficult to believe that man's transition from a cave-dwelling scavenger to the creator of modern civilization has been accomplished without some change in the dynamic operating characteristics of his brain. This intriguing hypothesis is unfortunately forever untestable.

The documentation of the changes in hominid brains in the last three or four million years provides some leads for hypotheses concerning global brain functions in man. Nevertheless, the question asked must be answered negatively: studies of brain evolution, like comparative studies of living mammals, have provided no knowledge of the function of intrinsic cortical microcircuits, nor of the dynamic operations of distributed cortical systems.

What Have Neuroanatomical Studies Contributed to Knowledge of the Cerebral Cortex?

One could hardly have guessed at midcentury that the then prosaic science of neuroanatomy would be one of the most successful of the subdisciplines of neuroscience in the decades that followed. Yet such is the case, for the invention and vigorous use of new methods have produced a picture of brain connectivity that would scarcely be recognized by our predecessors of two generations ago. The most productive of these methods come from the discovery of axoplasmic flow of molecules: after injection into the extracellular space, molecules are taken up by neuronal cell bodies and/or their terminals and transported throughout neurons, and in many cases they penetrate even their finest neurites. This has allowed the precise definition of the sources and targets of long-range connections between cortical areas, and between them and other brain structures. These labeling methods, now complemented by direct injection of molecular markers into cortical neurons, have revealed a neuronal morphology some steps beyond the best of the Golgi-era stains. Investigators are presently heavily engaged in working out the details of cell-to-cell connectivity, providing a prolegomenon for studies of the dynamic operations of intrinsic microcircuits.

A new and rapidly expanding area in neurobiology is the identification by biochemical and immunocytochemical methods of molecules on the surfaces of or within neurons that label selectively cytoarchitectural areas or, in several well-documented cases, subdivisions within those areas. Molecules have been identified that label in a restricted and selective way segments of neural systems (e.g., parts of the geniculocortical), but until now no case has been described in which an entire neuronal system has been labeled selectively across several system nodes. Further exploitation of these powerful methods will undoubtedly produce a new architecture of the brain, one that is based upon molecular differentiations.

For these large areas of neuroscience, anatomical studies have indeed advanced our understanding of the brain's circuitry, but in a special way. The astounding increments in knowledge of brain structure, from the level of molecules to that of neuronal systems, provide the essential base for the design of current and future studies of the dynamic intrinsic and distributed system activity in the nervous system; but in and of itself knowledge of structure provides no direct understanding of dynamic function. *Where is not how.*

What Have Studies of the Organization of the Neocortex Contributed to Understanding of Its Function?

The cerebral cortex of humans is a thin, extended, and convoluted sheet of tissue with a surface area of about 2,600 cm^2 and 3–4 mm thick. It contains about 28×10^9 neurons that are connected with each other and with neurons in other brain structures by axons that bear a large and uncertain number of synapses, perhaps as many as 10^{12}–10^{13}. The cortex contains about twice as many glial cells as neurons. The brain itself is connected to the outside world by a few million afferent and efferent nerve fibers.

Cortical neurons are arrayed in six layers, in some of which efferent pyramidal cells have laminar-specific targets external to the local area. They are also grouped into sets heavily interconnected in the vertical, translaminar direction; these are sparsely linked horizontally in the immediate surround, but they have horizontal intra-areal connections with more distant vertical groups of cells with similar functional properties (Chapters 4, 7). These vertical groups of neurons are called *columns;* they conform to the concept of modular organization, a widely documented principle of design for both vertebrate and invertebrate brains, of which columnar organization is an example. Columnar units vary little in cross-sectional measurement over a range of mammals whose cortical surface areas vary by three orders of magnitude.

Columns in heterotypical sensory and motor regions are defined and grouped into areas by dominating extrinsic connections, in the main by projections from and to the dorsal thalamus. Columnar defining factors in homotypical cortical areas are determined in part by dynamic operations within the area itself, in increasing degree the more distant the area from primary sensory and motor areas. The total set of columns within a defined cortical area may itself be fractionated into subsets by different patterns of extrinsic connections. Linkages between such sets in several larger cortical and subcortical regions compose distributed systems, whose observed and inferred functional properties I describe in a later section.

Columns are composed of 100–300 smaller units, called *minicolumns;* they have average transverse measurement of about 50 μm and contain about 100 neurons, including in usual proportions the various cortical cell phenotypes. Minicolumns are the mature product of the ontogenetic units generated in development by the temporal sequence of neurons that migrate to the cortical plate from a small polyclone in a local region of the germinal epithelium. The minicolumn is not an irreducible functional unit, for the pyramidal neurons within its layers III, V, and VI have different output targets. I infer, with no direct proof, that neuronal processing within intracolumnar microcircuits leading to those different outputs will produce different patterns of activity.

In sum, studies of the large-scale organization of the brain with anatomical and other methods have revealed an interconnected system of a hitherto unexpected complexity. A major result is support for the general hypothesis that cortical processing mechanisms in perception beyond primary sensory areas are carried out in re-entrantly connected distributed systems that bind together, in temporally changing functional arrays, activity in different cerebral structures that are frequently separated spatially. There is nothing diffuse or unspecific about a distributed system, for the intra-system connections between nodes are localized and highly specific and frequently project upon specific cell types, layers, or restricted columnar sets.

What Have Studies of the Ontogenetic and Secondary Histogenesis of the Cerebral Cortex Contributed to Understanding of Its Dynamic Actions?

The processes of neuronal histogenesis and the specification of cortical areas flow continuously through overlapping stages, controlled by a manifold of cell-autonomous and cell-extrinsic factors; both operate through gene expression and the synthesis of proteins important for axonal guidance, axon growth cone extension, the labeling of stop points, etc. We now have detailed phenomenological descriptions of this developmental saga for both monkey and rodent, and research programs under way aim to define the events at the molecular level. Although some uncertainty remains, I conclude that cortical areas are to a degree chemically specified within the germinal epithelium before migration begins, and that this—perhaps loose—specification is transferred to the developing subplate, forming there appropriately labeled targets for ingrowing thalamocortical fiber systems. It appears likely that it is only after these axonal systems reach the subplate and begin their secondary progress into the overlying cortex that areas in the latter are specified (Chapters 8 and 9). Even this specification is limited in degree, and is further refined in a dynamic way by activity in thalamocortical and intracortical systems to make areal boundaries precise and to guide development of subareal divisions and the details of intracortical connectivity. These dynamic processes of synapse specification and stabilization are achieved by processes similar to those accounting for plasticity in the developing and mature cortex (described in Chapter 6).

The major fields of neuroscience research I have just described in cursory fashion—the onto- and phylogenetic development of the cortex, the structure of the brains of living mammals, and the large-scale organization of the primate brain—have each contributed greatly to the fund of knowledge essential for current and future studies of the dynamic function of the cortex. However, my own experience has been that inferences concerning dynamic function drawn from knowledge of structure alone are hazardous; they are frequently simply wrong.

What Have Studies of Synaptic Transmission Contributed to Knowledge of Cortical Microcircuits?

We have witnessed in the last two decades a remarkable accumulation of knowledge, generated by the application of the methods and concepts of molecular and cellular neurobiology, of synaptic transmission between neurons. We are poised for what one can predict will follow, a quantum leap in understanding of the dynamic operations in cortical microcircuits and distributed systems, which are of course linked sets of microcircuits. I have described some of these discoveries in Chapters 5 and 6, with particular emphasis upon the following: the ionic hypothesis, the founding generality of cellular neurophysiology; the mechanisms of integrative action in single nerve cells; the discovery of chemical transmission between central neurons and the elucidation of the linked chain of molecular operations from transmitter synthesis to postsynaptic responses; the discovery of NMDA channels, synaptic plasticity, and the second-messenger systems that link presynaptic actions to gene expression in postsynaptic cells. Patch-clamp recordings and cortical slice preparations are important in the present context, for their use has provided descriptions of the biophysical properties of cortical neurons and correlation of those properties with cortical cell phenotype. It is only the isolatable microcircuits of invertebrates that until now have come under full experimental observation. Studies of those small-numbered neuronal circuits have yielded the remarkable discovery that the mode of operation of such a circuit can be changed quickly in a qualitative way, and as quickly reversed, by the brief action of modulatory inputs to the circuit. Given the dense innervation of the cerebral cortex by modulatory systems from the basal forebrain and brainstem reticular core, one can predict that similar qualitative modulations may also be imposed upon cortical microcircuits.

Studies in cortical slice preparations have yielded much of the knowledge of cortical synaptic mechanisms. Double intracellular recording-stimulation between pairs of neurons in cortical slice preparations has provided quantitative descriptions of the effective synaptic connections between identified neurons in the local circuits. It is important to emphasize that while intrinsic operations lead to different and segregated output channels from a microcircuit, there is no evidence that isolated processing pathways exist within such a microcircuit.

How Can We Study Microcircuits and Distributed Systems?

The discoveries noted above promise rapid progress in understanding the action of cerebral circuits when combined with methods for recording the electrical signs of neuronal activity in the cerebral cortices of waking nonhuman primates via large numbers of chronically implanted microelectrodes, each still movable in the transcortical dimension. To reveal the workings of local microcircuits, we need methods for recording from a substantial number of the 100 or so neurons of a cortical minicolumn in a waking monkey as he executes a perceptual task. This is now a doable experiment. Concerning opportunities for making progress in our knowledge of distributed systems, conjure up the image of 1,000 or so microelectrodes implanted to cover the several nodes of the parieto-frontal distributed system as a monkey reaches to a target he has selected from several in a perceptual decision. I emphasize that it is in the nodes that the essential system operations are carried out; internodal linkages carry but do not modify messages. Given average discharge rates of about 20/sec, a single behavioral trial of 10 seconds in length would require the collection, storage, and later analysis of several hundred action potential intervals during each trial on each of the 1,000 channels. Such an experiment will mark the transition of perceptual neuroscience from little science (one or a few investigators huddled about a minicomputer) to big science, with experiments executed and the results analyzed by an accomplished team of scientists who bring to the common effort a broad range of experience and skills. Such teams are already forming, struggling with the problems of making large enterprises work—ranging from the sociological challenges facing large working groups to obtaining the funding required. These problems can be solved; what could be more worthwhile, for the objectives are of transcendental importance. Presently no other experimental path is obvious, absent startlingly new technical developments.

Have Imaging Methods Contributed to Understanding of Cortical Functions?

The study of humans with brain lesions continues to reveal important aspects of altered cortical geography and the related functional impairments in the areas of motor control, language production and reception, hemispheric lateralization, and so on, as well as in perception. The present period is characterized by an explosion of several forms of imaging of the living, functioning human brain. These methods have revolutionized the diagnosis and localization of disease processes in the clinical neurological sciences; they are also important for the developing area of cognitive science. Their potential for contributing to knowledge of the dynamic function of the brain is limited, for they are geographic methods designed to answer "where" questions, and "where" answers reveal little of dynamic function. These new methods provide precise information about the locations within the cerebral cortex that are active in a wide range of cognitive and perceptual tasks. Some can trace changes in those locations in real time, and all can differentiate between global and local processing. A principal aim in the field now is to find a solution to the problem of how these changes in activity—e.g., those seen as changes in blood flow—can be translated into the neural actions that produce them. It is exactly the patterns of activity in large populations of cortical neurons that we need to know and analyze in order to reach a new comprehension of brain mechanisms.

What Do We Know of the Functions of Cortical Microcircuits?

The Properties of Microcircuits Are Emergent

I posed in Chapter 11 the questions: what transforms do cortical microcircuits impose upon their several inputs to produce their several outputs; and, what are the neuronal mechanisms of those transformations? Microcircuit properties are emergent—they are produced by the dynamic interactions of circuit elements. They are not predictable from knowledge of the functional properties of any single neuron or any single neuron class within the circuit. Moreover, given ubiquitous neuronal cell death, it seems likely that microcircuit operations will survive the loss of some—still uncertain—proportion of circuit elements.

Microcircuit Operations May Be Variable

There are reasons to suggest that the particular operation of a given cortical microcircuit is not constant. The example is before us of the dynamic qualitative changes in the operations of local circuits in invertebrates produced by modulatory controls. Given the established plasticity of synaptic operations in the mammalian neocortex, and its dense innervation by modulatory afferents, it is difficult to escape the idea that operations in local regions of cortex may vary over a range limited only by anatomical connectivity. Cortical neurons contain many voltage- and ligand-gated channels, and they receive dense synaptic inputs from the modulatory systems that operate with a number of small-molecule transmitters, as well as acetylcholine, the monamines, and polypeptides. If this variability exists in cortical circuits, the constancy of our perceptual operations must be explained; e.g., how do we recognize a familiar face or make a sensory discrimination over a wide range of levels of awareness from drowsiness to mania, states over which modulatory inputs are thought to have regulatory control? One hypothesis open for testing is that the variability of microcircuit operations, if true at all in the mammalian neocortex, is true only to a minimal extent at the entry levels of cortical systems.

Are Microcircuits Uniform throughout the Neocortex?

The uniformity of cell types and of their numerical proportions in different cortical areas, and the nearly uniform size of modules in mammalian cortices that vary greatly in surface area, have suggested to some that neocortical microcircuit operations may be more or less similar in all areas of the neocortex. Indeed, one of the most productive groups engaged in specifying the patterns of connectivity in cortical microcircuits describe their results in terms of a "canonical" circuit. Whether such a uniformity holds true for other cortical areas is a question awaiting experimental study. Some anatomical studies indicate that intracortical microcircuits may differ by some still undetermined degree between cortical areas that differ so strikingly in other respects, as do the striate and the prefrontal homotypical areas in the macaque monkey. It seems likely that there is a basically uniform microcircuit pattern throughout the neocortex upon which certain specializations unique to this or that cortical area are superimposed.

Transformations Executed in the Microcircuits of Primary Cortical Areas

Transformations in the primary visual cortex are of particular interest, for properties such as binocularity and orientation selectivity are either unknown, as for binocularity, or very weak, as for orientation selectivity, at precortical levels of the system. These properties are created early in the intracortical processing chain by combinations of trans-synaptic convergence and neuronal processing. The approach has been to define the functional properties of cortical neurons and then use neurophysiological methods to discover the mechanisms that produce them. The general result is that binocularity is produced by a simple convergence of monocular geniculocortical afferents upon cortical neurons. Orientation selectivity in the cat is produced by a combination of convergent summation of geniculocortical fibers with circular receptive fields, aligned along the angle of orientation of the cortical cells upon which they project; this property is then greatly sharpened by intracortical processing, including a powerful local excitatory loop at the level of entry. Moreover, in the monkey orientation selectivity appears to be generated entirely by intracortical processing mechanisms. The relative importance of inhibition in these processes is still uncertain. Some recent experiments in the monkey striate cortex show that orientation specificity is successively sharpened in the progression of activity from the input to the output cortical layers.

Many of the productive studies of cortical microcircuit connectivity and processing have been made on heterotypical cortical areas. Yet primary sensory and motor areas are poor general models of neocortex, for each is highly specialized, commonly matched to the requirements of the afferent or efferent system to which it is linked. This is particularly true for the striate cortex of cat and monkey, as well as for the primary somesthetic and auditory cortices; all are specialized transformation and distribution centers.

The Rodent Somesthetic Cortex

The rodent cortex has the advantages that it is readily available, that it may be isolated in a slice preparation with its thalamic afferents intact, and that a great deal is known of its structure, connectivity, and ontogenesis. The barrel cortex has been intensively studied in terms of the activity evoked in it by appropriate sensory stimuli and in terms of the successive translaminar processing of that activity that leads to its output channels. There is the disadvantage that the barrel is a highly specialized structure that evolved in animals who spend most of their lives in light-tight compartments, making their way by palpation of their spatial surrounds by synchronous sweeping movements of their whiskers. It is inferred that the output of each barrel—each one predominantly but not exclusively activated by movement of a single whisker—contributes to a population neural image of the spatial surround. This phenomenological description has not yet been explained at the level of mechanism.

Microcircuit Transformations in Homotypical Cortical Areas

The phenomenon of new feature construction is most fully developed in the microcircuit operations of the homotypical cortex of the posterior parietal, temporal, and frontal lobes of the brain. I have described some of these transformations in the cortex of the macaque monkey in Chapter 11. The results obtained in studies of the homotypical cortex in waking monkeys, although differing markedly in the qualitative nature of the properties constructed in different areas, have all revealed a common feature: it is not possible to predict the properties of homotypical cortical neurons from knowledge of those of afferent systems active during the particular task under study. Neurons of the posterior parietal cortex, e.g., display their full profiles of functional properties only if the behavioral task in which the animal is engaged has meaning for him, and only if he pays close attention to the relevant stimuli presented. This powerful modulatory control may be absolute, for many parietal neurons are simply inactive when the task stimuli are delivered to an inattentive animal, only to burst into activity when he attends! Little is known of the locations or the mechanisms of these powerful modulatory effects. Undoubtedly they act directly at the cortical level, but the possibility that they also act upon thalamocortical systems more generally considered should not be dismissed.

Rhythmicity and Synchronization in Neocortical Networks

A ubiquitous property of neural networks is a coherent periodicity of neuronal discharge and self-sustaining slow-wave oscillations in the frequency range of 1–100 Hz. These oscillations can be recorded from the surface of or within neural populations so diverse as the small-numbered networks of invertebrates and the mammalian neocortex. The discovery by Berger of the human electroencephalogram (EEG) initiated one of the most intense and prolonged research programs in the history of neuroscience. It appeared to the pioneers in the field that here was a method for assessing directly the dynamic activity of the brain, particularly of the cerebral cortex, and for correlating it with the behavior controlled by the brain, observed simultaneously (such as perceptual operations). The results obtained have been less than hoped for, but the method has been greatly elaborated and is now an essential tool in the clinical neurological sciences. The persisting studies of a relatively small group of investigators have defined some of the mechanisms that generate the EEG (described in Chapter 12). Oscillations characteristic of neuronal networks and seen in the EEG may either be produced by the activity of endogenously bursting neurons within the networks or by the interaction of synaptic actions within the networks, or they may be imposed by corticipetal systems. A major discovery is the dual role of the dorsal thalamus: it functions in its classical relay mode, and also as a neuronal oscillator that in many states drives and controls cortical rhythms.

The development of EEG recording with large numbers of surface electrodes, combined with new methods of analysis, has converted the EEG into what promises to be a useful tool for imaging the activity of the brain, with the advantage that changes in the electrical signs of brain activity are observed in real time and localized precisely.

The Complementary Paradigms of Hierarchy and Distribution

The traditional model of hierarchical processing within the nervous system has guided experimental design for a century. It is presently much less valuable, for it does not take into account the accumulating evidence that different features of external objects and events are transduced and encoded by different sets of primary afferent fibers. Activity in these sets is projected over afferent systems to and processed within different *cortical areas specialized for the appropriate processing, not functional localization.* These spatially separated areas are linked together in the large-scale distributed systems described in Chapter 10. Neurons in the separate nodes of distributed systems do not project convergently to any "higher-order" target in which an integrated perceptual image might be constructed. That image is thought to be embedded in the dynamic activity of the distributed system itself. The absence of convergence to an integrating center and the nature of distributed processing have raised again the well-known binding problem: how are the activities within and between the separate processing nodes bound together in momentary association to form a coherent representational state surmised to be the perception?

The Binding Hypothesis

The solution proposed is that the transition from the independent processing of different stimulus features in separate nodes of a re-entrantly linked system to a coherent neural image (of a perception) is enabled by a transient synchronization of the neuronal activity in the several nodes of the system. The hypothesis predicts that the coherent image is not located in any single node but is embedded within the dynamic activity of the system. That activity is labeled by a particular synchronized phase and/or frequency, and it can therefore be recognized and differentiated from other dynamic sets that may exist simultaneously within the same or partially overlapping distributed systems. The binding hypothesis is set at a limited range, for it proposes no solution for the problem that bedevils many formulations of the neural mechanisms in perception: what next? What neural mechanisms can be imagined to be sensitive to and recognize the presence of synchronization versus its absence? What mechanism can identify—i.e., *perceive*—the pattern of synchronized system activity as that of a particular external event? Whatever mechanism is proposed must function across a preconscious-conscious divide, still undefined in neural terms, for which no presently proposed paradigm presents a rational solution.

Experimental studies of the binding problem have been made in two quite different experimental designs. In the first, induced fast oscillations of the human EEG (described in Chapter 12) were recorded as subjects worked in cognitive or perceptual tasks. Induced oscillations are not limited to the "gamma band" around 40 Hz—they vary in frequency over the range of 10–100 Hz—although the peak power is frequently in that band. They also appear in slow-wave and REM sleep and are generated by local microzones of potential differences distributed through the vertical cortical columns, with limited horizontal coherence. Brief periods of fast oscillation evoked by sensory stimuli presented to perceiving humans are loosely linked to the evoking stimuli, with variable and sometimes long latencies. An identifying characteristic is that the frequencies of the fast oscillations are not imposed by any rhythm in the evoking stimuli but are generated by the neural networks activated by those stimuli. Synchronization of the fast oscillations occurs in cortical areas sometimes several centimeters apart. They have been observed in some experiments in humans making sensory discriminations, but the evidence that coherent fast oscillations are universal and necessary conditions for cortical perceptual operations is not compelling.

Many channel magnetoencephalographic recordings have been used to study the more global distributions of the fast oscillations in humans in waking and sleeping states and in perceptual operations. The widespread and intermittently coherent fast oscillations at about 40 Hz were reset by a brief auditory stimulus and were linked to an auditory discrimination. The results suggest that the fast oscillations (or what they represent) might function as a scanning or global binding mechanism for more general aspects of cognition. The idea that some component of the activity recorded by EEG might serve as a scanning device sweeping repetitively over the human cerebral cortex has been proposed in the field almost since its inception. On this new evidence, the hypothesis deserves further intensive study.

In the second set of experiments, the action potentials of cortical neurons and the local field potentials (LFPs) have been recorded in anesthetized cats and monkeys and in monkeys working in perceptual tasks. Coherent oscillations of the LFPs and synchronization of neuronal discharges are evoked in single columns in a cortical area in both anesthetized and waking animals, between separate columns in the same area, between different areas in the same hemisphere, between homologous areas in the two hemispheres, and in some cases between thalamic and cortical components of the same system. The synchronized neuronal activity is observed only in response to the stimuli that evoke it, and activities in two areas are synchronous only if linked by stimuli that contain features common to the processing specializations of the areas. It is synchronization that appears essential for the hypothesis. LFPs may or may not occur, but are the more important for synchronization the greater the distance between the two areas compared. Oscillatory activity of neuronal sets may be produced by bursting cells intrinsic to the cortical networks or by synaptic interactions within a distributed system.

These observations are by no means uniform, for a number of extensive and well-controlled experiments have not revealed coherent oscillations under conditions similar to those described above, and in other experiments coherent oscillations were observed only rarely. In only a few of these experiments, however, have analyses been made for both coherence of LFPs and synchronization of neuronal populations, and it is the latter that is thought essential for the binding operation.

I have given in Chapter 12 what I hope is a balanced account of the varieties of experimental evidence that bear upon the binding hypothesis. My own conclusion is that the evidence for synchronization between neuronal populations active in perceptual operations is reliable, but that the evidence that synchronization is a necessary event for cortical perceptual operations is not yet compelling. What is needed is an extensive set of experiments in which neural events are tested for synchronization in several nodes of a relevant distributed system and are compared on a trial-by-trial basis with the outcomes of the perceptual operations, recorded simultaneously. The aim will be to determine whether a necessary and dependent relation exists between a perceptual or sensory-motor operation and synchronized neural activity evoked in linked cortical areas by the same stimuli.

The Neocortex: A Synthesis

I give here a synthesis of some present ideas about the cerebral neocortex. The description is incomplete, contains assertions that while unproven may be of predictive value, and changes continually in the light of new discoveries. I retain a somewhat skeptical view of the current cortical zeitgeist.

The human cerebral cortex is an extended sheet of tissue with a surface area of about 2,600 cm^2 and thickness about 3–4 mm. It contains on the order of 28×10^9 neurons and perhaps twice that many glial cells. Cortical neurons are linked with each other and with neurons elsewhere in the brain by perhaps 10^{13} synapses. The mammalian neocortex is organized horizontally into six layers, and vertically into groups of cells linked synaptically across the layers. This vertical unit is the minicolumn, a narrow chain 30–50 μm in transverse measurement that contains about 100 cells, including the cortical neuronal phenotypes in the same proportions everywhere. Minicolumns are organized into larger units called modules or columns; each contains several hundred minicolumns. Columns are organized into areas, and areas are often categorized by lobe. Columns in different areas are linked together in nested and re-entrantly connected distributed systems in which hierarchy may obtain only at the entry level.

Studies of ontogenesis have revealed the mosaicism of the germinal epithelium and the molecular mechanisms guiding neuronal migration from the neuroepithelium to the developing cortical plate. A defined ontogenetic unit is inferred to be the precursor of the minicolumn in the mature cortex. Maturation of the cortex depends upon the interaction of genetically defined and experiential factors. Of the latter, neuronal activity plays a critical role in stabilizing synapses, establishing microcircuits, and defining cortical areas.

Surely few will doubt that the most important advances in neurobiology of the last half-century have been the elucidation of the molecular and cellular mechanisms of excitation and conduction in nerve axons, of neuromuscular transmission, and of synaptic transmission between nerve cells. I have described the latter in Chapters 5 and 6, where I emphasized that this mature model of synaptic transmission, derived in the main from study of neurons in simpler structures, has been tested and found directly applicable to transmission between cortical neurons, both as pertains to general principles and a great mass of detail of the biochemical and biophysical mechanisms involved. This base of knowledge is now used intensively in studies of dynamic actions in cortical microcircuits, with the aim to discover the operations they execute. I summarized what is known of those operational principles in Chapter 11.

Slow-wave electrical events generated by the brain remain subjects of intensive enquiry. Leaving aside their obvious usefulness in the clinical neurological sciences and in defining behavioral states, it remains uncertain whether slow waves are more than epiphenomenal signs of the action of large populations of neurons; or are active agents; or function as signal carriers; or serve as a mechanism for binding together the actions of different neuronal populations. A major problem is how to devolve the electrical oscillations of the EEG into the underlying patterns of neuronal activity. Presently no unique solution has been found, and the EEG remains an ambiguous indicator of that activity.

The present synthesis includes what is useful from nearly two centuries of study of humans with brain lesions and the purported "localization of function" that resulted, but it avoids defining function in terms of the defects produced by lesions. Where nodes are funnels at entry or exit from systems, lesions will destroy or seriously degrade function, but this is weak evidence that the function is normally localized in the area lesioned. Higher-order perceptual and cognitive processes are thought to be embedded in the dynamic neuronal activity in distributed systems. This conjecture has stimulated study of neuronal populations with the aim to discover how such complex processes are signaled in distributed neural codes. Cortical areas are specialized for modes of processing, not for strict localization of function.

Application of the methods of cellular and molecular neurobiology has yielded precise descriptions of the biophysical properties of cortical neurons and revealed the complex variety of transmitters, channels, and postsynaptic receptors, which differ in their modes of action and operate on time scales from milliseconds to hours or days. Long-term changes in synaptic efficacy are effected by molecular chains that link presynaptic actions to gene expression, protein synthesis, and structural change. These capacities are present during embryonic and neonatal life and persist in the mature cortex. They are proposed as the cellular mechanisms of learning and memory. How those local changes might effect those more global classes of cognitive function in distributed systems is an object of intense study.

Descriptions of models of cortical operations flood the neuroscience scene. Many are based upon the known properties of neurons and neuronal systems. I believe that these studies can be, and often are, of great value, for there appears to be no other ready way in which one can conceptualize or test the operations of such a large-numbered, nonlinear system as the cerebral cortex. It may be possible to establish in this way the range and mode of those operations; it may also turn out that such models will yield precisely designed experiments to test them. We need global theories of brain function, but perhaps especially at the present time we need models of part functions that can be brought to experimental study with presently available methods. For examples, among many: the exact neural mechanisms of an association, the role of re-entrant connections in establishing the perceptual image, a solution to the binding problem, how complex activity is coupled between parallel maps, or the sensory-motor linkage at the cortical level.

The decline of dualism has freed us to consider the relation between brain and mind in a rational way. The dominant theme among neuroscientists—with many variations—is that all behaviors, including those we regard as mental, are externally observed and/or internally experienced aspects of brain processes. The functional state of consciousness is regarded as the more complex of those behaviors, not one of a unique class; it is also thought to be the expression of dynamic activity in some but not all brain systems. The linking mechanisms between brain activity and subjective experience are unknown. What that linkage may be presents a major unsolved problem in neuroscience that will be a fertile field for future theoretical and experimental studies. It is not possible at present to predict or even imagine the nature of such a linking mechanism. Briefly put, how do we come to recognize and interpret patterns of neuronal activity within our own brains? How does a brain come to know itself?

Brain processes are, on the large scale, emergent in nature, for they are embedded in the activity patterns of large numbers of heavily interconnected populations of neurons located in the nodes of distributed systems of the cerebral cortex and its linked appendages. The dynamic patterns of activity in those systems are described as "emergent" because they depend upon ("emerge from") the cooperative activity of neurons located in many nodes—sometimes widely separated—within the system. They can seldom be predicted from knowledge of the activity patterns of any single class of neurons, or of the population in any single node of a distributed system.

Thus a major task for neuroscience is to devise ways to study and to analyze the activity in distributed systems in waking brains, including particularly human brains, and to seek direct correlations and explanations of the relevant behavior observed in terms of those patterns of neuronal activity.

References

Abeles M. 1982. *Local Cortical Circuits*. Berlin and New York: Springer-Verlag.

Abeles M, H Bergman, I Gat, I Meilijson, E Seidemann, N Tishby, and E Vaadia. 1995. Cortical activity flips among quasi-stationary states. *Proc. Natl. Acad. Sci. USA* 92: 8616–8620.

Abeles M, H Bergman, E Margalit, and E Vaadia. 1993a. Spatiotemporal firing patterns in the frontal cortex of behaving monkeys. *J. Neurophysiol.* 70: 1629–1638.

Abeles M, Y Prut, H Bergman, and E Vaadia. 1994. Synchronization in neuronal transmission and its importance for information processing. *Prog. Brain Res.* 102: 395–404.

Abeles M, E Vaadia, H Bergman, Y Prut, I Haalman, and H Slovin. 1993b. Dynamics of neuronal interactions in the frontal cortex of behaving monkeys. *Concepts Neurosci.* 4: 131–158.

Abeliovich A, R Paylor, C Chen, JJ Kim, JM Wehner, and S Tonegawa. 1993. PKC mutant mice exhibit mild deficits in spatial and contextual learning. *Cell* 75: 1263–1275.

Abraham WC, BR Christie, B Logan, P Lawlor, and M Dragunow. 1994. Immediate early gene expression associated with persistence of heterosynaptic long-term depression in the hippocampus. *Proc. Natl. Acad. Sci. USA* 91: 10049–10053.

Adrian ED and BHC Matthews. 1934. The Berger rhythm: Potential changes from the occipital lobes in man. *Brain* 57: 356–385.

Adrian ED and K Yamigawa. 1935. The origin of the Berger rhythm. *Brain* 58: 323–351.

Aertsen A, M Erb, G Palm, and A Schuz. 1994. Coherent assembly dynamics in the cortex: Multineuronal recordings, network simulations, and anatomical considerations. In *Oscillatory Event-related Brain Dynamics,* ed. C Pantev, T Elbert, and B Lutkenhoner, pp. 59–84. Nato ISI Series A; Life Sciences Vol. 271. New York: Plenum.

Aertsen A, E Vaadia, M Abeles, E Ahissar, H Bergman, B Karmon, Y Lavner, E Margalit, I Nelken, and S Rotter. 1991. Neural interactions in frontal cortex of a behaving monkey: Signs of dependence on stimulus context and behavioral state. *J. Hirnforschung* 32: 735–743.

Agmon A and BW Connors. 1991. Thalamocortical responses of mouse somatosensory (barrel) cortex in vitro. *Neurosci.* 41: 365–379.

Ahissar M, E Ahissar, H Bergman, and E Vaadia. 1992. Encoding of sound-source location and movement: Activity of single neurons and interactions between adjacent neurons in the monkey auditory cortex. *J. Neurophysiol.* 67: 203–215.

Ahissar E and E Vaadia. 1990. Oscillatory activity of single units in the somatosensory cortex of an awake monkey and their possible role in texture analysis. *Proc. Natl. Acad. Sci. USA* 87: 8935–8939.

Ahmed B, JC Anderson, RJ Douglas, KAC Martin, and JC Nelson. 1994. Polyneuronal innervation of spiny stellate neurons in cat visual cortex. *J. Comp. Neurol.* 341: 39–49.

Akil M and DA Lewis. 1992. Differential distribution of parvalbumin-immunoreactive pericellular clusters of terminal boutons in developing and adult monkey neocortex. *Exp. Neurol.* 115: 239–249.

Albright TD, R Desimone, and CG Gross. 1984. Columnar organization of directionally selective cells in visual area MT of the macaque. *J. Neurophysiol.* 51: 16–31.

Allendoerfer KL and CJ Shatz. 1994. The subplate, a transient neocortical structure: Its role in the development of connections between thalamus and cortex. *Annu. Rev. Neurosci.* 17: 185–218.

Allendoerfer KL, DL Shelton, EM Shooter, and CJ Shatz. 1990. Nerve growth factor receptor immunoreactivity is transiently associated with subplate neurons of the mammalian cerebral cortex. *Proc. Natl. Acad. Sci. USA* 87: 187–190.

Alloway KD and H Burton. 1985. Submodality and columnar organization of the second somatic sensory area in cats. *Exp. Brain Res.* 61: 128–140.

——— 1986. Bicuculline-induced alterations in neuronal responses to controlled tactile stimuli in the second somatosensory cortex of the cat: A microiontophoretic study. *Somatosensory Research* 3: 197–211.

——— 1991. Differential effects of GABA and bicuculline on rapidly- and slowly-adapting neurons in primary somatosensory cortex of primates. *Exp. Brain Res.* 85: 598–610.

Almers W and FW Tse. 1990. Transmitter release from synapses: Does a preassembled fusion pore initiate exocytosis? *Neuron* 4: 813–818.

Altman J and SA Bayer. 1990. Vertical compartmentalization and cellular transformations in the germinal matrices of the embryonic rat cerebral cortex. *Exp. Neurol.* 107: 23–35.

Amir Y, M Harel, and R Malach. 1993. Cortical hierarchy reflected in the organization of intrinsic connections in macaque monkey visual cortex. *J. Comp. Neurol.* 334: 198–246.

Amitai Y and BW Connors. 1995. Intrinsic physiology and morphology of single neurons in neocortex. In *Cerebral Cortex,* Volume 11: *The Barrel Cortex of Rodents,* ed. EG Jones and A Peters, pp. 299–331. New York: Plenum.

Amitai Y, A Friedman, BW Connors, and MJ Gutnick. 1993. Regenerative activity in apical dendrites of pyramidal cells in neocortex. *Cerebral Cortex* 3: 26–38.

Andersen RA and VB Mountcastle. 1983. The influence of the angle of gaze upon the excitability of the light-sensitive neurons of the posterior parietal cortex. *J. Neurosci.* 3: 532–548.

Anderson JC, RJ Douglas, KA Martin, and JC Nelson. 1994a. Synaptic output of physiologically identified spiny stellate neurons in cat visual cortex. *J. Comp. Neurol.* 341: 16–24.

——— 1994b. Polyneuronal innervation of spiny stellate neurons in cat visual cortex. *J. Comp. Neurol.* 341: 39–49.

Anderson KD, RF Alderson, CA Altar, PS DiStefano, TL Corcoran, RM Lindsay, and SJ Wiegand. 1995. Differential distribution of exogenous BDNF, NGF, and NT-3 in the brain corresponds to the relative abundance and distribution of high-affinity and low-affinity neurotrophin receptors. *J. Comp. Neurol.* 357: 296–317.

Angevine JB and RL Sidman. 1961. Autoradiographic study of cell migration during histogenesis of the cerebral cortex in the mouse. *Nature* 192: 766–768.

Ariens-Kappers CU, GC Huber, and EC Crosby. 1936. *The Comparative Anatomy of the Nervous System of Vertebrates, Including Man,* vol I. New York: Macmillan.

Arimatsu Y, M Miyamoto, I Nihonmatsu, K Hirata, Y Uratani, Y Hatanaka, and K Takiguchi-Hayashi. 1992. Early regional specification for molecular neuronal phenotype in the rat neocortex. *Proc. Natl. Acad. Sci. USA* 89: 8879–8883.

Armstrong RC and MR Montminy. 1993. Transsynaptic control of gene expression. *Annu. Rev. Neurosci.* 16: 17–29.

Armstrong-James M. 1975. The functional status and columnar organization of single cells responding to cutaneous stimulation in neonatal rat somatosensory cortex S-1. *J. Physiol. Lond.* 246: 501–538.

Armstrong-James M and CA Callahan. 1991. Thalamo-cortical processing of vibrissal information in the rat. II. Spatiotemporal convergence in the thalamic ventro-posterior medial nucleus (VPm) and its relevance to generation of receptive fields of S1 cortical "barrel" neurons. *J. Comp. Neurol.* 303: 211–224.

Armstrong-James M, CA Callahan, and M Friedman. 1991. Thalamo-cortical processing of vibrissal information in the rat. I. Intracortical origins of surround but not centre-receptive fields of layer IV neurones in the rat S1 barrel field cortex. *J. Comp. Neurol.* 303: 193–210.

Armstrong-James M and K Fox. 1987. Spatiotemporal convergence and divergence in the rat S1 "barrel" cortex. *J. Comp. Neurol.* 263: 265–281.

Armstrong-James M, K Fox, and A Das-Gupta. 1992. Flow of excitation within rat barrel cortex on striking a single vibrissa. *J. Neurophysiol.* 68: 1345–1358.

Aroniadou AV and A Keller. 1993. The pattern and synaptic properties of horizontal connections in the motor cortex. *J. Neurophysiol.* 70: 1553–1569.

Aroniadou VA and TJ Teyler. 1991. The role of NMDA receptors in long-term potentiation (LTP) and depression (LTD) in rat visual cortex. *Brain Res.* 562: 136–143.

———— 1992. Induction of NMDA receptor-independent long-term potentiation in visual cortex in adult rats. *Brain Res.* 584: 169–173.

Artola A. 1994. Homosynaptic long-term depression and its relation to long-term potentiation in the rat neocortex in vitro. In *Long-term Potentiation,* vol II, ed. M Baudry and JL Davis, pp. 207–226. Cambridge, MA: MIT Press.

Artola A, S Brocher, and W Singer. 1990. Different voltage-dependent thresholds for inducing long-term depression and long-term potentiation in slices of rat visual cortex. *Nature* 347: 69–72.

Artola A and W Singer. 1993. Long-term depression of excitatory synaptic transmission and its relationship to long-term potentiation. *Trends Neurosci.* 16: 480–487.

Asanuma H. 1975. Recent developments in the study of the columnar organization of neurons within the motor cortex. *Physiol. Rev.* 55: 143–156.

———— 1981. Functional role of sensory inputs to the motor cortex. *Prog. Neurobiol.* 16: 241–262.

Asanuma H and I Rosen. 1972. Topographical organization of cortical efferent zones projecting to distal forelimb muscles in the monkey. *Exp. Brain Res.* 14: 243–256.

Ashton EH. 1981. Primate locomotion: Some problems in analysis and interpretation. *Phil. Trans. Roy. Soc. Lond.* B292: 77–87.

Ayala FJ. 1995. The myth of Eve: Molecular biology and human origins. *Science* 270: 1930–1936.

Bach ME, RD Hawking, M Osman, ER Kandel, and M Mayford. 1995. Impairment of spatial but not contextual memory in CaMKII mutant mice with a selective loss of hippocampal LTP in the range of theta frequency. *Cell* 81: 905–915.

Baier H and F Bonhoeffer. 1992. Axon guidance by gradients of a target-derived component. *Science* 255: 472–475.

Baimbridge KG, MR Celio, and JH Rogers. 1992. Calcium-binding proteins in the nervous system. *Trends Neurosci.* 15: 303–308.

Bair W, C Koch, W Newsome, and K Britten. 1994. Power spectrum analysis of bursting cells in area MT in the behaving monkey. *J. Neurosci.* 14: 2870–2892.

Baloyannis SJ, S Manolides, L Arzoglou, V Costa, and L Manolides. 1993. The structual organization of layer I in the adult human acoustic cortex. A golgi and electron microscopy study. *Acta Oto-Laryngologica* 113: 502–506.

Baranyi A, BM Szente, and CD Woody. 1991. Properties of associative long-term potentiation induced by cellular conditioning in the motor cortex of conscious cats. *Neurosci.* 42: 321–334.

—— 1993a. Electrophysiological characterization of different types of neurons recorded in vivo in the motor cortex of the cat. I. Patterns of firing activity and synaptic responses. *J. Neurophysiol.* 69: 1850–1864.

—— 1993b. Electrophysiological characterization of different types of neurons recorded in vivo in the motor cortex of the cat. II. Membrane parameters, action potentials, current-induced voltage responses and electrotonic structures. *J. Neurophysiol.* 69: 1865–1879.

Barbas H. 1986. Pattern in the laminar origin of cortico-cortical connections. *J. Comp. Neurol.* 252: 415–422.

Barbas H and DN Pandya. 1989. Architecture and intrinsic connections of the prefrontal cortex in the rhesus monkey. *J. Comp. Neurol.* 286: 353–375.

Barbe MF and P Levitt. 1991. The early commitment of fetal neurons to the limbic cortex. *J. Neurosci.* 11: 519–533.

—— 1992. Attraction of specific thalamic input by cerebral grafts depends on the molecular identity of the implant. *Proc. Natl. Acad. Sci. USA* 89: 3706–3710.

Barlow HB. 1972. Single units and cognition: A neurone doctrine for perceptual psychology. *Perception* 1: 371–394.

—— 1995. The neuron doctrine in perception. In *The Cognitive Neurosciences,* ed. M Gazzaniga, pp. 415–436. Cambridge, MA: MIT Press.

Barlow HB, C Blakemore, and JD Pettigrew. 1967. The neural mechanism of binocular depth discrimination. *J. Physiol. Lond.* 216: 39–68.

Barlow JS. 1993. *The Electroencephalogram: Its Patterns and Origins.* Cambridge, MA: MIT Press.

Barnes CA. 1995. Involvement of LTP in memory: Are we "searching under the street light"? *Neuron* 15: 751–754.

Barnes CA, MW Jung, BL McNaughton, KL Karol, K Andreasson, and PF Worley. 1994. LTP saturation and spatial learning disruption: Effects of task variables and saturation levels. *J. Neurosci.* 14: 5793–5806.

Barth TM and BB Stanfield. 1994. Homotopic, but not heterotopic, fetal cortical transplants can result in functional sparing following neonatal damage to frontal cortex in rats. *Cerebral Cortex* 4: 271–278.

Basar E. 1992. Brain natural frequencies are causal factors for resonances and induced rhythms. In *Induced Rhythms in the Brain,* ed. E Basar and TH Bullock. Boston: Birkhauser.

Basar E and TH Bullock, eds. 1992. *Induced Rhythms in the Brain.* Boston: Birkhauser.

Bassler U. 1986. On the definition of central pattern generator and its sensory control. *Biol. Cyber.* 54: 65–69.

Bayer SA and J Altman. 1991. *Neocortical Development.* New York: Raven.

Bear MF. 1995. Mechanism for a sliding synaptic modification threshold. *Neuron* 15: 1–4.

Bear MF and RC Malenka. 1994. Synaptic plasticity: LTP and LTD. *Current Opinion in Neurobiology* 4: 389–399.

Beaulieu C and M Colonnier. 1985. A laminar analysis of the number of round-asymmetric and flat-symmetric synapses on spines, dendritic trunks and cell bodies in area 17 of the cat. *J. Comp. Neurol.* 231: 180–189.

Beaulieu C, Z Kisvarday, P Somoygi, M Cynader, and A Cowey. 1992. Quantitative distribution of GABA-immunopositive and -immunonegative neurons and synapses in the monkey striate cortex (area 17). *Cerebral Cortex* 2: 295–309.

Bekkers JM. 1994. Quantal analysis of synaptic transmission in the central nervous system. *Current Opinion in Neurobiology* 4: 360–366.

Belinchenko PV, DMV Weisenhorn, J Myuklossy, and MR Cellio. 1995. Calretinin-positive Cajal-Retzius cells persist in the adult human neocortex. *Neuroreport* 6: 1869–1874.

Ben-Ari Y and L Aniksztejn. 1995. Role of glutamate metabotropic receptors in long-term potentiation in the hippocampus. *Sem. Neurosci.* 7: 127–135.

Bennett MVL, KC Barrio, TA Bargiello, DC Spray, E Herzberg, and JC Saez. 1991. Gap junctions, new tools, new answers, new questions. *Neuron* 6: 305–320.

Berman NJ, RJ Douglas, KA Martin, and D Whitteridge. 1991. Mechanisms of inhibition in the cat visual cortex. *J. Physiol. Lond.* 440: 697–722.

Bernard O, J Drago, and H Sheng. 1992. L-myc and N-myc influence lineage determination in the central nervous system. *Neuron* 9: 1217–1224.

Bicknese AR, AM Shepard, DD O'Leary, and AL Pearlman. 1994. Thalamocortical axons extend along a chondroitin sulfate proteoglycan-enriched pathway coincident with the neocortical subplate and distinct from the efferent path. *J. Neurosci.* 14: 3500–3510.

Bienenstock E, L Cooper, and P Munro. 1982. Theory for the development of neuron specificity and binocular interaction in visual cortex. *J. Neurosci.* 2: 32–48.

Bishop PO, JS Combs, and GH Henry. 1973. Receptive fields of simple cells in cat striate cortex. *J. Physiol. Lond.* 231: 31–60.

Blakemore C and Z Molnar. 1990. Factors involved in the establishment of specific interconnections between thalamus and cerebral cortex. *Cold Spring Harb. Symp. Quant. Biol.* 55: 491–504.

Blaschke AJ, K Stanley, and J Chun. 1996. Widespread programmed cell death in proliferative and postmitotic regions of fetal cerebral cortex. *Development* 122: 1165–1174.

Blasdel GG. 1992a. Differential imaging of ocular dominance and orientation selectivities in monkey striate cortex. *J. Neurosci.* 12: 3115–3138.

——— 1992b. Orientation selectivity, preference, and continuity in monkey striate cortex. *J. Neurosci.* 12: 3139–3161.

Blasdel GG and D Fitzpatrick. 1984. Physiological organization of layer 4 in macaque striate cortex. *J. Neurosci.* 4: 880–895.

Bleakman D, RJ Miller, and WF Colmers. 1993. In *The Biology of Neuropeptide Y and Related Peptides,* ed. WF Colmers and C Wahlestedt, pp. 241–272. Totowa, NJ: Humana.

Blinkov SM and II Glezer. 1968. *The Human Brain in Figures and Tables.* New York: Plenum.

Bliss TVP and GL Collingridge. 1993. A synaptic model of memory: Long-term potentiation in the hippocampus. *Nature* 361: 31–38.

Bliss TVP and AR Gardner-Medwin. 1973. Long-lasting potentiation of synaptic transmission in the dentate area of the unanesthetized rabbit following stimulation of the perforant path. *J. Physiol. Lond.* 232: 357–374.

Bliss TVP and T Lomo. 1973. Long-lasting potentiation of synaptic transmission in the dentate area of the anaesthetized rabbit following stimulation of the perforant path. *J. Physiol. Lond.* 232: 331–356.

Bloom FR. 1986. In *Handbook of Physiology, Section I: The Nervous System, Vol. 4: Intrinsic Regulatory Systems of the Brain,* ed. FR Bloom, VB Mountcastle, and SM Geiger. Bethesda, MD: American Physiological Society.

Bolshakov VY and SA Siegelbaum. 1994. Postsynaptic induction and presynaptic expression of hippocampal long-term depression. *Science* 264: 1148–1152.

Bolz J, N Novak, and V Staiger. 1992. Formation of specific afferent connections in organotypic slice cultures of rat visual cortex cocultured with lateral geniculate nucleus. *J. Neurosci.* 12: 3054–3070.

Bonin G von and P Bailey. 1947. *The Neocortex of Macaca mulatta.* Illinois Monographs in Medical Sciences. Urbana, IL: Univ. of Illinois Press.

Bopyapati J and GH Henry. 1985. The character and influence of the claustral pathway to the striate cortex of the cat. *Exp. Brain Res.* 61: 141–152.

Boring EG. 1952. *Sensation and Perception in the History of Experimental Psychology.* New York: Appleton-Century Crofts.

Bortolotto ZA and GL Collingridge. 1993. Characterization of LTP induced by the activation of metabotropic receptors in area CA1 of the hippocampus. *Neuropharmacology* 32: 1–9.

Bourgeois JP, PS Goldman-Rakic, and P Rakic. 1994. Synaptogenesis in the prefrontal cortex in rhesus monkeys. *Cerebral Cortex* 4: 78–96.

Bourgeois JP and P Rakic. 1993. Changes in synaptic density in the primary visual cortex of the macaque monkey from fetal to adult stage. *J. Neurosci.* 13: 2801–2820.

Bourne HR and R Nicoll. 1993. Molecular machines integrate coincident synaptic signals. *Cell* 71/*Neuron* 10 (suppl.): 65–76.

Bouyer JJ, MF Montaron, and A Rougeul. 1981. Fast fronto-parietal rhythms during combined focused attentive behavior and immobility in cat: Cortical and thalamic localizations. *Electroencephalogr. Clin. Neurophysiol.* 51: 244–252.

Bowcock AM, A Ruiz-Linares, J Tomfohrde, E Minch, JR Kidd, and LL Cavilla-Sforza. 1994. High resolution of human evolutionary trees with polymorphic microsatellites. *Nature* 368: 455–457.

Bowe MA and JR Fallon. 1995. The role of agrin in synapse formation. *Annu. Rev. Neurosci.* 18: 443–462.

Braak H. 1980. Architectonics as seen in lipofuscin stains. In *Cerebral Cortex, Volume I: Cellular Components of the Cerebral Cortex,* ed. A Peters and EG Jones. New York: Plenum.

——— 1984. *The Architectonics of the Human Telencephalic Cortex.* Berlin and New York: Springer-Verlag.

Braengaard J, SM Evans, CV Howard, and HJ Gundersen. 1990. The total number of neurons in the human neocortex unbiasedly estimated using optical dissectors. *J. Microsc.* 157: 285–304.

Bredt DS, CE Glatt, PM Hwang, M Fotuhi, TM Dawson, and SH Snyder. 1991. Nitric oxide synthase protein and mRNA are discretely localized in neuronal populations of the mammalian CNS together with NADPH diaphorase. *Neuron* 7: 615–624.

Bredt DS and SH Snyder. 1992. Nitric oxide, a novel neuronal messenger. *Neuron* 8: 3–11.

Bregman BS, E Kunkel-Bagden, L Schnell, HN Dai, D Gao, and ME Schwab. 1995. Recovery from spinal cord injury mediated by antibodies to neurite growth factors. *Nature* 378: 498–501.

Bressler SL. 1995. Large-scale cortical networks and cognition. *Brain Res. Rev.* 20: 288–304.

Bressler SL, R Coppola, and R Nakamura. 1993. Episodic multiregional cortical coherence at multiple frequencies during visual task performance. *Nature* 366: 153–156.

Brocher S, A Artola, and W Singer. 1992. Intracellular injection of Ca^{2+} chelators blocks induction of long-term depression in rat visual cortex. *Proc. Natl. Acad. Sci. USA* 89: 123–127.

Brodmann K. 1905. Beitrage zur histologischen Lokalisation der Grosshirnrinde: Die Rindenfeldern der niederen Affen. *J. Psychol. Neurol.* 4: 177–226.

———— 1914. Physiologie des Gehirns. In *Neue Deutsche Chirurgie,* vol. 11, ed. P. von Brun, pp. 85–426. Stuttgart: Enke.

Brosch M, R Bauer, and R Eckhorn. 1995. Synchronous high-frequency oscillations in cat area 18. *Eur. J. Neurosci.* 7: 86–95.

Brown F, J Harris, R Leakey, and A Walker. 1985. Early *H. erectus* skeleton from west Lake Turkana, Kenya. *Nature* 316: 788–792.

Brown TH, EW Kairiss, and CL Keenan. 1990. Hebbian synapses: Biophysical mechanisms and algorithms. *Annu. Rev. Neurosci.* 13: 475–512.

Brugge JF, NA Dubrowsky, LM Aitkin, and DJ Anderson. 1969. Sensitivity of single neurons in auditory cortex of cat to binaural tonal stimulation; effects of varying interaural time and intensity. *J. Neurophysiol.* 32: 1005–1024.

Brugge JF and MM Merzenich. 1973. Responses of neurons in auditory cortex of the macaque monkey to monaural and binaural stimulation. *J. Neurophysiol.* 36: 1138–1158.

Buchs P-A and D Muller. 1996. Induction of long-term potentiation is associated with major ultrastructural changes of activated synapses. *Proc. Natl. Acad. Sci. USA* 93: 8040–8045.

Bugbee NM and P Goldman-Rakic. 1983. Columnar organization of corticocortical projections in squirrel and rhesus monkeys: Similarities of columnar width in species with different cortical volumes. *J. Comp. Neurol.* 220: 355–364.

Bulfone A, L Puelles, MH Porteus, MA Frohman, GR Martin, and JLR Rubenstein. 1993. Spatially restricted expression of Dlx-1, Dlx-2 (TYES-1), GBX-2 and Wnt-3 in the embryonic day 12.5 mouse forebrain defines potential transverse and longitudinal segmental boundaries. *J. Neurosci.* 13: 3155–3172.

Bullier J and LG Nowak. 1995. Parallel versus serial processing: New vistas on the distributed organization of the visual system. *Current Opinion in Neurobiology* 5: 497–503.

Bullock TH. 1986. Some principles in the brain analysis of important signals: Mapping and stimulus recognition. *Brain Behav. Evol.* 28: 145–156.

———— 1989. The micro-EEG represents varied degrees of cooperativity among wide-band generators: Spatial and temporal microstructure of field potentials. In *Brain Dynamics: Progress and Perspectives,* ed. E Basar and TH Bullock, pp. 5–12. Berlin and New York: Springer-Verlag.

———— 1992. Introduction to induced rhythms: A widespread, heterogeneous class of oscillations. In *Induced Rhythms in the Brain,* ed. E Basar and TH Bullock. Boston: Birkhauser.

———— 1993. How are more complex brains different? *Brain Behav. Evol.* 41: 88–96.

Bullock TH and JZ Abramowicz. 1994. A comparative study of event related brain oscillations. In *Oscillatory Event-related Brain Dynamics,* ed. C Pantev, T Elbert, and B Lukenhoner, pp. 11–26. New York: Plenum.

Bullock TH and MC McClune. 1989. Lateral coherence of the electrocorticogram: A new measure of brain synchrony. *Electroencephalogr. Clin. Neurophysiol.* 73: 479–498.

Bullock TH, MC McClune, JZ Abramowicz, VJ Iragui-Madoz, RB Duckrow, and SS Spencer. 1995a. EEG coherence has structure in the millimeter domain: Subdural and hippocampal recordings from epileptic patients. *Electroencephalogr. Clin. Neurophysiol.* 95: 161–177.

———— 1995b. Temporal fluctuations in coherence of brain waves. *Proc. Natl. Acad. Sci. USA* 92: 11568–11572.

Bunge M. 1980. *The Mind-Body Problem: A Psychobiological Approach.* Oxford, Pergamon.

Bunge M and R Ardila. 1987. *Philosophy of Psychology.* Berlin and New York: Springer-Verlag.

Burkhalter A, KL Bernbardo and V Charles. 1989. Postnatal development of intracortical connections in the human visual cortex. *Proc. Natl. Acad. Sci. USA* 86: 1071–1075.

———— 1993. Development of local circuits in human visual cortex. *J. Neurosci.* 13: 1916–1931.

Burt DR and GL Kamatchi. 1991. GABA$_A$ receptor subtypes: From pharmacology to molecular biology. *FASEB J.* 5: 2916–2923.

Cabelli RJ, A Hohn, and CJ Shatz. 1995. Inhibition of ocular dominance column formation by infusion of NT-4/5 or BDNF. *Science* 167: 1662–1666.

Calloway EM and LC Katz. 1992. Development of axonal arbors of layer 4 spiny neurons in cat striate cortex. *J. Neurosci.* 12: 570–582.

Caminiti R and GM Innocenti. 1981. The postnatal development of somatosensory callosal connections after partial lesions of somatosensory areas. *Exp. Brain Res.* 42: 53–62.

Cann RL, M Stoneking, and AC Wilson. 1987. Mitochondrial DNA and human evolution. *Nature* 325: 31–36.

Carreras M and SA Andersson. 1963. Functional properties of neurons of the anterior ectosylvian gyrus of the cat. *J. Neurophysiol.* 26: 100–126.

Cases O, T Vitalis, I Seif, E De Maeyer, C Sotelo, and P Gaspar. 1996. Lack of barrels in the somatosensory cortex of monamine oxidase A-deficient mice: Role of a serotonin excess during the critical period. *Neuron* 16: 297–307.

Castelo-Branco M, S Neuenschwander, S Hereculano, and W Singer. 1996. Synchronization of visual responses between the cortex, LGN and retina in the anesthetized cat. *Neurosci. Abs.* 23: 643.

Castro-Alamancos MA and BW Connors. 1996. Short-term synaptic enhancement and long-term potentiation in the neocortex. *Proc. Natl. Acad. Sci. USA* 93: 1335–1339.

Castro-Alamancos MA, JP Donoghue, and BW Connors. 1995. Different forms of synaptic plasticity in somatosensory and motor areas of the neocortex. *J. Neurosci.* 15: 5324–5333.

Caton R. 1875. The electric currents of the brain. *Brit. Med. J.* 2: 278.

Cauller LJ and BW Connors. 1994. Synaptic physiology of horizontal afferents to layer I of primary somatosensory cortex in rats. *J. Neurosci.* 14: 751–762.

Caviness VS jr. 1976. Patterns of cell and fiber distribution in neocortex of the reeler mutant mouse. *J. Comp. Neurol.* 170: 435–448.

———— 1982. Neocortical histogenesis in normal and reeler mice: A developmental study based upon 3H-thymidine autoradiography. *Dev. Brain Res.* 4: 293–302.

Caviness VS jr, JE Crandall, and MA Edwards. 1988. The reeler malformation: Implications for neocortical histogenesis. In *Cerebral Cortex, Vol. 7: Development and Maturation of Cerebral Cortex,* ed. A Peters and EG Jones, pp. 59–90. New York: Plenum.

Caviness VS jr, T Takahashi, and RS Nowakowski. 1995. Numbers, time and neocortical neurogenesis: A general developmental and evolutionary model. *Trends Neurosci.* 18: 379–383.

Cepko CL. 1989. Immortalization of neural cells via retrovirus-mediated oncogene transduction. *Annu. Rev. Neurosci.* 12: 47–65.

Cepko CL, CP Austin, C Walsh, EF Ryder, A Halliday, and SF Berry. 1990. Studies of cortical development using retrovirus vectors. *Cold Spring Harbor Symp. Quant. Biol.* 55: 265–278.

Chagnac-Amitai Y and BW Connors. 1989. Horizontal spread of synchronized activity in neocortex and its control by GABA mediated inhibition. *J. Neurophysiol.* 61: 747–758.

Chagnac-Amitai Y, HJ Luhmann, and DA Prince. 1990. Burst generating and regular spiking layer 5 pyramidal neurons of rat neocortex have different morphological features. *J. Comp. Neurol.* 296: 598–613.

Chaiai NL, SE Fish, WR Barnes, CA Bennett-Clarke, and RW Rhoades. 1992. Postnatal blockade of cortical activity by tetrodotoxin does not disrupt the formation of vibrissae-related patterns in the cat's somatosensory cortex. *Dev. Brain Res.* 665: 244–250.

Chalupa LM and HP Killackey. 1989. Process elimination underlies ontogenetic change in the distribution of callosal projection neurons in the postcentral gyrus of the fetal rhesus monkey. *Proc. Natl. Acad. Sci. USA* 86: 1076–1079.

Changeux J-P. 1996. Neurotransmitter receptors in the changing brain; allosteric transitions, gene expression and pathology. In *The Lifespan Development of Individuals: Behavioral, Neurobiological, and Psychosocial Perspectives,* ed. D Magnuson, T Greitzk, LG Nilsson, B Winblad, T Hokfeld, and L Terenius. Cambridge, UK: Cambridge U. Press.

Changeux J-P and A Danchin. 1976. Selective stabilization of developing synapses as a mechanism for the specification of neuronal networks. *Nature* 264: 705–711.

Chapman B, KR Zahs, and MP Stryker. 1991. Relation of cortical cell orientation selectivity to alignment of receptive fields of the geniculocortical afferents that arborize within a single orientation column in ferret visual cortex. *J. Neurosci.* 11: 1347–1358.

Chen W, GY Hu, YD Zhou, and CP Wu. 1994. Two mechanisms underlying the induction of long-term potentiation in motor cortex of adult cat in vitro. *Exp. Brain Res.* 100: 149–154.

Chen WR, S Lee, K Kato, D Spencer, GM Shepherd, and A Williamson. 1996. Long-term modification of synaptic efficiencey in the human inferior and middle temporal cortex. *Proc. Natl. Acad. Sci. USA* 93: 8011–8015.

Chmielowska J, M Kossut, and M Chmielowski. 1986. Single vibrissal cortical columns in the mouse labeled with 2-deoxyglucose. *Exp. Brain Res.* 63: 607–619.

Chun JJ and CJ Shatz. 1989. Interstitial cells of the adult neocortical white matter are remnants of the early generated subplate neuron population. *J. Comp. Neurol.* 282: 555–569.

Clapham DE. 1994. Direct G protein activation of ion channels? *Annu. Rev. Neurosci.* 17: 441–464.

Cleland TA and AI Selverston. 1995. Glutamate-gated inhibitory currents of central pattern generator neurons in the lobster stomatogastric ganglion. *J. Neurosci.* 15: 6631–6639.

Clements JD. 1996. Transmitter time course in the synaptic cleft; its role in central synaptic function. *Trends Neurosci.* 19: 163–171.

Cohen AH, S Rossignol, and S Grillner. 1988. *Neural Control of Rhythmic Movements in Vertebrates.* New York: Wiley-Interscience.

Cohen-Tannoudji M, C Babinet, and M Wassef. 1994. Early determination of a mouse somatosensory cortex marker. *Nature* 31: 460–462.

Collingridge GL, SJ Kehl, and H McLennan. 1983. Excitatory amino acids in synaptic transmission in the Schaffer collateral-commissural pathway in the rat hippocampus. *J. Physiol. Lond.* 334: 33–46.

Colmers WF and C Wahlestedt, eds. 1993. *The Biology of Neuropeptide Y and Related Peptides.* Totowa, NJ: Humana.

Colonnier M. 1968. Synaptic patterns on different cell types in different laminae of the cat visual cortex. *Brain Res.* 9: 268–287.

———— 1981. The electron-microscopic analysis of the neuronal organization of the cerebral cortex. In *The Organization of the Cerebral Cortex*, ed. FO Schmitt, FG Worden, G Adelman, and SG Dennis, pp. 125–152. Cambridge, MA: MIT Press.

Connors BW and Y Amitai. 1995. Function of local circuits in neocortex: Synchrony and laminae. In *The Cortical Neuron*, ed. MJ Gutnick and I Mody. Oxford: Oxford U. Press.

Connors BW, LS Benardo, and DA Prince. 1983. Coupling between neurons in the developing rat neocortex. *J. Neurosci.* 3: 773–782.

Connors BW and MJ Gutnick. 1990. Intrinsic firing patterns of diverse neocortical neurons. *Trends Neurosci.* 13: 99–104.

Connors BW, MJ Gutnick, and DA Prince. 1982. Electrophysiological properties of neocortical neurons in vitro. *J. Neurophysiol.* 48: 1302–1320.

Connors BW, RC Malenka, and LR Silva. 1988. Two inhibitory postsynaptic potentials, and GABA$_A$ and GABA$_B$ receptor-mediated responses in neocortex of rat and cat. *J. Physiol. Lond.* 406: 443–468.

Conti F, J DeFilipe, I Farinas, and T Manzoni. 1989. Glutamate-positive neurons and axon terminals in cat sensory cortex. A correlative light and electron microscopic study. *J. Comp. Neurol.* 290: 141–153.

Contreras D and M Steriade. 1995. Cellular basis of EEG slow rhythms: A study of dynamic corticothalamic relationships. *J. Neurosci.* 15: 604–622.

Coombs JS, DR Curtis, and JC Eccles. 1957. The generation of impulses in motoneurons. *J. Physiol.* 139: 232–249.

Coombs JS, JC Eccles, and P Fatt. 1955a. The specific ionic conductances and the ionic movements across the motoneuron membrane that produce the inhibitory post-synaptic potential. *J. Physiol.* 130: 326–373.

———— 1955b. Excitatory synaptic actions in motoneurons. *J. Physiol.* 130: 374–395.

Corkin S. 1984. Lasting consequences of bilateral medial temporal lobectomy: Clinical course and experimental findings in H.M. *Sem. Neurol.* 4: 249–259.

Cowan WM, JW Fawcett, DDM O'Leary, et al. 1985. Regressive phenomena in the development of the vertebrate nervous system. *Science* 225: 1258–1265.

Crair MC and RC Malenka. 1995. A critical period for long-term potentiation at thalamocortical synapses. *Nature* 375: 325–328.

Crandell JE, J-P Misson, and D Butler. 1990. Functional organization in cortical barrels of normal and vibrissae-damaged mice: A (3-H) 2-deoxyglucose study. *J. Comp. Neurol.* 235: 97–110.

Creutzfeldt O. 1995. *Cortex cerebri: Performance, Structural and Functional Organization of the Cortex*. Oxford: Oxford U. Press.

Creutzfeldt OD and J Houchin. 1976. Neuronal basis of EEG-waves. In *Handbook of Electroencephalography and Clinical Neurophysiology,* vol. 2, ed. O Creutzfeldt, pp. 2C/3–2C/55. Amsterdam: Elsevier.

———— 1984. Neuronal basis of EEG-waves. In *Handbook of Electroencephalography and Clinical Neurophysiology,* vol. 2, ed. A Remond, pp. 2/C/3–2/C/55. Amsterdam: Elsevier.

Creutzfeldt OD, U Kuhnt, and LA Benevento. 1974. An intracellular analysis of visual cortical neurons to moving stimuli: Responses of a co-operative neuronal network. *Exp. Brain Res.* 21: 251–274.

Creutzfeldt OD, S Watanabe, and HD Lux. 1966. Relation between EEG-phenomena and potentials in single cells. Parts I and II. *Electroencephalogr. Clin. Neurophysiol.* 20: 1–37.

Crick F and C Koch. 1990a. Towards a neurological theory of consciousness. *Sem. Neurosci.* 2: 263–275.

———— 1990b. Some reflections on visual awareness. *Cold Spring Harbor Symp. Quant. Biol.* 55: 953–962.

Crombie AC. 1952. *From Augustine to Galileo, Vol. I: Science in the Later Middle Ages and Modern Times, XIII–XVII Centuries.* London: Heineman.

Cronin JE, NT Boaz, CB Stringer, and Y Rak. 1981. Tempo and mode in hominid evolution. *Nature* 292: 113–122.

Crook JM and UT Eysel. 1992. GABA-induced inactivation of functional characterized sites in cat visual cortex (area 18): Effects on orientation tuning. *J. Neurosci.* 12: 1816–1825.

Crook JM, UT Eysel, and HF Machemer. 1991. Influence of GABA-induced remote inactivation on the orientation tuning of cells in area 18 of feline visual cortex: A comparison with area 17. *Neurosci.* 40: 1–12.

Culican SM, NL Baumrind, M Yamamoto, and AL Pearlman. 1990. Cortical radial glia: Identification in tissue culture and evidence for their transformation into astrocytes. *J. Neurosci.* 10: 684–692.

Curtis DR, JW Phillis, and JC Watkins. 1960. The chemical excitation of spinal neurones by certain acidic amino acids. *J. Physiol. Lond.* 150: 656–582.

D'Arcangelo G, GG Miao, SC Chen, HD Soares, JI Morgan, and T Curran. 1995. A protein related to extracellular matrix proteins deleted in the mouse mutant reeler. *Nature* 374: 719–723.

Darian-Smith I, MP Galea, C Darian-Smith, M Sugitani, A Tan, and K Buirman. 1997. The anatomy of manual dexterity. The new connectivity of the primate sensorimotor thalamus and cerebral cortex. *Adv. Anat. Embryol. Cell Biol.* 133: 1–142.

Darian-Smith I, AW Goodwin, M Sugitani, and J Heywood. 1984. The tangible features of textured surfaces: Their representation in the monkey's somatosensory cortex. In *Dynamic Aspects of Neocortical Function,* ed. GM Edelman, WM Cowan, and WE Gall, pp. 475–500. New York: Wiley.

Dart RA. 1925. *Australopithecus africanus,* the man-ape of South Africa. *Nature* 115: 195.

Davies AM. 1994. Intrinsic programs of growth and survival in developing vertebrate neurons. *Trends Neurosci.* 17: 195–198.

Davies CH, SJ Starkey, MF Pozza, and GL Collingridge. 1991. GABA autoreceptors regulate the induction of LTP. *Nature* 349: 609–611.

Davies MF, RA Deisz, DA Prince, and SJ Perouka. 1987. Two distinct effects of 5-hydroxytryptamine on single cortical neurons. *Brain Res.* 423: 347–352.

Davies PW, AL Berman, and VB Mountcastle. 1955. Functional analysis of first somatic area of cat's cerebral cortex in terms of activity of single neurons. *Am. J. Physiol.* 183: 646.

Davis S, SP Butcher, and RGM Morris. 1992. The NMDA receptor antagonist D-2-amino-5-phosphonopentanoate (D-AP5) impairs spatial learning and LTP *in vivo* at intracerebral concentrations comparable to those that block LTP *in vitro. J. Neurosci.* 12: 21–34.

Dawson TM and VL Dawson. 1995. Nitric oxide: Actions and pathological roles. *Neuroscientist* 1: 7–18.

Deacon T. 1990. Rethinking mammalian brain evolution. *Am. Zool.* 30: 629–705.

DeCarlos JA and DDM O'Leary. 1992. Growth and targeting of subplate axons and establishment of major cortical pathways. *J. Neurosci.* 10: 684–692.

DeFelipe J. 1993. Neocortical neuronal diversity: Chemical heterogeneity revealed by co-localization studies of classic transmitters, neuropeptides, calcium-binding proteins and cell surface molecules. *Cerebral Cortex* 3: 273–289.

DeFelipe J, J Conley, and EG Jones. 1986. Long-range focal collateralization of axons arising from corticocortical cells in monkey sensory-motor cortex. *J. Neurosci.* 6: 3749–3766.

DeFelipe J and I Farinas. 1992. The pyramidal neuron of the cerebral cortex: Morphological and chemical characteristics of the synaptic inputs. *Prog. Neurobiol.* 39: 563–607.

DeFelipe J, SCH Hendry, T Hashikawa, M Molinari, and EG Jones. 1990. A microcolumnar structure of monkey cerebral cortex revealed by immunocytochemical studies of double bouquet cell axons. *Neurosci.* 37: 655–673.

DeFelipe J, SHC Hendry, and EG Jones. 1986. A correlative electron microscopic study of basket cells and large GABAergic neurons in the monkey sensory-motor cortex. *Neurosci.* 17: 991–1009.

——— 1989a. Synapses on double bouquet cells in monkey cerebral cortex visualized by calbindin immunoreactivity. *Brain Res.* 503: 49–54.

——— 1989b. Visualization of chandelier cell axons by parvalbumin immunoreactivity in monkey cerebral cortex. *Proc. Natl. Acad. Sci. USA* 86: 2093–2097.

DeFelipe J, SHC Hendry, EG Jones, and D Schmechel. 1985. Variability in the terminations of GABAergic chandelier cell axons on initial segments of pyramidal cell axons in the monkey sensory-motor cortex. *J. Comp. Neurol.* 231: 364–384.

DeFelipe J and EG Jones. 1988a. *Cajal on the Cerebral Cortex: An Annotated Translation of the Complete Writings.* Oxford: Oxford U. Press.

———— 1988b. A light and electron microscopic study of serotonin-immunoreactive fibers and terminals in the monkey sensory-motor cortex. *Exp. Brain Res.* 71: 171–182.

———— 1992. High resolution light and electron microscopic immunocytochemistry of co-localized GABA and calbindin D-28k in somata and double bouquet cell axons of monkey somatosensory cortex. *Eur. J. Neurosci.* 4: 46–60.

DeHay C, P Giraud, M Berland, H Killackey, and H Kennedy. 1996a. Contribution of thalamic input to the specification of cytoarchitectonic cortical fields in primate: Effects of bilateral enucleation in the fetal monkey on the boundaries, dimensions and gyrification of striate and extrastriate cortex. *J. Comp. Neurol.* 367: 70–89.

DeHay C, P Giraud, M Berland, HP Killackey, and H Kennedy. 1996b. Phenotypic characterisation of respecified visual cortex subsequent to prenatal enucleation in the monkey. Development of acetylcholinesterase and cytochrome oxidase patterns. *J. Comp. Neurol.* 3l7: 1–17.

DeHay C, P Giraud, M Berland, I Smart, and H Kennedy. 1993. Modulation of the cell cycle contributes to the parcellation of the primate visual cortex. *Nature* 366: 464–466.

DeHay C, G Horsburgh, M Berland, H Killacky, and H Kennedy. 1989. Maturation and connectivity of the visual cortex in monkey is altered by prenatal removal of the retinal input. *Nature* 337: 265–267.

DeHay C, G Horsburgh, M Berland, H Killacky, and H Kennedy. 1991. The effects of bilateral enucleation in the primate fetus on the parcellation of visual cortex. *Dev. Brain Res.* 62: 137–141.

Del Castillo J and B Katz. 1954. Quantal components of the end plate potential. *J. Physiol. Lond.* 124: 560–573.

del Rio MR and J DeFelipe. 1995. A light and electron microscopic study of calbinden d-28K immunoreactive double bouquet cells in human temporal cortex. *Brain Res.* 690: 133–140.

DeMenocal PB. 1995. Plio-pleistocene African climate. *Science* 270: 53–59.

Denk W, M Sugimori, and R Llinas. 1995. Two types of calcium response limited to single spines of cerebellar Purkinje cells. *Proc. Natl. Acad. Sci. USA* 92: 8279–8282.

De Robertis E, A Pelligrino de Iraldi, G Rodruguez, and C Gomez. 1961. On the isolation of nerve endings and synaptic vesicles. *J. Biophys. Biochem. Cytol.* 9: 229–235.

Derrick BE, SB Weinberger, and JL Martinez jr. 1991. Opioid receptors are involved in an NMDA receptor independent mechanism of LTP induction at hippocampal mossy fiber-CA3 synapses. *Brain Res. Bull.* 27: 219–223.

Descartes R. 1965 [1637]. *Discourse on Method, Optics, Geometry, and Meteorology.* Trans. PJ Olscamp. Indianapolis, IN: Bobbs-Merrill.

Desmedt JE and C Tomberg. 1994. Transient phase-locking of 40 Hz electrical oscillations in prefrontal and parietal human cortex reflects the process of conscious somatic perception. *Neurosci. Lett.* 168: 126–129.

Deuchars J and AM Thomson. 1995. Single axon fast inhibitory postsynaptic potentials elicited by a sparsely spiny interneuron in rat neocortex. *Neurosci.* 65: 935–942.

Deuchars J, DC West, and AM Thomson. 1994. Relationships between morphology and physiology of pyramid-pyramid single axon connections in rat neocortex *in vitro. J. Physiol. Lond.* 478: 423–435.

Devoto SH. 1990. Neuronal growth cone migration. *Experientia* 46: 916–922.

DeYoe EA, S Hochfield, H Garren, and D Van Essen. 1990. Antibody labelling functional divisions in visual cortex. Cat-301 immunoreactivity in striate and extrastriate cortex of the macaque monkey. *Vis. Neurosci.* 5: 67–76.

DiDiego I, A Smith-Fernandez, and A Fairen. 1994. Cortical cells that migrate beyond area boundaries: Characterization of an early neuronal population in the lower intermediate zone of prenatal rats. *Eur. J. Neurosci.* 6: 983–997.

Dingledine R, ed. 1984. *Brain Slices.* New York: Plenum.

Distler C, D Boussaoud, R Desimone, and LG Ungerleider. 1993. Cortical connections of inferior temporal area TEO in macaque monkeys. *J. Comp. Neurol.* 334: 125–150.

Dodd J and TM Jessell. 1988. Axon guidance and the patterning of neuronal projections in vertebrates. *Science* 242: 692–699.

Doherty P and FS Walsh. 1994. Signal transduction events underlying neurite outgrowth stimulated by cell adhesion molecules. *Current Opinion in Neurobiol.* 4: 49–55.

Douglas RJ, C Koch, M Mahowald, KA Martin, and HH Suarez. 1995. Recurrent excitation in neocortical circuits. *Science* 269: 981–985.

Douglas RJ and KA Martin. 1991. A functional microcircuit for cat visual cortex. *J. Physiol. Lond.* 440: 735–769.

Douglas RJ, KAC Martin, and D Whitteridge. 1988. Selective responses of visual cortical cells do not depend on shunting inhibition. *Nature* 332: 642–644.

——— 1989. A canonical microcircuit for neocortex. *Neural Computation* 1: 480–488.

——— 1991. An intracellular analysis of the visual responses of neurones in cat visual cortex. *J. Physiol. Lond.* 440: 659–696.

Drager U. 1981. Observations on the organization of the visual cortex in the reeler mouse. *J. Comp. Neurol.* 201: 555–570.

Dudek SM and M Bear. 1992. Homosynaptic long-term depression in area CA1 of hippocampus and effects of *N*-methyl-D-aspartate receptor blockade. *Proc. Natl. Acad. Sci. USA* 89: 4363–4367.

——— 1993. Bi-directional long-term modification of synaptic effectiveness in the adult and immature hippocampus. *J. Neurosci.* 13: 2910–2918.

Durham D and TA Woolsey. 1985. Functional organization in cortical barrels of normal and vibrissae-damaged mice: A (3H) 2-deoxyglucose study. *J. Comp. Neurol.* 235: 97–110.

Dykes RW, P Landry, R Metherate, and TYP Hicks. 1984. Functional role of GABA in cat primary somatosensory cortex: Shaping receptive fields of cortical neurons. *J. Neurophysiol.* 52: 1066–1093.

Eccles JC. 1949. Modes of communication between nerve cells. In *Australian Yearbook of Science.* Sydney: White and Bull.

——— 1952. *The Neurophysiological Basis of Mind: The Principles of Neurophysiology.* Oxford: Clarendon Press.

——— 1955. The central action of antidromic impulses in motor nerve fibers. *Pflug. Arch. Ges. Physiol.* 260: 385–415.

——— 1964. *The Physiology of Synapses.* Berlin and New York: Springer-Verlag.

Eckenstein F and RW Baughman. 1987. Cholinergic innervation in cerebral cortex. In *Cerebral Cortex, Vol. 6: Further Aspects of Cortical Function, Including Hippocampus,* ed. EG Jones and A Peters, pp. 129–160. New York: Plenum.

Eckhorn R. 1994. Oscillatory and non-oscillatory synchronizations in the cortex and their possible roles in associations of visual features. *Prog. Brain Res.* 102: 405–426.

Eckhorn R, R Bauer, W Jordan, M Brosch, W Kruse, M Munk, and HJ Reitboeck. 1988. Coherent oscillations: A mechanism for feature linking in the visual cortex? Multiple electrode and correlation analysis in the cat. *Biol. Cyber.* 60: 121–130.

Eckhorn R, A Frien, R Bauer, T Woelbern, and H Kehr. 1993. High frequency (60–90 Hz) oscillations in primary visual cortex of awake monkey. *Neuroreport* 4: 243–246.

Eckhorn R and HJ Reitboeck. 1988. Assessment of cooperative firing in groups of neurons: Special concepts for multiunit recordings from the visual system. In *Dynamics of Sensory and Cognitive Processing by the Brain,* ed. E Basar. Berlin and New York: Springer-Verlag.

Eckhorn R, HJ Reitboeck, M Arndt, and P Dicke. 1990. Feature linking via synchronization among distributed assemblies: Simulations of results from cat visual cortex. *Network* 2: 293–307.

Eckhorn R, T Schanze, M Brosch, W Salem, and R Bauer. 1992. Stimulus specific synchronizations in cat visual cortex: Multiple microelectrode and correlation studies from several cortical areas. In *Induced Rhythms in the Brain,* ed. TH Bullock and E Basar. Boston: Birkhauser.

Edelman GM. 1978. Group selection and phasic re-entrant signalling: A theory of higher brain function. In *The Mindful Brain,* ed. GM Edelman and VB Mountcastle. Cambridge, MA: MIT Press.

———— 1983. Cell adhesion molecules. *Science* 219: 450–457.

———— 1984. Modulation of cell adhesion during induction, histogenesis, and perinatal development of the nervous system. *Annu. Rev. Neurosci.* 7: 339–375.

———— 1987. *Neural Darwinism: The Theory of Neuronal Group Selection.* New York: Basic Books.

———— 1988. *Topobiology: An Introduction to Molecular Embryology.* New York: Basic Books.

———— 1989. *The Remembered Present: A Biological Theory of Consciousness.* New York: Basic Books.

———— 1992. Morphoregulation. *Develop. Dynamics* 193: 2–10.

———— 1993. Neural Darwinism: Selection and reentrant signalling in higher brain function. *Neuron* 10: 115–125.

Edelman GM, BA Cunningham, and JP Thiery. 1990. *Morphological Molecules.* New York: Wiley.

Edelman GM, E Gall, and WM Cowan. 1985. *Molecular Basis of Neural Development.* New York: Wiley.

Edelman GM and JA Gally. 1992. Nitric oxide: Linking space and time in the brain. *Proc. Natl. Acad. Sci. USA* 89: 11651–11652.

Edmondson JC, RK Liem, JE Kuster, and ME Hatten. 1988. Astrotactin: A novel neuronal cell surface antigen that mediates neuron-astroglial interactions in cerebellar microcultures. *J. Cell. Biol.* 106: 505–517.

Eggermont JJ. 1991. Rate and synchronization measures of periodicity coding in cat primary auditory cortex. *Hear. Res.* 56: 153–167.

Eldredge N and SJ Gould. 1972. Punctuated equilibrium: An alternative to phyletic gradualism. In *Models in Paleobiology,* ed. TJM Schopf, pp. 82–115. San Francisco: Freeman.

Eldredge N and I Tattersall. 1975. Evolutionary models, phylogenetic reconstruction, and another look at hominid phylogeny. *Contrib. Primat.* 5: 218–242.

Elias H and D Schwartz. 1971. Cerebro-cortical surface areas, volumes, lengths of gyri and their interdependence in mammals, including man. *Z. Saugetierekunde* 36: 147–163.

Elson RC and AI Selverston. 1992. Mechanism of gastric rhythm generation in the isolated stomatogastric ganglion of spiny lobsters: Bursting pacemaker potentials, synaptic interactions, and muscarinic modulation. *J. Neurophysiol.* 68: 890–907.

Engel AK, P Konig, CM Gray, and W Singer. 1990. Stimulus-dependent neuronal oscillations in cat visual cortex: Inter-columnar interaction as determined by cross-correlation analysis. *Eur. J. Neurosci.* 2: 588–606.

Engel AK, P Konig, AK Kreiter, TB Schillen, and W Singer. 1992. Temporal coding in the visual cortex: New vistas on integration in the nervous system. *Trends Neurosci.* 15: 218–226.

Engel AK, P Konig, AK Kreiter, and W Singer. 1991a. Interhemispheric synchronization of oscillatory neuronal responses in cat visual cortex. *Science* 252: 1177–1179.

Engel AK, AK Kreiter, P Konig, and W Singer. 1991b. Synchronization of oscillatory neuronal responses between striate and extrastriate visual cortical areas of the cat. *Proc. Natl. Acad. Sci. USA* 88: 6048–6052.

Erwin E, K Obermeyer, and K Schulten. 1995. Models of orientation and ocular dominance columns in the visual cortex: A critical comparison. *Neural Computation* 7: 425–468.

Escobar MI, H Pimienta, VS Caviness jr, M Jacobson, JE Crandall, and KS Kosik. 1986. Architecture of apical dendrites in the murine neocortex: Dual apical dendritic systems. *Neurosci.* 17: 975–989.

Evarts EV. 1966. Methods for recording activity of individual neurons in moving animals. In *Methods in Medical Research,* vol. II, ed. RF Rushmer, pp. 241–250. Chicago: Yearbook.

Evarts EV, Y Shinoda, and SP Wise. 1984. *Neurophysiological Approaches to Higher Brain Functions.* New York: Wiley.

Eysel UT and IA Shevelev. 1994. Time-slice analysis of inhibition in cat striate cortical neurones. *Neuroreport* 5: 2033–2036.

Fairen A, J DeFelipe, and J Regidor. 1984. Nonpyramidal neurons: General account. In *Cerebral Cortex, Vol. 1: Cellular Components of the Cerebral Cortex,* ed. A Peters and EG Jones, pp. 251–254. New York: Plenum.

Fallon JH and SE Loughlin. 1987. Monamine innervation of cerebral cortex and a theory of the role of monoamines in cerebral cortex and basal ganglia. In *Cerebral Cortex, Vol. 6: Further Aspects of Cortical Function, Including Hippocampus,* ed. EG Jones and A Peters, pp. 41–128. New York: Plenum.

Fatt P and B Katz. 1952. Spontaneous subthreshold activity at motor nerve endings. *J. Physiol.* 117: 109–128.

Favorov OV. 1991. Detection and characterization of the mosaic body representation in SI cortex. In *Information Processing in the Somatosensory Cortex,* ed. O Franzen and J Westman, pp. 221–232. London: Macmillan.

Favorov OV and ME Diamond. 1990. Demonstration of discrete place-defined columns—segregates—in the cat SI. *J. Comp. Neurol.* 298: 97–112.

Favorov OV, ME Diamond, and BL Whitsel. 1987. Evidence for a mosaic representation of the body surface in area 3b of the somatic cortex of cat. *Proc. Natl. Acad. Sci. USA* 84: 6606–6610.

Favorov OV and BL Whitsel. 1988a. Spatial organization of the peripheral input to area 1 cell columns: I. The detection of "segregates." *Brain Res. Rev.* 13: 25–42.

——— 1988b. Spatial organization of the peripheral input to area 1 cell columns: II. The forelimb representation achieved by a mosaic of segregates. *Brain Res. Rev.* 13: 43–56.

Fechner GT. 1966 [1860]. *Elements of Psychophysics,* vol. 1. Trans. HE Adler. New York: Rinehart and Winston.

Feldman ML. 1984. Morphology of the neocortical pyramidal neuron. In *Cerebral Cortex, Vol. 1: Cellular Components of the Cerebral Cortex,* ed. A Peters and EG Jones, pp. 123–200. New York: Plenum.

Felleman DJ and DC Van Essen. 1991. Distributed hierarchical processing in the primate cerebral cortex. *Cerebral Cortex* 1: 1–47.

Feng TP. 1941. Studies on the neuromuscular junction. XXVI. The changes in the end-plate potential during and after prolonged stimulation. *Chin. J. Physiol.* 16: 341–372.

Ferrer I, E Soriano, JA Del Rio, S Alcantara, and C Auladell. 1992. Cell death and removal in the cerebral cortex during development. *Prog. Neurobiol.* 39: 1–43.

Ferster D, S Chung, and H Wheat. 1996. Orientation selectivity of thalamic input to simple cells in cat visual cortex. *Nature* 380: 249–252.

Ferster D and B Jagadeesh. 1992. EPSP-IPSP interactions in cat visual cortex studied in vivo with whole-cell patch recording. *J. Neurosci.* 12: 1262–1274.

Filapek PA, C Richemme, DN Kennedy, and VA Caviness jr. 1994. The young adult human brain: An MRI-based morphometric analysis. *Cerebral Cortex* 4: 344–361.

Finger S. 1994. *Origins of Neuroscience: A History of Explorations into Brain Function.* Oxford: Oxford U. Press.

Finlay BL. 1992. Cell death and the creation of regional differences in neuronal numbers. *J. Neurobiol.* 23: 1159–1171.

Finlay BL and RB Darlington. 1995. Linked regularities in the development and evolution of mammalian brains. *Science* 268: 1578–1584.

Fischbach GD and KM Rosen. 1997. ARIA: A neuromuscular junction neuregulin. *Annu. Rev. Neurosci.* 20: 429–458.

Fishell G and ME Hatten. 1991. Astrotactin provides a receptor system for CNS neuronal migration. *Development* 113: 755–765.

Fishell G, CA Mason, and ME Hatten. 1993. Dispersion of neural progenitors within the germinal zones of the forebrain. *Nature* 362: 636–638.

Fisken RA, LJ Garey, and TPS Powell. 1973. Patterns of degeneration after intrinsic lesions of the visual cortex (area 17) of the monkey. *Brain Res.* 208–213.

——— 1975. The intrinsic, association and commissural connections of area 17 of the visual cortex. *Phil. Trans. Roy. Soc. Lond.* B272: 487–536.

Flechsig P. 1920. *Anatomie des menschlichen Gehirns und Ruckenmarks.* Leipzig: Thieme.

Fleischauer K, H Pesche, and W Wittkoniski. 1972. Vertical bundles of dendrites in the neocortex. *Z. Anat. Entw. Gesch.* 136: 213–233.

Fonnum F. 1984. Glutamate: A neurotransmitter in mammalian brain. *J. Neurochem.* 42: 1–11.

Fox K. 1995. The critical period for long-term potentiation in primary sensory cortex. *Neuron* 15: 485–488.

Frahm HD, H Stephan, and M Stephan. 1982. Comparison of brain structure volumes in Insectivora and Primates. I. Neocortex. *J. Hirnforschung* 23: 375–389.

Freeman WJ. 1975. *Mass Action in the Nervous System: Examination of the Neurophysiogical Basis of Adaptive Behavior through the EEG.* New York: Academic.

——— 1994a. Characterization of state transitions in spatially distributed, chaotic, nonlinear, dynamical systems in cerebral cortex. *Integr. Physiol. Behav. Sci.* 29: 294–306.

——— 1994b. Neural networks and chaos. *J. Theor. Biol.* 171: 13–18.

Freinwald WA, AK Kreiter, and W Singer. 1995. Stimulus dependent intercolumnar synchronization of single unit responses in cat area 17. *Neuroreport* 6: 2348–2352.

Friauf E, SK McConnell, and CJ Shatz. 1990. Functional synaptic circuits in the subplate during fetal and early postnatal development of cat visual cortex. *J. Neurosci.* 10: 2601–2613.

Friauf E and CJ Shatz. 1991. Changing patterns of synaptic input to subplate and cortical plate during development of visual cortex. *J. Neurophysiol.* 66: 2059–2071.

Friedman HR and PS Goldman-Rakic. 1995. Coactivation of prefrontal cortex and inferior parietal cortex in working memory tasks revealed by 2DG functional mapping in rhesus monkey. *J. Neurosci.* 14: 2775–2788.

Frien A, R Eckhorn, R Bauer, T Woelbern, and H Kehr. 1994. Stimulus specific fast oscillations at zero phase between visual areas V1 and V2 of awake monkey. *Neuroreport* 5: 2273–2277.

Fries P, PE Roelfsema, AE Engel, P Konig, and W Singer. 1996. Synchronized gamma frequency oscillations correlated with perception during binocular rivalry in awake squinting cats. *Neurosci. Abstr.* 23: 262.

Fujita I, K Tanaka, M Ito, and K Cheng. 1992. Columns for visual features of objects in monkey inferotemporal cortex. *Nature* 360: 343–346.

Fuxe K and LF Agnati, eds. 1991. *Volume Transmission in the Brain: Novel Mechanisms for Neural Transmission. Advances in Neuroscience,* vol. 1. New York: Raven.

Gadisseux JF, P Evrard, JP Mission, and VS Caviness jr. 1989. Dynamic structure of the radial glial fiber system of the developing murine cerebral wall. An immunocytochemical analysis. *Brain. Res. Dev.* 50: 55–67.

———— 1992. Dynamic changes in the density of radial glial fibers of the developing murine cerebral wall: A quantitative immunohistological analysis. *J. Comp. Neurol.* 322: 246–254.

Gadisseux JF, HJ Kadhim, P van den Bosch de Aguilar, VS Caviness jr, and P Evrard. 1990. Neuron migration within the radial glial fiber system of the developing murine cerebrum: An electron microscopic autoradiographic analysis. *Dev. Brain Res.* 52: 39–56.

Galambos R. 1989. Electrogenesis of evoked potentials. In *Brain Dynamics: Progress and Perspectives,* ed. E Basar and TH Bullock, pp. 13–25. Berlin and New York: Springer-Verlag.

Galambos R, S Makieg, and P Talmachoff. 1981. A 40 Hz auditory potential recorded from the human scalp. *Proc. Natl. Acad. Sci. USA* 78: 2643–2647.

Galanter E. 1984. Detection and discrimination of environmental change. In *Handbook of Physiology, Section I: The Nervous System, Vol. III: Sensory Processes, Part 1,* ed. JM Brookhart, I Darian-Smith, VB Mountcastle and SR Geigers. Bethesda MD: American Physiological Society.

Galea MP and I Darian-Smith. 1994. Multiple corticospinal neuron populations in macaque monkey are specified by their unique cortical origins, spinal terminations, and connections. *Cerebral Cortex* 4: 166–194.

Gally JA, PR Montague, GN Reeke, and GM Edelman. 1990. The NO hypothesis: Possible effects of a short-lived rapidly diffusible signal in the development and function of the nervous system. *Proc. Natl. Acad. Sci. USA* 87: 3547–3551.

Galuske RA and W Singer. 1996. The origin and topography of long-range intrinsic projections in cat visual cortex: A developmental study. *Cerebral Cortex* 6: 417–430.

Garthwaite J, SL Charles, and R Chess-Williams. 1988. Endothelial-derived relaxing factor released on activation of NMDA receptors suggests role as an intercellular messenger in the brain. *Nature* 336: 385–388.

Georgopoulos AP. 1991. Higher order motor control. *Annu. Rev. Neurosci.* 14: 361–377.

———— 1995. Current issues in directional motor control. *Trends Neurosci.* 11: 506–510.

Georgopoulos AP and G Pelizzer. 1995. The mental and the neural. Psychological and neural studies of mental rotation and memory scanning. *Neuropsychologia* 33: 1531–1547.

Georgopoulos AP, M Taira, and A Lukashin. 1993. Cognitive neurophysiology and motor control. *Science* 260: 47–52.

Gerstein GL and AMHJ Aertsen. 1985. Representation of cooperative firing activity among simultaneously recorded neurons. *J. Neurophysiol.* 54: 1513–1528.

Gerstein GL, P Bedenburgh, and AMHJ Aertsen. 1989. Neuronal assemblies. *IEEE Trans. Biomedical Engineering* 36: 4–14.

Gerstein GL, D Perkel, and J Dayhoff. 1985. Cooperative firing activity in simultaneously recorded populations of neurons: Detection and measurement. *J. Neurosci.* 5: 881–889.

Gerstner W, R Ritz, and LA Hemmen. 1993. A biologically motivated and analytically soluble model of collective oscillation in the cortex. *Biol. Cyber.* 68: 363–374.

Getting P. 1989. Emerging principles governing the operation of neural networks. *Annu. Rev. Neurosci.* 12: 185–204.

Gevins A. 1995. High-resolution electroencephalographic studies of cognition. *Adv. Neurol.* 66: 181–195.

Gevins A, B Cutillo, J Desmond, M Ward, S Bressler, N Barbero, and K Laxer. 1994a. Subdural grid recordings of distributed neocortical networks involved with somatosensory discrimination. *Electroencephalogr. Clin. Neurophysiol.* 92: 282–290.

Gevins A, J Le, NK Martin, P Brickett, J Desmond, and B Reutter. 1994b. High resolution EEG: 124 channel recording, spatial deblurring and MRI integration methods. *Electroencephalogr. Clin. Neurophysiol.* 90: 337–358.

Gevins A, H Leong, R Du, ME Smith, J Le, D DuRousseau, J Zhang, and J Libove. 1995. Towards measurement of brain function in operational environments. *Biol. Psychol.* 40: 169–186.

Gevins A, H Leong, ME Smith, J Le, and R Du. 1996. Mapping cognitive brain function with modern high-resolution electroencephalography. *Trends Neurosci.* 18: 429–436.

Ghose GM and RD Freeman. 1992. Oscillatory discharge in the visual system: Does it have a functional role? *J. Neurophysiol.* 68: 1558–1574.

Ghosh A, A Antonini, SK McConnell, and CJ Shatz. 1990. Requirement for subplate neurons in the formation of thalamocortical connections. *Nature* 347: 179–181.

Ghosh A and CJ Shatz. 1992. Involvement of subplate neurons in the formation of ocular dominance columns. *Science* 255: 1441–1443.

Gibbs FA and EL Gibbs. 1950. *Atlas of Electroencephalography: I. Methodology and Controls.* 2d ed. Cambridge, MA: Addison-Wesley.

Gibson EJ. 1966. *The Senses Considered as Perceptual Systems.* Boston: Houghton Miflin.

Gilbert CD. 1983. Microcircuitry of the visual cortex. *Annu. Rev. Neurosci.* 6: 217–248.

———— 1992. Horizontal integration and cortical dynamics. *Neuron* 9: 1–13.

———— 1993. Circuitry, architecture, and functional dynamics of visual cortex. *Cerebral Cortex* 3: 373–386.

Gilbert CD and JP Kelly. 1975. The projection of cells in different layers of the cat's visual cortex. *J. Comp. Neurol.* 163: 81–106.

Gilbert CD and TN Wiesel. 1979. Morphology and intracortical projections of functionally characterized neurons in the cat visual cortex. *Nature* 290: 120–125.

———— 1983. Clustered intrinsic connections in cat visual cortex. *J. Neurosci.* 3: 1116–1133.

———— 1989. Columnar specificity of intrinsic horizontal and corticocortical connections in cat visual cortex. *J. Neurosci.* 9: 2432–2442.

Gloor P. 1969. Hans Berger and the electroencephalogram: The fourteen original reports on the human electroncephalogram. *Electroencephalogr. Clin. Neurophysiol.,* Suppl 28.

———— 1975. Contributions of electroencephalography and electrocorticography to the neurosurgical treatment of epilepsy. *Adv. Neurol.* 8: 59–105.

Goffinet AM. 1984. Phylogenetic determinants of radial organization in the cerebral cortex. *Z. mikrosk. Anat. Forsch. Leipsig* 98: 909–925.

Gold JI and MF Bear. 1994. A model of dendritic spine Ca^{2+} concentration exploring possible bases for a sliding synaptic modification threshold. *Proc. Natl. Acad. Sci. USA* 91: 3941–3945.

Goldman PS and WJH Nauta. 1977. Columnar distribution of cortico-cortical fibers in the frontal association, limbic, and motor cortex of the developing rhesus monkey. *Brain Res.* 122: 393–413.

Goldman-Rakic PS. 1988. Topography of cognition: Parallel distributed networks in primate association cortex. *Annu. Rev. Neurosci.* 11: 137–156.

Goldman-Rakic PS, MS Lidov, and DW Gallager. 1990. Overlap of dopaminergic, adrenergic and serotonergic receptors and complementarity of their subtypes in primate prefrontal cortex. *J. Neurosci.* 10: 2125–2138.

Goldman-Rakic PS, MS Lidov, JF Smiley, and MS Williams. 1992. The anatomy of dopamine in monkey and human prefrontal cortex. *J. Neural. Trans.* Suppl. 36: 163–177.

Goldman-Rakic PS and WJH Nauta. 1977. Columnar organization of association and motor cortex: Autoradiographic evidence for cortico-cortical and commissural columns in frontal lobe of the newborn rhesus monkey. *Brain Res.* 122: 369–385.

Goldman-Rakic PS and ML Schwartz. 1982. Interdigitation of contralateral and ipsilateral columnar projections to frontal association cortex in primates. *Science* 216: 755–757.

Goldstein DB, A Ruiz Linares, C Cavilla-Sforza, and MW Feldman. 1995. Genetic absolute dating based on microsatellites and the origin of modern humans. *Proc. Natl. Acad. Sci. USA* 92: 6723–6727.

Golowasch J and E Marder. 1992. Ionic currents of the lateral pyloric neurons of the stomatogastric ganglion of the crab. *J. Neurophysiol.* 67: 318–331.

Gorski RA. 1985. Sexual dimorphisms of the brain. *J. Anim. Sci.* 61 (Suppl. 3): 38–61.

Gould SJ and N Eldredge. 1977. Punctuated equilibrium: Tempo and mode of evolution reconsidered. *Paleobiology* 3: 115–151.

———— 1993. Punctuated equilibrium comes of age. *Nature* 366: 223–227.

Goy RW and BS McEwen. 1980. *Sexual Differentiation of the Brain.* Cambridge, MA: MIT Press.

Grant G, S Landgren, and H Silvenius. 1975. Columnar distribution of U-fibres from the postcruciate cerebral projection area of the cat's group-I muscle afferent. *Exp. Brain Res.* 24: 57–74.

Grant SGN and TJ O'Dell. 1994. Targeting tyrosine kinase genes and long-term potentiation. *Sem. Neurosci.* 6: 45–52.

Gray CM, AK Engel, P Konig, and W Singer. 1990. Stimulus-dependent neuronal oscillations in cat visual cortex: Receptive field properties and feature dependence. *Eur. J. Neurosci.* 2: 607–619.

Gray CM, AK Engel, P Konig, and W Singer. 1992. Synchronization of oscillatory neuronal responses in cat striate cortex: Temporal properties. *Vis. Neurosci.* 8: 337–347.

Gray CM, P Konig, AK Engel, and W Singer. 1989. Oscillatory responses in cat visual cortex exhibit inter-columnar synchronization which reflects global stimulus properties. *Nature* 338: 334–337.

Gray CM and DA McCormick. 1996. Chattering cells: Superficial pyramidal neurons contributing to generation of synchronous oscillations in the visual cortex. *Science* 274: 109–113.

Gray CM and W Singer. 1989. Stimulus-specific neuronal oscillations in orientation columns of cat visual cortex. *Proc. Natl. Acad. Sci. USA* 86: 1698–1702.

Gray EG. 1959. Axo-somatic and axo-dendritic synapses in the cerebral cortex: An electron microscopic study. *J. Anat.* 93: 420–433.

Gray EG and VP Whittaker. 1960. The isolation of synaptic vesicles from the central nervous system. *J. Physiol. Lond.* 153: 35–37.

———— 1962. The isolation of nerve endings from brain: An electron microscopic study of cell fragments derived by homogenization and centrifugation. *J. Anat.* 96: 79–88.

Gregory RA, ed. 1996. *Perception,* vol. 25, part 10. London: Pion.

Gressens P, F Gofflot, G Van Maele Fabry, JP Misson, JF Gadisseux, P Evrard, and JJ Picard. 1992a. Early neurogenesis and teratogenesis in whole mouse embryo cultures. Histochemical, immunocytological and ultrastructural study of the premigratory neuronal-glial units in normal mouse embryo and in mouse embryos influenced by cocaine and retinoic acid. *J. Neuropathol. Exp. Neurol.* 51: 206–219.

Gressens P, C Richelme, HJ Kadheim, JF Gadisseux, and P Evrard. 1992b. The germinative zone produces the most cortical astrocytes after neuronal migration in the developing mammalian brain. *Biol. Neonate* 61: 4–24.

Groenewegen H and HW Berendse. 1994. The specificity of the "nonspecific" midline and intralaminar thalamic nuclei. *Trends Neurosci.* 17: 52–57.

Gross CG, DB Bender, and CE Rocha-Miranda. 1969. Visual receptive fields of neurons in the inferotemporal cortex of the monkey. *Science* 166: 1303–1306.

Gross CG, CE Rocha-Miranda, and DB Bender. 1972. Visual properties of neurons in the inferotemporal cortex of the macaque. *J. Neurophysiol.* 35: 96–111.

Grumet M, S Hoffman, and GM Edelman. 1984. Two antigenetically related neuronal CAMs of different specificities mediate neuron-neuron and neuron-glia adhesion. *Proc. Natl. Acad. Sci. USA* 81: 267–271.

Gunderson HJG. 1986. Stereology of arbitrary particles. A review of unbiased number and size estimates and presentation of some new ones, in memory of William R. Thompson. *J. Microsc.* 143: 3–45.

Guthrie A. 1992. Lineage in the cerebral cortex: When is a clone not a clone? *Trends Neurosci.* 15: 273–275.

Guthrie PB, M Segal, and SB Kater. 1991. Independent regulation of calcium revealed by imaging dendritic spines. *Nature* 354: 76–80.

Gutnick MJ and I Mody, eds. 1995. *The Cortical Neuron.* Oxford: Oxford U. Press.

Gutnick MJ and DA Prince. 1981. Dye coupling and possible electrotonic coupling in the guinea pig neocortical slice. *Science* 211: 67–70.

Haberland C and M Perou. 1969. Primary bilateral anophthalmia. *J. Neuropath. Exp. Neurol.* 28: 337–351.

Haley JE and EM Schuman. 1994. Involvement of nitric oxide in synaptic plasticity and learning. *Sem. Neurosci.* 6: 11–20.

Hamburger A and RW Oppenheim. 1982. Naturally occurring neuronal death in vertebrates. *Neuroscience Commentaries* 2: 39–55.

Hand P. 1981. The deoxyglucose method. In *Neuroanatomical Tracking Methods,* ed. R Heimer and MJ Robards. New York: Plenum.

Hari R and R Samelin. 1997. Human cortical oscillations: A neuromagnetic view through the skull. *Trends Neurosci.* 20: 44–49.

Harmori J, J Takacs, and P Petruz. 1990. Immunogold electronmicroscopic demonstration of glutamate and GABA in normal and deafferented cerebellar cortex: Correlation between transmitter content and synaptic size. *J. Histochem. Cytochem.* 389: 1767–1777.

Harris KM and SB Kater. 1994. Dendritic spines: Cellular specializations imparting both stability and flexibility to synaptic function. *Annu. Rev. Neurosci.* 17: 341–371.

Harris-Warwick RM and E Marder. 1991. Modulation of neural networks for behavior. *Annu. Rev. Neurosci.* 14: 39–57.

Harris-Warwick RM, F Nagy, and MP Nusbaum. 1992. Neuromodulation of stomatogastric networks of identified neurons and transmitters. In *Dynamic Neural Networks,* ed. RM Harris-Warwick, E Marder, AI Selverston, and M Moulins, pp. 87–137. Cambridge, MA: MIT Press.

Hartley D. 1749. *Observations on Man.* London: Legate and Frederick.

Hatten ME. 1985. Neuronal regulation of astroglial morphology and proliferation in vitro. *J. Cell Biol.* 100: 384–396.

———— 1990. Riding the glial monorail: A common mechanism for glial-guided neuronal migration in different regions of the developing mammalian brain. *Trends Neurosci.* 13: 179–184.

———— 1993. The role of migration in central nervous system development. *Current Opinion in Neurobiology* 3: 38–44.

Hatten ME and CA Mason. 1990. Mechanisms of glia-guided neuronal migration in vitro and in vivo. *Experientia* 46: 907–916.

Haug H. 1987. Brain sizes, surfaces, and neuronal sizes of the cortex cerebri: A stereological investigation of man and his variablility and a comparison with some mammals (primates, whales, marsupials, insectivores, and one elephant). *Am. J. Anat.* 180: 126–142.

Haug H, S Kuhl, E Mecke, N-L Sass, and K Wasner. 1984. The significance of morphometric procedures in the investigation of age changes in cytoarchitectonic structures of the human brain. *Int. J. Brain Res. Neurobiol.* 25: 353–374.

Hawkins RD, ER Kandel, and SA Siegelbaum. 1993. Learning to modulate transmitter release. Themes and variations in synaptic plasticity. *Annu. Rev. Neurosci.* 16: 615–665.

Haydon PG and F Drapeau. 1995. From contact to connection: Early events during synaptogenesis. *Trends Neurosci.* 18: 196–201.

Hayes TL, JL Cameron, JD Fernstrom, and DA Lewis. 1991. A comparative analysis of the distribution of prosomatostatin-derived peptides in human and monkey neocortex. *J. Comp. Neurol.* 303: 585–599.

Hebb DO. 1949. *The Organization of Behavior: A Neuropsychological Theory.* New York: Wiley.

Hedlich A, HJ Luth, L Werner, B Bar, U Hanisch, and E Winklemann. 1990. Gabaergic NADPH-diaphorase-positive Martinotti cells in the visual cortex of rats. *J. Hirnforsch.* 31: 681–687.

Heffner CD, AGS Lumsden, and DDM O'Leary. 1990. Target control of collateral extension and directional axon growth in the mammalian brain. *Science* 247: 217–220.

Heil P, R Rajan, and DR Irvine. 1992a. Sensitivity of neurons in cat primary auditory cortex to tones and frequency-modulated stimuli. II. Organization of response properties along the 'isofrequency' dimension. *Hear. Res.* 63: 135–156.

———— 1992b. Sensitivity of neurons in cat primary auditory cortex to tones and frequency-modulated stimuli. I. Effects of variation of stimulus parameters. *Hear. Res.* 63: 108–134.

———— 1994. Topographic representation of tone intensity along the isofrequency axis of cat primary auditory cortex. *Hear. Res.* 76: 188–202.

Helmholtz H von. 1962. *Handbook of Physiological Optics,* New York: Dover. Translation of *Handbuch der physiologischen Optik,* 3 vols. Ed. and trans. JPC Southall. Hamburg: Voss, 1856, 1860, 1866.

Henderson TA, TA Woolsey, and MF Jacquin. 1992. Infraorbital nerve blockade from birth does not disrupt central trigeminal pattern formation in the rat. *Brain Res. Dev.* 66: 146–152.

Hendrickson AE and JR Wilson. 1979. A difference in [14C]deoxyglucose autoradiographic patterns in striate cortex between *Macaca* and *Saimiri* monkeys. *Brain* 170: 353–358.

Hendry SHC. 1993. Organization of neuropeptide Y neurons in the mammalian central nervous system. In *The Biology of Neuropeptide Y and Related Peptides,* ed. WF Colmeers and C Wahlstedt, pp. 65–156. Totowa, NJ: Humana.

Hendry SHC, S Hochfield, EG Jones, and RDG McKay. 1984. Monoclonal antibody that identified subsets of neurons in the visual systeam of the monkey and cat. *Nature* 307: 267–271.

Hendry SH, CR Houser, EG Jones, and JE Vaughan. 1983. Synaptic organization of the immunocytochemically identified GABA neurons in the monkey sensory-motor cortex. *J. Neurocytol.* 12: 639–660.

Hendry SH and EG Jones. 1981. Sizes and distributions of intrinsic neurons incorporating tritiated GABA in the monkey sensory-motor cortex. *J. Neurosci.* 1: 390–408.

———— 1983. The organization of pyramidal and non-pyramidal cell dendrites in relation to thalamic afferent terminations in the monkey somatic sensory cortex. *J. Neurocytol.* 12: 277–298.

Hendry SHC, EG Jones, and MC Beinfeld. 1983. Cholecystokinin-immunoreactive neurons in rat and monkey cerebral cortex make symmetric synapses and have intimate associations with blood vessels. *Proc. Natl. Acad. Sci. USA* 80: 2400–2404.

Hendry SHC, EG Jones, J DeFelipe, J Schmechel, C Brandon, and PC Emson. 1984a. Neuropeptide-containing neurons of the cerebral cortex are also GABA-ergic. *Proc. Natl. Acad. Sci. USA* 81: 6526–6530.

Hendry SHC, EG Jones, and PC Emson. 1984b. Morphology, distribution and synaptic relations of somatostatin- and neuropeptide Y-immunoreactive neurons in rat and monkey neocortex. *J. Neurosci.* 4: 2497–2517.

Hendry SHC, EG Jones, PC Emson, DEM Lawson, CW Heizmann, and P Streit. 1989. Two classes of cortical GABA neurons defined by differential calcium binding protein immunoreactivities. *Exp. Brain Res.* 76: 467–472.

Hendry SHC, HD Schwark, EG Jones, and J Yan. 1987. Numbers and proportions of GABA-immunoreactive neurons in different areas of the monkey cerebral cortex. *J. Neurosci.* 7: 1503–1519.

Henry GH, PO Bishop, and B Dreher. 1974. Orientation, axis and direction as stimulus parameters for striate cells. *Vision Res.* 14: 767–777.

Hepler JR, CS Toomin, KD McCarthy, F Conti, G Battaglia, A Rustioni, and P Petrusz. 1988. Characterization of antisera to glutamate and aspartate. *J. Histochem. Cytochem.* 36: 13–22.

Hestrin S, RA Nicoll, DJ Perkel, and P Sah. 1990. Analysis of excitatory synaptic action in pyramidal cells using whole-cell recording from rat hippocampal slices. *J. Physiol. Lond.* 422: 205–222.

Hirotsune S, T Takahara, S Sasaki, K Hirose, A Yoshida, T Ohashi, M Kusakabe, M Muramatsu, S Watanabe, et al. 1995. The reeler gene encodes a protein with an EGF-like motif expressed by pioneer neurons. *Nature Genetics* 10: 77–83.

Hobbes T. 1651. *Leviathan, or the Matter, Form and Power of a Commonwealth.* London.

Hockfield S, RG Kalb, S Zaremba, and H Fryer. 1990. Expression of neural proteoglycans correlated with the acquisition of mature neuronal properties in the mammalian brain. *Cold Spring Harbor Symp. Quant. Biol.* 55: 505–514.

Hockfield S, RDG McKay, SHC Hendry, and EG Jones. 1983. A surface antigen that identifies ocular dominance columns in cortical area 17 and laminar features in the internal geniculate nucleus. *Cold Spring Harbor Symp. Quant. Biol.* 48: 837–890.

Hockfield S and M Sur. 1990. Monoclonal antibody Cat-301 identified Y-cells in the dorsal lateral geniculate nucleus of the cat. *J. Comp. Neurol.* 30: 320–330.

Hodgkin AL. 1964. *The Conduction of the Nerve Impulse.* Liverpool: Liverpool U. Press.

Hodgkin AL and AF Huxley. 1952. A quantitative description of membrane current and its application to conduction and excitation in nerve. *J. Physiol. Lond.* 117: 500–544.

Hofman MA. 1982. Encephalization in mammals in relation to the size of the cerebral cortex. *Brain Behav. Evol.* 20: 84–96.

———— 1983. Encephalization in hominids: Evidence for the model of punctualism. *Brain Behav. Evol.* 22: 102–117.

———— 1985a. Neuronal correlates of corticalization in mammals: A theory. *J. Theor. Biol.* 7: 77–95.

———— 1985b. Size and shape of the cerebral cortex in mammals. I. The cortical surface. *Brain Behav. Evol.* 27: 28–40.

———— 1988. Size and shape of the cerebral cortex in mammals. II. The cortical volume. *Brain Behav. Evol.* 32: 17–26.

———— 1989. On the evolution and geometry of the brain in mammals. *Prog. Neurobiol.* 32: 137–158.

Hohn A, J Liebrock, K Bailey, and Y-A Barde. 1990. Identification and characterization of a novel member of the nerve growth factor/brain derived neurotrophic factor family. *Nature* 344: 339–341.

Hollmann M and S Heinemann. 1994. Cloned glutamate receptors. *Annu. Rev. Neurosci.* 17: 31–108.

Holloway RL. 1982. Human brain evolution: A search for units, models, and synthesis. *Canad. J. Anthropol.* 3: 215–230.

———— 1983. Human paleontological evidence relevant to language behavior. *Hum. Neurobiol.* 2: 105–114.

———— 1995. Toward a synthetic theory of brain evolution. In *Origins of the Human Brain,* ed. J-P Changeux and J Chavaillon, pp. 52–44. Oxford: Clarendon Press.

Horai S, K Hayasaka, R Kondo, K Tsugane, and N Takahata. 1995. Recent African origin of modern humans revealed by complete sequences of hominoid mitochondrial DNAs. *Proc. Natl. Acad. Sci. USA* 2: 532–536.

Horton HL and P Levitt. 1988. A unique membrane protein is expressed on early developing limbic system axons and cortical targets. *J. Neurosci.* 8: 4652–4661.

Horton JC. 1984. Cytochrome oxidase patches: A new cytoarchitectonic feature of monkey visual cortex. *Phil. Trans. Roy. Soc. Lond.* B304: 199–253.

Horton JC and DH Hubel. 1981. Regular patchy distribution of cytochrome oxidase staining in primary visual cortex of macaque monkey. *Nature* 292: 762–764.

Houser CR, SHC Hendry, EG Jones, and JE Vaughan. 1983. Morphological diversity of immunocytochemically identified GABA neurons in the monkey sensory-motor cortex. *J. Neurocytol.* 12: 617–638.

Huang W, R Ciochon, G Yumin, R Larrick, F Qiren, H Schwarz, C Yonge, J de Vos, and W Rink. 1995. Early *Homo* and associated artefacts from Asia. *Nature* 378: 275–278.

Huang Y-Y, PV Nguyen, T Abel, and ER Kandel. 1996. Long-lasting forms of synaptic potentiation in the mammalian hippocampus. *Learning and Memory* 3: 74–85.

Hubel DH and MS Livingstone. 1987. Segregation of form, color and stereopsis in primate area 18. *J. Neurosci.* 7: 3378–3415.

Hubel D and TN Wiesel. 1962. Receptive fields, binocular interaction and functional architecture in the cat's visual cortex. *J. Physiol. Lond.* 160: 106–154.

———— 1968. Receptive fields and functional architecture of monkey striate cortex. *J. Physiol. Lond.* 195: 215–243.

———— 1977. Functional architecture of macaque monkey cortex. *Proc. Roy. Soc. Lond.* B198: 1–559.

Hume D. 1977. *An Enquiry Concerning Human Understanding.* Reprint of the posthumous edition of *Philosophical Essays Concerning Human Understanding* (1748), ed. LZ Selby-Bigge and PH Nidditch. Oxford: Clarendon.

Hummel JE and I Biederman. 1992. Dynamic binding in a neural network for shape recognition. *Psychol. Rev.* 99: 480–517.

Hunter KE and ME Hatten. 1995. Radial glial cell transformation to astrocytes is bidirectional: Regulation by a diffusible factor in embryonic forebrain. *Proc. Natl. Acad. Sci. USA* 92: 2061–2065.

Huntley GW and EG Jones. 1991a. Relationship of intrinsic connections of forelimb movement representations in monkey motor cortex: A correlative anatomic and physiological study. *J. Neurophysiol.* 66: 390–413.

———— 1991b. The emergence of architectural field structure and area boundaries in the developing monkey sensorimotor cortex. *Neurosci.* 44: 287–310.

Hvalby O, HC Hemmings jr, O Paulsen, AJ Czernik, AC Nairn, JM Godfriend, V Jensen, M Raastad, JF Storm, P Andersen, and P Greengard. 1994. Specificity of protein kinase inhibitor peptide and induction of long-term potentiation. *Proc. Natl. Acad. Sci. USA* 91: 4761–4765.

Imig TJ and HO Adrian. 1977. Binaural columns in the primary field (A1) of cat auditory cortex. *Brain Res.* 138: 241–257.

Imig TJ and JF Brugge. 1978. Sources and terminations of callosal axons related to binaural and frequency maps in primary auditory cortex of the cat. *J. Comp. Neurol.* 182: 637–660.

Innocenti GM and R Caminiti. 1980. Postnatal shaping of callosal connections from sensory areas. *Exp. Brain Res.* 38: 381–394.

Innocenti GM, L Fiore, and R Caminiti. 1977. Exuberant projection into the corpus callosum from the visual cortex of newborn cats. *Neurosci. Lett.* 4: 237–242.

Ioannides AA, PB Fenwick, J Lumsden, MJ Liu, PD Bamidis, KC Squires, D Lawson, and GW Fenton. 1994. Activation sequence of discrete brain areas during cognitive processes: Results from magnetic field tomography. *Electroencephalogr. Clin. Neurophysiol.* 91: 399–402.

Ioannides AA, KD Singh, R Hasson, SB Baumann, RL Rogers, FC Guito jr, and AC Papanicolaou. 1993. Comparison of single current dipole and magnetic field tomography analyses of the cortical response to auditory stimuli. *Brain Tomog.* 6: 27–34.

Isaac JTR, RA Nicoll, and RC Malenka. 1995. Evidence for silent synapses: Implications for the expression of LTP. *Neuron* 15: 427–434.

Ito M. 1989. Long-term depression. *Annu. Rev. Neurosci.* 12: 85–102.

Iwamura Y, M Tanaka, and O Hikosaka. 1980. Overlapping representation of fingers in the somatosensory cortex (area 2) of the conscious monkey. *Brain Res.* 187: 516–520.

Jacklet JW, ed. 1989. *Neuronal and Cellular Oscillations.* New York: Dekker.

Jackson CA, JD Peduzzi, and TL Hickey. 1989. Visual cortex development in the ferret. I. Genesis and migration of visual cortical neurons. *J. Neurosci.* 9: 1242–1253.

Jacobsen S and JQ Trojanowski. 1977. Prefrontal granular cortex of the rhesus monkey. II. Interhemispheric cortical afferents. *Brain Res.* 132: 235–246.

Jagadeesh B, CM Gray, and D Ferster. 1992. Visually evoked oscillations of membrane potential in cells of cat visual cortex. *Science* 257: 552–554.

Jahn R and TC Sudhoff. 1994. Synaptic vesicles and exocytosis. *Annu. Rev. Neurosci.* 17: 2219–2246.

Jahnsen H and R Llinas. 1984a. Electrophysiological properties of guinea-pig thalamic neurones: An *in vitro* study. *J. Physiol. Lond.* 349: 205–226.

——— 1984b. Ionic basis for the electroresponsiveness and oscillatory properties of guinea-pig thalamic neurones *in vitro*. *J. Physiol. Lond.* 349: 227–247.

Jaslove SW. 1992. The integrative properties of spiny distal dendrites. *Neurosci.* 47: 495–519.

Jasper HH. 1981. Problems in relating cellular and modular specificity to cognitive function: Importance of state-dependent reactions. In *The Organization of the Cerebral Cortex,* ed. FO Schmitt, FG Worden, G Adelman, amd SG Dennis. Cambridge, MA: MIT Press.

Jasper HH, G Ricci, and B Doane. 1960. Microelectrode analysis of cortical cell discharge during avoidance conditioning in the monkey. *Int. J. Electroencephalogr. Clin. Neurophysiol.* Suppl. 131: 137–156.

Jeffreys JGR, RD Traub, and MA Whittington. 1996. Neuronal networks for induced "40 Hz" rhythms. *Trends Neurosci.* 19: 202–208.

Jerrison HJ. 1991. Brain size and the evolution of mind. *Am. Mus. Nat. Hist.* pp. 1–99.

Jessell TM and ER Kandel. 1993. Synaptic transmission: A bi-directional and self-modifiable form of cell-cell communication. *Cell* 72/*Neuron* 10 (Suppl.): 1–30.

Johanson D and L Johanson. 1994. *Ancestors: In Search of Human Origins.* New York: Villard Books, Random House.

Johanson DC and TD White. 1979. A systematic assessment of early African hominids. *Science* 203: 321–330.

Johnston J and D Van der Kooy. 1988. Protooncogene expression identifies a columnar organization of the ventricular zone. *Proc. Natl. Acad. Sci. USA* 86: 1066–1070.

Joliot M, U Ribary, and R Llinas. 1994. Human oscillatory brain activity near 40 Hz co-exists with cognitive temporal binding. *Proc. Natl. Acad. Sci. USA* 91: 11748–51.

Jones EG. 1975. Varieties and distributions of non-pyramidal cells in the somatic sensory cortex of the squirrel monkey. *J. Comp. Neurol.* 160: 205–268.

———— 1981. Anatomy of the cerebral cortex: Columnar input-output organization. In *The Organization of the Cerebral Cortex,* ed. FO Schmitt, FG Worden, G Adelman, and SG Dennis, pp. 199–236. Cambridge, MA: MIT Press.

———— 1983. The columnar basis of cortical circuitry. In *The Clinical Neurosciences,* vol. 5, pp. 257–383. London: Churchill-Livingstone.

———— 1984a. Neurogliaform or spiderweb cells. In *Cerebral Cortex, Vol. 1: Cellular Components of the Cerebral Cortex,* ed. A Peters and EG Jones, pp. 409–418. New York: Plenum.

———— 1984b. Laminar distribution of cortical efferent cells. *Cerebral Cortex, Vol. 1: Cellular Components of the Cerebral Cortex,* ed. A Peters and EG Jones, pp. 521–553. New York: Plenum.

———— 1985. *The Thalamus.* New York: Plenum.

———— 1990a. Modulatory events in the development and evolution of the primate neocortex. In *Cerebral Cortex, Vol. 8a: Comparative Structure and Evolution of Cerebral Cortex, Part I,* ed. EG Jones and A Peters, pp. 311–362. New York: Plenum.

———— 1990b. The role of afferent activity in the maintenance of primate neocortical function. *J. Exp. Biol.* 153: 155–176.

———— 1991. Cellular organization in the primate postcentral gyrus. In *Information Processing in the Somatosensory System,* ed. O Franzen and J Westman, pp. 95–107. New York: Macmillan.

———— 1993. GABAergic neurons and their role in cortical plasticity in primates. *Cerebral Cortex* 3: 361–372.

———— 1995. Extent of intracortical arborizations of thalamocortical axons as a determinant of representational plasticity in the monkey somatic sensory cortex. *J. Neurosci.* 15: 4270–4288.

Jones EG, H Burton, and R Porter. 1975. Commissural and cortico-cortical "columns" in the somatic sensory cortex of primates. *Science* 190: 572–574.

Jones EG, JD Coulter, and SP Wise. 1979. Commissural columns in the sensory-motor cortex of monkeys. *J. Comp. Neurol.* 188: 113–135.

Jones EG, J DeFelipe, SH Hendry, and JE Maggio. 1988. A study of tachykinin-immunoreactive neurons in monkey cerebral cortex. *J. Neurosci.* 8: 1206–1224.

Jones EG and IT Diamond, eds. 1995. *Cerebral Cortex, Vol. 11: The Barrel Cortex of Rodents.* New York: Plenum.

Jones EG and SHC Hendry. 1984. Basket cells. In *Cerebral Cortex, Vol. 1: Cellular Components of the Cerebral Cortex,* ed. A Peters and EG Jones, pp. 309–336. New York: Plenum.

———— 1986. Co-localization of GABA and neuropeptides in neocortical neurons. *Trends Neurosci.* 9: 71–76.

Jones EG, SHC Hendry, and J DeFelipe. 1987. GABA-peptide neurons of the primate cerebral cortex: A limited cell class. In *Cerebral Cortex, Vol. 6: Further Aspects of Cortical Function, Including Hippocampus,* ed. A Peters and EG Jones, pp. 237–256. New York: Plenum.

Jones EG, SHC Hendry, J DeFelipe, and DL Benson. 1994. GABA neurons and their role in activity dependent plasticity in adult primate visual cortex. In *Cerebral Cortex, Vol. 6: Further Aspects of Cortical Function, Including Hippocampus,* ed. A Peters and EG Jones, pp. 237–266. New York: Plenum.

Jones EG, GW Huntley, and DL Benson. 1993. Alpha calcium/calmodulin dependent protein kinase II selectively expressed in a subpopulation of excitatory neurons in monkey sensory motor cortex: Comparison with GAB-67 expression. *J. Neurosci.* 14: 611–629.

Jones EG and SP Wise. 1975. Size, laminar and columnar distribution of efferent cells in the sensory-motor cortex of monkeys. *J. Comp. Neurol.* 175: 391–437.

Jones HE and AM Sillito. 1994. Directional asymmetries in length-response profiles of cells in the feline dorsal lateral geniculate nucleus. *J. Physiol. Lond.* 479: 475–486.

Juliano SL, P Hand, and BL Whitsel. 1981. Patterns of increased metabolic activity in somatosensory cortex of monkeys (*Macaca fascicularis*) subjected to controlled cutaneous stimulation: A 2-deoxyglucose study. *J. Neurophysiol.* 46: 1260–1284.

Juliano SL and BL Whitsel. 1987. A combined 2-deoxyglucose and neurophysiological study of primate somatosensory cortex. *J. Comp. Neurol.* 263: 514–525.

Juliano SL, BL Whitsel, M Tommerdahl, and SS Cheema. 1989. Determinants of patchy metabolic labeling in the somatosensory cortex of cats: A possible role for intrinsic inhibitory circuitry. *J. Neurosci.* 9: 1–12.

Jung R. 1963. Hans Berger und die Entdeckung des EEG nach seineer Tagebuchern und Protokollen. In *Jenenser EEG-Symposium 30, Jahre Electroenzephalographie,* ed. R Werner. Berlin: Volk und Gesundheit.

———— 1965. Some European neuroscientists. A personal tribute. In *The*

Neurosciences: Paths of Discovery, ed. EG Worden, JP Swazey, and G Adelman. Cambridge, MA: MIT Press.

———— 1984. Sensory research in historical perspective; some philosophical foundations of perception. In *Handbook of Physiology, Section I: The Nervous System, Vol. III: Sensory Processes, Part I,* ed. I Darian-Smith, JM Brookhart, VB Mountcastle, and SR Geiger, pp. 1–74. Bethesda, MD: American Physiological Society.

Kaas JH. 1991. The parcellations of somatosensory cortex: Modules, columns, and somatotopic segregates. In *Information Processing in the Somatosensory Cortex,* ed. O Franzen and J Westman, pp. 211–218. London: Macmillan.

Kaas JH, RJ Nelson, M Sur, and MM Merzenich. 1981. Organization of somatosensory cortex of primates. In *Organization of the Cerebral Cortex in Primates,* ed. FO Schmitt, WG Worden, G Adelman, and SG Denis. Cambridge, MA: MIT Press.

Kaas JH and TP Pons. 1988. The somatosensory system in primates. In *Comparative Primate Biology, Vol. 4: The Neurosciences,* ed. JP Steklis, pp. 421–468. New York: Liss.

Kaczmarek LK and IB Levitan. 1987. *Neuromodulation: The Biochemical Control of Neuronal Excitability.* Oxford: Oxford U. Press.

Kalb RG. 1995. Current excitement about the glutamate receptor family. *Neuroscientist* 1: 60–63.

Kandel ER and WA Spencer. 1968. Cellular neurophysiological approaches in the study of learning. *Physiol. Rev.* 48: 665–134.

Kasai H and OH Peterson. 1994. Spatial dynamics of second messengers: IP$_3$ and cAMP long-range and associative messengers. *Trends Neurosci.* 17: 95–101.

Kasper E, AU Larkman, J Lubke, and C Blakemore. 1994. Pyramidal neurons in layer 5 of the rat visual cortex. I. Correlation between cell morphology, intrinsic electrophysiological properties and axon targets. *J. Comp. Neurol.* 339: 458–474.

Katz B. 1969. *The Release of Neural Transmitter Substances.* Springfield, IL: CC Thomas.

Katz B and R Miledi. 1965. The effect of calcium upon acetylcholine release from motor nerve terminals. *Proc. Roy. Soc. Lond.* B161: 496–503.

Katz LC and EM Calloway. 1992. Development of local circuits in the mammalian cortex. *Annu. Rev. Neurosci.* 15: 31–56.

Katz LC and MP Dalva. 1994. Scanning laser photostimulation: A new approach for analyzing brain circuits. *J. Neurosci. Methods* 54: 205–218.

Katz PS and RM Harris-Warwick. 1990. Actions of identified modulatory neurons in a simple motor system. *Trends Neurosci.* 13: 367–373.

Keller, A. 1993. Intrinsic synaptic organization of the motor cortex. *Cerebral Cortex* 3: 430–441.

Keller A, A Iriki, and H Asanuma. 1990. Identification of neurons producing long-term potentiation in the cat motor cortex: Intracellular recordings and labeling. *J. Comp. Neurol.* 300: 47–60.

Kelly RB. 1993. Storage and release of neurotransmitters. *Cell 72/Neuron* 10 (suppl.): 43–55.

Kennedy H and C DeHay. 1993a. Cortical specification of mice and men. *Cerebral Cortex* 3: 171–186.

——— 1993b. The importance of developmental timing in cortical specification. *Per. Dev. Neurobiol.* 1: 93–99.

——— 1997. The nature and nurture of cortical development. In *Normal and Abnormal Development of the Cortex,* ed. A Galaburda and Y Cristien. Berlin and New York: Springer-Verlag.

Kennedy H, C DeHay, M Berland, P Savatier, and V Cortay. 1995. In vitro proliferation of primate cortical precursors and specification of cortical areas. *Abstr. Soc. Neurosci.* 21: 593.1.

Kennedy, MB. 1992. Second messengers and neuronal function. In *An Introduction to Molecular Neurobiology,* ed. ZW Hall, pp. 207–246. Sunderland, MA: Sinauer Associates.

Kennedy MB and E Marder. 1992. Cellular and molecular mechanisms of neuronal plasticity. In *An Introduction to Molecular Neurobiology,* ed. ZW Hall, pp. 463–495. Sunderland, MA: Sinauer Associates.

Kerkut GA and HV Wheal, eds. 1981. *Electrophysiology of Isolated Mammalian CNS Preparations.* London: Academic Press.

Kertesz A, M Polk, SE Black, and J Howell. 1990. Sex, handedness and the morphometry of cerebral asymmmetries of magnetic resonance imaging. *Brain Res.* 15: 40–48.

Kim GJ, CJ Shatz, and SK McConnell. 1991. Morphology of pioneer and follower growth cones in the developing cerebral cortex. *J. Neurobiol.* 22: 629–642.

Kim HG and BW Connors. 1993. Apical dendrites of the neocortex: Correlation between sodium- and calcium-dependent spiking and pyramidal morphology. *J. Neurosci.* 13: 5301–5311.

Kimbel WH, DC Johanson, and Y Rak. 1994. The first skull and other discoveries of *Australopithecus afarensis* at Hadar, Ethiopia. *Nature* 368: 449–451.

Kimura D. 1992. Sexual differences in the brain. *Sci. Am.* 267: 118–125.

Kirkwood A, MF Lee, and MF Bear. 1995. Co-regulation of long-term potentiation and experience-dependent synaptic plasticity in visual cortex by age and experience. *Nature* 375: 328–331.

Kirkwood BL, J Price, and EA Grove. 1992. Technical comment. *Science* 258: 317–319.

Kisvarday ZF, A Cowey, DA Smith, and P Somogyi. 1989. Interlaminar and lateral excitatory aminoacid connections in the striate cortex of the monkey. *J. Neurosci.* 9: 667–682.

Kisvarday ZF, KAC Martin, TF Freund, ZS Maglocsky, D Whitteridge, and P

Somogyi. 1986. Synaptic targets of HRP-filled layer III pyramidal cells in the cat striate cortex. *Exp. Brain Res.* 64: 541–552.

Klein RG. 1988. The causes of "robust" Australopithecine extinction. In *Evolutionary History of the "Robust" Australopithecines,* ed. FE Grinik, pp. 490–505. New York: Gruter.

Koch C and F Crick. 1994. Some further ideas regarding the neuronal basis of awareness. In *Large-Scale Neuronal Theories of the Brain,* ed. C Koch and JL Davis, pp. 93–109. Cambridge, MA: MIT Press.

Koch C and A Zador. 1993. The function of dendritic spines: Devices subserving biochemical rather than electrical compartmentalization. *J. Neurosci.* 13: 413–422.

Koester SE and DD O'Leary. 1993. Connectional distinction between callosal and subcortically projecting neurons is determined prior to axon extension. *Dev. Biol.* 160: 1–14.

Koffka K. 1935. *Principles of Gestalt Psychology.* New York: Harcourt.

Kolodkin AL. 1996. Growth cones and the cues that repel them. *Trends Neurosci.* 19: 507–513.

Konig P, AK Engel, S Lowel, and W Singer. 1993. Squint affects synchronization of oscillatory responses in cat visual cortex. *Eur. J. Neurosci.* 5: 501–508.

Konig P, AK Engel, and W Singer. 1995. Relation between oscillatory activity and long-range synchronization in cat visual cortex. *Proc. Natl. Acad. Sci. USA* 92: 290–294.

Konig P and TB Schillen. 1991. Stimulus-dependent assembly formation of oscillatory responses: I. Synchronization. *Neural Comp.* 3: 155–166.

Kornack DR and P Rakic. 1995. Radial and horizontal deployment of clonally related cells in primate neocortex: Relationship to distinct mitotic lineages. *Neuron* 15: 311–321.

Kornorski J. 1948. *Conditioned Reflexes and Neuron Organization.* Cambridge: Cambridge U. Press.

Korsching S. 1993. The neurotropic factor concept: A reexamination. *J. Neurosci.* 13: 2739–2748.

Kossut M, PJ Hand, J Greenberg, and CL Hand. 1988. Single vibrissal cortical column in SAI cortex of rat and its alterations in neonatal and adult vibrissa-deafferented animals: A quantitative 2DG study. *J. Neurophysiol.* 60: 829–852.

Kostovic I, M Judas, L Kostovic Knezevic, G Simic, I Delalle, D Chudy, B Sajin, and Z Petanjek. 1991. Zagreb collection of human brains for developmental neurobiologists and clinical neuroscientists. *Int. J. Dev. Biol.* 35: 215–230.

Kostovic I, N Lukinovic, M Judas, N Bogdanovic, L Mrzljak, N Zecevic, and M Kubat. 1989. Structural basis of the developmental plasticity in the human cerebral cortex: The role of the transient subplate zone. *Metab. Brain Dis.* 4: 17–23.

Kostovic I and ME Molliver. 1974. A new interpretation of the laminar development of cerebral cortex: Synaptogenesis in different layers of neopallium in the human fetus. *Anat. Red.* 178: 395.

Kostovic I and P Rakic. 1980. Cytology and time of origin of interstitial neurons in the white matter in infant and adult human and monkey telencephalon. *J. Neurocytol.* 9: 219–242.

———— 1990. Developmental history of the transient subplate zone in the visual and somatosensory cortex of the macaque monkey and human brain. *J. Comp. Neurol.* 297: 441–470.

Kreiter AK and W Singer. 1992. Oscillatory neuronal responses in the visual cortex of the awake macaque monkey. *Eur. J. Neurosci.* 4: 369–375.

———— 1996. Stimulus-dependent synchronization of neuronal responses in the visual cortex of the awake macaque monkey. *J. Neurosci.* 16: 2381–2396.

Kretschmann H-J, A Schleicher, F Wingert, K Zilles, and H-J Loblich. 1979. Human brain growth in the 19th and 20th century. *J. Neurol. Sci.* 40: 169–188.

Kritzer MF and P Goldman-Rakic. 1995. Intrinsic circuit organization of the major layers and sublayers of the dorsolateral prefrontal cortex in the macaque monkey. *J. Comp. Neurol.* 359: 131–143.

Krmpoti'c-Nemani'c J, I Kostovi'c, and D Nemani'c. 1984. Prenatal and perinatal development of radial cell columns in the human auditory cortex. *Acta Otolaryngol. Stockh.* 97: 4898–4950.

Krnjevic K and JW Phillis. 1963. Iontophoretic studies of neurones in the mammalian cerebral cortex. *J. Physiol. Lond.* 165: 274–304.

Krueger LE. 1989. Reconciling Fechner and Stevens: Toward a unified psychophysical law. *Behav. Brain Sci.* 12: 251–320.

Kruse W and R Eckhorn. 1996. Inhibition of sustained gamma oscillations (35–80 Hz) by fast transient responses in cat visual cortex. *Proc. Natl. Acad. Sci. USA* 93: 6112–6117.

Kuhnt U and LL Vorinin. 1994. Interaction between paired-pulse facilitation and long-term potentiation in area CA1 of guinea-pig hippocampal slices: Application of quantal analysis. *Neurosci.* 62: 391–397.

Kuljis RO and P Rakic. 1989. Multiple types of neuropeptide Y-containing neurons in the primate neocortex. *J. Comp. Neurol.* 280: 393–409.

Kullmann DM, DJ Perkel, T Manabe, and RA Nicoll. 1992. Ca^{2+} entry via postsynaptic voltage-sensitive CA^{2+} channels can transiently potentiate excitatory synaptic transmission in the hippocampus. *Neuron* 9: 1175–1183.

Kullmann DM and SA Siegelbaum. 1995. The site of expression of NMDA receptor-dependent LTP: New fuel for an old flame. *Neuron* 15: 997–1002.

Kunzle H. 1976. Alternating afferent zones of high and low axon terminal density within the macaque motor cortex. *Brain Res.* 106: 365–370.

———— 1978. An autoradiographic analysis of the efferent connections from premotor and adjacent prefrontal regions (areas 6 and 9) in *Macaca fascicularis. Brain Behav. Evol.* 15: 185–234.

Lamport L. 1978. Time, clocks, and the ordering of events in a distributed system. *Communications of ACM* 21: 558–565.

Larkman AU and JJB Jack. 1995. Synaptic plasticity: Hippocampal LTP. *Current Opinion Neurobiol.* 5: 324–334.

Larkman A and A Mason. 1990. Correlations between morphology and electrophysiology of pyramidal neurons in slices of rat visual cortex. *J. Neurosci.* 10: 1407–1414.

Larrabee MG and DW Bronk. 1947. Prolonged facilitation of synaptic excitation in sympathetic ganglia. *J. Neurophysiol.* 10: 139–154.

Lashley KS and G Clark. 1946. The cytoarchitecture of the cerebral cortex of *Ateles.* A critical examination of architectonic studies. *J. Comp. Neurol.* 85: 223–305.

Law SK, PL Nunez, and RS Wijesinghe. 1993. High-resolution EEG using spline generated surface Laplacians on spherical and ellipsoidal surfaces. *IEEE Trans. Biomed. Eng.* 40: 145–153.

Le J, V Menon, and A Gevins. 1994. Local estimate of surface Laplacian derivation on a realistically shaped scalp surface and its performance on noisy data. *Electroencephalogr. Clin. Neurophysiol.* 92: 433–441.

Leakey MG. 1981. Tracks and tools. *Phil. Trans. Roy. Soc. Lond.* B292: 95–102.

Leakey MG, CS Feibel, I McDougall, and A Walker. 1995. New four-million-year-old hominid species from Kanapoi and Allia Bay, Kenya. *Nature* 376: 565–571.

Leakey MG and RL Hay. 1979. Pliocene footprints in the Laetoli beds in Laetoli, northern Tanzania. *Nature* 278: 317–323.

Lemmon V and AL Pearlman. 1981. Does laminar position determine the receptive field properties of cortical neurons? A study of corticotectal cells in area 17 of the normal mouse and reeler mutant. *J. Neurosci.* 1: 83–93.

LeVay S and SB Nelson. 1991. Columnar organization of the visual cortex. In *Vision and Visual Dysfunction, Vol. 4: The Neural Basis of Visual Function,* ed. JP Cronley-Dillon, pp. 266–315. London: Macmillan.

LeVay S and H Sherk. 1981. The visual claustrum of the cat. II. The visual field map. *J. Neurosci.* 1: 981–992.

Levick WR and LN Thibos. 1982. Analysis of orientation bias in cat retina. *J. Physiol. Lond.* 329: 243–261.

Levi-Montalcini R. 1987. The nerve growth factor: Thirty-five years later. *EMBO* 6: 1145–1154.

Levitt P. 1984. A monoclonal antibody to limbic system neurons. *Science* 233: 299–401.

Levitt P, MF Barbe, and KL Eagleson. 1997. Patterning and specification of the cerebral cortex. *Annu. Rev. Neurosci.* 20: 1–24.

Levitt P, ML Cooper, and P Rakic. 1983. Early divergence and changing proportions of neuronal and glial precursor cells in the primate cerebral ventricular zone. *Dev. Biol.* 96: 472–484.

Lewis DA, MJ Campbell, SL Foote, M Goldstein, and JH Morrison. 1987. The distribution of tyrosine hydroxylase-immunoreactive fibers in primate neocortex is widespread but regionally specific. *J. Neurosci.* 7: 279–290.

Lewis DA, MJ Campbell, SL Foote, and JH Morrison. 1986. The monoaminergic innervation of primate neocortex. *Hum. Neurobiol.* 5: 181–188.

Li CH and H McIlwain. 1957. Maintenance of resting membrane potentials in slices of mammalian cerebral cortex and other tissues. *J. Physiol. Lond.* 139: 178–190.

Liao D, NA Hessler, and R Malinow. 1995. Activation of postsynaptically silent synapses during pairing-induced LTP in CA1 region of hippocampal slice. *Nature* 375: 400–405.

Lichtman JW and RJ Balice-Gordon. 1990. Understanding synaptic competition in theory and in practice. *J. Neurobiol.* 21: 99–106.

Liese M. 1990. Modular construction of nervous systems: A basic principle of design for invertebrates and vertebrates. *Brain Res. Rev.* 15: 1–23.

Liesi P. 1990. Extracellular matrix and neuronal movement. *Experientia* 46: 907–916.

Linden DJ. 1994. Long-term synaptic depression in the mammalian brain. *Neuron* 12: 457–472.

Linden DJ and JA Connor. 1995. Long term synaptic depression. *Annu. Rev. Neurosci.* 18: 319–357.

Linden R. 1994. The survival of developing neurons: A review of afferent control. *Neurosci.* 58: 671–682.

Lisman JE and KM Harris. 1993. Quantal analysis and synaptic anatomy—integrating two views of hippocampal plasticity. *Trends Neurosci.* 16: 142–147.

Livingstone MS and DH Hubel. 1983. Specificity of cortico-cortical connections in monkey visual system. *Nature* 304: 531–534.

——— 1984. Specificity of intrinsic connections in primate visual cortex. *J. Neurosci.* 4: 2830–2835.

Lledo P-M, GO Hejelmstad, S Mukeriji, TR Soderling, RD Malenka, and RA Nicoll. 1995. Calcium/calmodulin-dependent kinase II and long-term potentiation enhance synaptic transmission by the same mechanism. *Proc. Natl. Acad. Sci. USA* 92: 11175–11179.

Llinas RR. 1990. Intrinsic electrical properties of mammalian neurons and CNS function. In *Fidia Research Foundation Prize Lectures*, pp. 175–194. New York: Raven Press.

Llinas R and H Jahnsen. 1982. Electrophysiology of mammalian thalamic neurones *in vitro*. *Nature* 297: 406–408.

Llinas R and D Pare. 1996. The brain as a closed system modulated by the senses. In *The Mind-Brain Continuum,* ed. R Llinas and PS Churchland, pp. 1–18. Cambridge, MA: MIT Press.

Llinas R and U Ribary. 1993. Coherent 40-Hz oscillation characterizes dream state in man. *Proc. Natl. Acad. Sci. USA* 90: 2078–2081.

———— 1994. Perception as an oneiric-like state modulated by the senses. In *Large-scale Neuronal Theories of the Brain,* ed. C Koch and JL Davis, pp. 111–124. Cambridge, MA: MIT Press.

Llinas R, U Ribary, M Joliot, and X-J Wang. 1994. Content and context in temporal thalamocortical binding. In *Temporal Coding in the Brain,* ed. G Busaki, R Llinas, W Singer, A Berthoz, and Y Cristien, pp. 251–272. Berlin and New York: Springer-Verlag.

Lloyd DPC. 1949. Post-tetanic potentiation of response in monosynaptic pathways of the spinal cord. *J. Gen. Physiol.* 33: 147–170.

Locke J. 1690. *An Essay Concerning Human Understanding.* London: George Rutledge and Sons. Also, an unabridged edition collated and annotated by AC Fraser, New York, Dover, 1959.

Lois C, J-M Garcia-Verdugo, and A Alvarez-Buylla. 1996. Chain migration of neuronal precursors. *Science* 271: 978–981.

Lomo T. 1966. Frequency potentiation of excitatory synaptic activity in the dentate area of the hippocampal formation. *Acta Physiol. Scand.* 68 (suppl. 277): 128.

Lorento de No R. 1922. La corteza cerebral del ratón. *Trab. Lab. Invest. Biol. Univ. Madrid* 20: 1–38.

———— 1938. Cerebral cortex: Architecture, intracortical connections, motor projections. In *Physiology of the Nervous System,* ed. JF Fulton. Oxford: Oxford U. Press.

Lotto RB and DJ Price. 1995. The stimulation of thalamic neurite outgrowth by cortex-derived growth factors in vitro: The influence of cortical age and activity. *Eur. J. Neurosci.* 7: 318–328.

Lo-Turco JJ and AR Kriegstein. 1991. Clusters of coupled neuroblasts in embryonic neocortex. *Science* 252: 563–566.

Loughlin SE and JH Fallon, eds. 1993. *Neurotrophic Factors.* New York: Academic Press.

Lund JS, RG Booth, and RD Lund. 1977. Development of neurons in the visual cortex of the monkey *(Macaca nemestrima):* A Golgi study from fetal day 127 to postnatal maturity. *J. Comp. Neurol.* 176: 149–188.

Lund JS, RD Lund, AE Hendrickson, AH Bunt, and AF Fuchs. 1975. The origin of efferent pathways from the primary visual cortex, area 17, of the macaque monkey as shown by retrograde transport of horseradish peroxidase. *J. Comp. Neurol.* 163: 287–304.

Lund JS and T Yoshioka. 1991. Local circuit neurons of macaque monkey striate cortex: III. Neurons of laminae 4B, 4A and 3B. *J. Comp. Neurol.* 311: 234–258.

Lund JS, T Yoshioka, and JB Levitt. 1993. Comparison of intrinsic connectivity in different areas of monkey cerebral cortex. *Cerebral Cortex* 3: 148–162.

——— 1994. Substrates for interlaminar connections in area V1 of macaque monkey cerebral cortex. In *Cerebral Cortex, Vol. 10: Primary Visual Cortex in Primates,* ed. A Peters and KS Rockland, pp. 37–60. New York: Plenum.

Luskin MB. 1993. Restricted proliferation and migration of postnatally generated neuron derived from the forebrain subventricular zone. *Neuron* 11: 173–189.

——— 1996. Neural cell lineage in the vertebrate central nervous system. *FASEB Journal* 8: 722–730.

Luskin MB, JG Parnavelas, and JA Barfield. 1993. Neurons, astrocytes and oligodendrocytes of the rat cerebral cortex originate from separate progenitor cells: An ultrastructural analysis. *J. Neurosci.* 13: 1730–1750.

Luskin MB and CJ Shatz. 1985. Studies of the earliest generated cells of the cat's visual cortex: Cogeneration of subplate and marginal zones. *J. Neurosci.* 5: 1062–1075.

Luskin MB, T Zigova, R Betarbet, and BJ Soteres. 1997. Characterization of neuronal progenitor cells of the neonatal forebrain. In *Isolation, Characterization and Utilization of CNS Stem Cells,* ed. FH Gage and Y Cristien, pp. 67–86. Berlin: Springer-Verlag.

Macchi G. 1993. The intralaminar system revisited. In *Thalamic Relay and Modulation,* ed. D Minciacchi, M Molinarr, G Maachi, and EG Jones. London: Pergamon.

Macchi G and M Bentivoglio. 1988. The intralaminar nuclei and the cerebral cortex. In *Cerebral Cortex, Vol. 5: Sensory-Motor Areas and Aspects of Cortical Connectivity,* ed. EG Jones and A Peters. New York: Plenum.

Mackay DM. 1970. Perception and brain function. In *The Neurosciences. Second Study Program,* ed. FO Schmitt, pp. 30303–316. New York: Rockefeller U. Press.

——— 1984. Source density mapping of human visual receptive fields using scalp electrodes. *Exp. Brain Res.* 54: 579–581.

MacPhail EM. 1982. *Brain and Intelligence in Vertebrates.* Oxford: Clarendon.

Mainen ZF, JR Joerges, JR Huguenard, and TJ Sejnowsky. 1995. A model of spike initiation by neocortical pyramidal neurons. *Neuron* 15: 1427–1439.

Malenka RC. 1991. Postsynaptic factors control the duration of synaptic enhancement in area CA1 of the hippocampus. *Neuron* 6: 53–60.

——— 1995. LTP and LTD: Dynamic and interactive processes of synaptic plasticity. *Neuroscientist* 1: 35–42.

Malenka RC and RA Nicoll. 1993. NMDA-receptor-dependent synaptic plasticity: Multiple forms and mechanisms. *Trends Neurosci.* 16: 521–527.

Malgaroli A, AE Ting, B Wentland, A Bergamanischi, A Villa, RQ Tsien, and

RH Scheller. 1995. Presynaptic component of long-term potentiation visualized at individual hippocampal synapses. *Science* 268: 1624–1628.

Manabe T and RA Nicoll. 1994. Long-term potentiation: Evidence against an increase in transmitter release probability in the CA1 region of the hippocampus. *Science* 265: 1888–1892.

Marder E. 1994. Invertebrate neurobiology. Polymorphic neural networks. *Current Biol.* 4: 752–754.

Maren S and M Baudry. 1995. Properties and mechanisms of long-term synaptic plasticity in the mammalian brain: Relationships to learning and memory. *Neurobiol. Learn. Mem.* 63: 1–18.

Marin-Padilla M. 1974. Three-dimensional reconstruction of the pericellular nests (baskets) of the motor area (area 4) and visual (area 17) areas of the human cerebral cortex: A Golgi study. *Z. Anat. Entwicklungsgesch.* 144: 123–135.

——— 1978. Dual origin of the mammalian neocortex and evolution of the cortical plate. *Anat. Embryol.* 152: 109–126.

——— 1984. Neurons of layer I. A developmental analsysis. In *Cerebral Cortex, Vol. 1: Cellular Components of the Cerebral Cortex,* ed. A Peters and EG Jones, pp. 447–478. New York: Plenum.

——— 1987. The chandelier cell of the human visual cortex: A Golgi study. *J. Comp. Neurol.* 256: 61–70.

Marin-Padilla M and MT Marin-Padilla. 1982. Origin, prenatal development and structural organization of layer 1 of the human cerebral (motor) cortex: A Golgi study. *Anat. Embryol.* 164: 161–206.

Marshack A. 1985. Hierarchical evolution of the human capacity: The paleolithic evidence. *54th James Arthur Lecture on the Evolution of the Human Brain.* New York: American Museum of Natural History.

Martin KAC. 1988. From single cells to simple circuits in the cerebral cortex. *Quart. J. Exp. Physiol.* 73: 637–702.

——— 1994. A brief history of the "feature detector." *Cerebral Cortex* 4: 1–7.

Martin KAC and D Whitteridge. 1984. Form, function and intracortical projections of spiny neurons in the striate visual cortex of the cat. *J. Physiol. Lond.* 353: 463–504.

Martin RD. 1982. Allometric approaches to the evolution of the primate nervous system. In *Primate Brain Evolution: Methods and Concepts,* ed. E Armstrong and D Falk, pp. 36–56. New York: Plenum.

——— 1990. *Primate Origin and Evolution. A Phylogenetic Reconstruction.* Princeton, NJ: Princeton U. Press.

Martin RD and PH Harvey. 1985. Brain size allometry: Ontogeny and phylogeny. In *Size and Scaling in Primate Biology,* ed. EL Jungens, pp. 147–173. New York: Plenum.

Martinez JL and BE Derrick. 1966. Long-term potentiation and learning. *Annu. Rev. Psychol.* 47: 173–203.

Mason A and A Larkman. 1990. Correlations between morphology and electrophysiology of pyramidal neurons in slices of rat visual cortex. II. Electrophysiology. *J. Neurosci.* 10: 1415–1428.

Mason A, A Nicoll, and K Stratford. 1991. Synaptic transmission between individual pyramidal neurons of the rat visual cortex in vitro. *J. Neurosci.* 11: 72–84.

Mason CA, JC Edmondson, and ME Hatten. 1988. The extending astroglial process: Development of glial cell shape, the growing tip, and interactions with neurons. *J. Neurosci.* 8: 3124–3134.

Matthews G. 1996. Neurotransmitter release. *Annu. Rev. Neurosci.* 19: 219–233.

Maunsell JHR and DC Van Essen. 1983. The connections of the middle temporal visual area (MT) and their relationship to a cortical hierarchy in the macaque monkey. *J. Neurosci.* 3: 2563–2586.

Maycox PR, JW Hell, and R Jahn. 1990. Amino acid neurotransmission: Spotlight on synaptic vesicles. *Trends Neurosci.* 13: 83–87.

Mayford M, T Abel, and ER Kandel. 1995a. Transgenic approaches to cognition. *Current Opinion in Neurobiology* 5: 141–148.

Mayford M, J Wang, ER Kandel, and T O'Dell. 1995b. CaMKII regulates the frequency-response function of hippocampal synapses for the production of both LTD and LTP. *Cell* 81: 891–904.

McAllister AK, DC Lo, and LC Katz. 1995. Neurotrophins regulate dendritic growth in developing visual cortex. *Neuron* 15: 791–803.

McCasland JS and TA Woolsey. 1988. High-resolution 2-deoxyglucose mapping of functional cortical columns in mouse barrel cortex. *J. Comp. Neurol.* 278: 555–569.

McConnell SK. 1988. Fates of visual cortical neurons in the ferret after isochronic and heterochronic transplantation. *J. Neurosci.* 8: 945–974.

——— 1990. The specification of neuronal identity in the mammalian cerebral cortex. *Experientia* 46: 922–929.

——— 1991. The generation of neuronal diversity in the central nervous system. *Annu. Rev. Neurosci.* 14: 922–929.

McConnell SK, A Ghosh, and CJ Shatz. 1989. Subplate neurons pioneer the first axon pathway from the cerebral cortex. *Science* 245: 978–982.

McConnell SK and CE Kaznowski. 1991. Cell cycle dependence of laminar determination in developing neocortex. *Science* 254: 282–285.

McCormick DA. 1989. GABA as an inhibitory neurotransmitter in human cerebral cortex. *J. Neurophysiol.* 62: 1018–1027.

——— 1992. Neurotransmitter actions in the thalamus and cerebral cortex. *J. Clin. Neurophysiol.* 9: 212–223.

McCormick DA, BW Connors, JW Lighthall, and DA Prince. 1985. Comparative electrophysiology of pyramidal and sparsely spiny stellate neurons of the neocortex. *J. Neurophysiol.* 54: 782–806.

McCormick DA, Z Wang, and J Huguenard. 1993. Neurotransmitter control of neocortical neuronal activity and excitability. *Cerebral Cortex* 3: 367–399.

McHenry HM. 1982. The pattern of human evolution: Studies on bipedalism, mastication and encephalization. *Annu. Rev. Anthrop.* 11: 151–173.

———— 1994. Tempo and mode in human evolution. *Proc. Natl. Acad. Sci. USA* 91: 6780–6787.

McHugh TJ, KL Blum, JZ Tsien, S Tonegawa, and MA Wilson. 1996. Impaired hippocampal representation of space in CA1-specific knockout mice. *Cell* 87: 1339–1349.

McIlwain H. 1984. Cerebral subsystems and isolated tissues. In *Handbook of Neurochemistry,* ed. A Lajtha, pp. 315–341. New York: Plenum.

McKay RDG and S Hockfield. 1982. Monoclonal antibodies distinguish antigenetically discrete neuronal types in the vertebrate central nervous system. *Proc. Natl. Acad. Sci. USA* 79: 6747–6750.

McKenna TM, BL Whitsel, DA Dryer, and CB Metz. 1981. Organization of cat anterior parietal cortex: Relations among cytoarchitecture, single neuron functional properties, and interhemispheric connectivity. *J. Neurophysiol.* 45: 667–697.

McKernan RM and PJ Whiting. 1996. Which GABA$_A$ receptor subtypes really occur in the brain? *Trends Neurosci.* 19: 139–143.

McMahon J. 1990. The agrin hypothesis. *Cold Spring Harbor Symp. Quant. Biol.* 55: 407–418.

McMahon HT and DG Nicholls. 1991. The bio-energetics of neurotransmitter release. *Biochemica et Biophysica Acta* 1059: 243–264.

Meffert MK, NC Calakos, RH Scheller, and H Schulman. 1996. Nitric oxide modulates synaptic vesicle docking/fusion reactions. *Neuron* 16: 1229–1236.

Meller K and W Tetzlaff. 1975. Neuronal migration during early development of the cerebral cortex: A scaning electron microscopic study. *Cell Tissue Res.* 163: 313–325.

Mellers P and C Stringer, eds. 1989. *The Human Revolution: Behavioral and Biological Perspectives on the Origin of Modern Humans.* Princeton, NJ: Princeton U. Press.

Mendelson JR and KL Grasse. 1992. A comparison of monaural and binaural responses to frequency modulated (FM) sweeps in cat primary auditory cortex. *Exp. Brain Res.* 91: 435–454.

Mendelson JR, CE Schreiner, ML Sutter, and KL Grasse. 1993. Functional topography of cat primary auditory cortex: Responses to frequency-modulated sweeps. *Exp. Brain Res.* 94: 65–87.

Menon V, WJ Freeman, BA Cutillo, JE Desmond, MF Ward, SL Bressler, KD Laxer, N Barbaro, and AS Gevins. 1996. Spatio-temporal correlations in human gamma band electrocorticograms. *Electroencephalogr. Clin. Neurophysiol.* 98: 89–102.

Merzenich MM and JF Brugge. 1973. Representation of the cochlear partition on the superior temporal plane of the macaque monkey. *Brain Res.* 50: 275–296.

Merzenich MM, SA Colwell, and RA Andersen. 1982. Thalamocortical and corticothalamic connections in the auditory system of cat. In *Cortical Sensory Organization, Vol. 3: Multiple Auditory Areas,* ed. CN Woolsey, pp. 43–57. Clifton, NJ: Humana Press.

Mesulam MM, AD Rosen, and EJ Mufson. 1984. Regional variations in cortical cholinergic innervation: Chemoarchitectonics of acetylcholinesterase-containing fibers in the macaque brain. *Brain Res.* 311: 245–258.

Meyer A. 1981. Paul Flechsig's system of myelogenetic cortical localization in the light of recent research in neuroanatomy and neurophysiology. Parts I and II. *Le Journal Canadien des Sciences Neurologique* 8: 1–6, 95–104.

Meyer G. 1987. Forms and spatial arrangement of neurons in the primary motor cortex of man. *J. Comp. Neurol.* 262: 402–428.

Meyer G and T Gonzalez-Hernandez. 1993. Developmental changes in layer I of the human neocortex during prenatal life: A DiI-tracing and AChE and NADPH-d histochemistry study. *J. Comp. Neurol.* 338: 317–336.

Meyer G, P Wahle, A Castaneyra-Perdomo, and R Ferres-Torres. 1992. Morphology of neurons in the white matter of the adult human neocortex. *Exp. Brain Res.* 88: 204–212.

Meyer RL and RW Sperry. 1973. Tests for neuroplasticity in the anuran retinotectal system. *Exp. Neurol.* 40: 525–539.

Michaelis EK. 1996. Glutamate neurotransmission: Characteristics of NMDA receptors in the mammalian brain. *Neural Notes* 2: 3–7.

Middlebrooks JC, RW Dykes, and MM Merzenich. 1980. Binaural response-specific bands in primary auditory cortex (A1) of the cat: Topographical organization orthogonal to isofrequency contours. *Brain Res.* 181: 31–48.

Middlebrooks JC and JD Pettigrew. 1981. Functional classes of neurons in primary auditory cortex of the cat distinguished by sensitivity to sound location. *J. Neurosci.* 1: 107–120.

Mikoshiba K, Y Nishimura, and Y Tsukada. 1983. Absence of bundle structure in the neocortex of the reeler mouse at the embryonic stage. Studies by scanning electron microscopic fractography. *Dev. Neurosci.* 6: 18–25.

Miller GA. 1956. The magical number seven plus or minus two: Some limits on our capacity for processing information. *Psychol. Rev.* 63: 81–97.

Milner B. 1966. Amnesia following operation on the temporal lobes. In *Amnesia,* ed. CWM Whitty and O Zangwill, pp. 109–133. London: Butterworth.

Milner P. 1974. A model for visual shape recognition. *Psychol. Rev.* 81: 521–535.

Mione, MC, D Danevic, P Boardman, H Harris, and PG Parnavelas. 1994. Lineage analysis reveals neurotransmitter (GABA or glutamate) but not calcium-binding protein homogeneity in clonally related cortical neurons. *J. Neurosci.* 14: 107–123.

Misson JP, MA Edwards, M Yamamoto, and VS Caviness jr. 1988. Identification of radial glial cells within the developing murine central nervous system: Studies based upon a new immunohistochemical marker. *Brain Res. Dev.* 44: 95–108.

Misson JP, T Takahashi, and VS Caviness jr. 1991. Ontogeny of radial and other astroglial cells in murine cerebral cortex. *Glia* 4: 138–148.

Molliver ME. 1987. Serotonergic neuronal systems: What their anatomic organization tells us about function. *J. Clin. Psychopharm.* 7: 3S–23S.

Molnar Z and C Blakemore. 1991. Lack of regional specificity for connections formed between thalamus and cortex in coculture. *Nature* 351: 475–477.

Monaghan DT and CW Cotman. 1985. Distribution of *N*-Methyl-D-aspartate sensitive L-[^{2}H] glutamate-binding sites in rat brain. *J. Neurosci.* 5: 2909–2919.

Moore R and J Price. 1992. The distribution of cones of neurons in the rat somatosensory cortex. *J. Neurocytol.* 21: 737–743.

Morel A, PE Garraghty, and JH Kaas. 1993. Tonotopic organization, architectonic fields, and connections of auditory cortex in macaque monkeys. *J. Comp. Neurol.* 335: 437–459.

Morgan JI and T Curran. 1989. Stimulus-transcription coupling in neurons: Role of cellular immediate early genes. *Trends Neurosci.* 12: 459–462.

Morris RGM, E Anderson, GS Lynch, and M Baudry. 1986. Selective impairment of learning and blockade of long-term potentiation by an *N*-methyl-D-aspartate receptor antagonist. *Nature* 319: 774–776.

Morrison JH, SL Foote, ME Molliver, FE Bloom, and HG Lidov. 1982. Noradrenergic and serotonergic fibers innervate complementary layers in monkey primary visual cortex: An immunohistochemical study. *Proc. Natl. Acad. Sci. USA* 79: 2401–2405.

Morrison JH, SL Foote, D O'Connor, and FE Bloom. 1992. Laminar, tangential and regional organization of the noradrenergic innervation of monkey cortex: Dopamine-beta-hydroxylase immunohistochemistry. *Brain Res. Bull.* 9: 309–319.

Morrison JH and PR Hot. 1992. The organization of the cerebral cortex: From molecules to circuits. *Discussion Neurosci.* 9: 10–79.

Morrone MC, DC Burr, and L Maffei. 1991. Functional implications of cross-orientation inhibition of cortical visual cells. *Proc. Roy. Soc. Lond.* B216: 335–354.

Motter BC, MA Steinmetz, CJ Duffy, and VB Mountcastle. 1987. Functional properties of parietal visual neurons: Mechanisms of directionality along a single axis. *J. Neurosci.* 7: 154–176.

Mountcastle VB. 1957. Modality and topographic properties of single neurons of cat's somatic sensory cortex. *J. Neurophysiol.* 20: 408–434.

———— 1967. The problem of sensing and the neural coding of sensory events. In *The Neurosciences: A Study Program,* ed. GC Quarton, T Melnechuk, and FO Schmitt. New York: Rockefeller U. Press.

———— 1978. An organizing principle for cerebral function. In *The Mindful Brain,* ed. GM Edelman and VB Mountcastle. Cambridge, MA: MIT Press. Also printed in *The Neurosciences: A Fourth Study Program,* ed. FO Schmitt and FG Worden. Cambridge, MA: MIT Press.

———— 1984. Central nervous mechanisms in mechanoreceptive sensibility. In *Handbook of Physiology, Section I: The Nervous System, Vol. III: Sensory Processes, Part 2,* ed. JM Brookhart, VB Mountcastle, SR Geiger, and I Darian-Smith, pp. 789–878. Bethesda, MD: Am Physiol Soc.

———— 1995. The parietal system and some higher brain functions. *Cerebral Cortex* 5: 377–390.

Mountcastle VB, RA Andersen, and BC Motter. 1981. The influence of attentive fixation upon the excitability of the light sensitive neurons of the posterior parietal cortex. *J. Neurosci.* 1: 1218–1235.

Mountcastle VB, AL Berman, and PW Davies. 1955. Topographic organization and modality representation in first somatic area of cat's cerebral cortex by method of single unit analysis. *Am. J. Physiol.* 183: 646.

Mountcastle VB, JC Lynch, AP Georgopoulos, H Sakata, and C Acuna. 1975. The posterior parietal association cortex of the monkey: Command functions for operations in extrapersonal space. *J. Neurophysiol.* 38: 871–908.

Mountcastle VB and BC Motter. 1981. The functional properties of the light-sensitive neurons of the posterior parietal cortex studied in waking monkeys: Foveal sparing and opponent vector organization. *J. Neurosci.* 1: 3–26.

Mountcastle VB, BC Motter, MA Steinmetz, and CJ Duffy. 1984. Looking and seeing: The visual functions of the parietal lobe system. In *Dynamic Aspects of Neocortical Function,* ed. GM Edelman, WE Gall, and WM Cowan, pp. 159–193. New York: Wiley Interscience.

Mountcastle VB and TPS Powell. 1959a. Central nervous mechanisms subserving position sense and kinesthesis. *Bull. Johns Hopkins Hosp.* 105: 173–200.

———— 1959b. Neural mechanisms subserving cutaneous sensibility, with special reference to the role of afferent inhibition in sensory perception and discrimination. *Bull. Johns Hopkins Hosp.* 105: 201–232.

Mountcastle VB, HJ Reitboeck, GF Poggio, and MA Steinmetz. 1991. Adaptation of the Reitboeck method of multiple microelectrode recording to the neocortex of the waking monkey. *J. Neurosci. Methods* 36: 77–84.

Mountcastle VB, WH Talbot, H Sakata, and J Hyvarinen. 1969. Cortical neuronal mechanisms studied in unanesthetized monkeys. Neuronal periodicity and frequency discrimination. *J. Neurophysiol.* 32: 452–484.

Mulkey RN, CE Herron, and RC Malenka. 1993. An essential role for protein phosphatases in hippocampal long-term depression. *Science* 261: 1051–1058.

Mulkey RM and RC Malenka. 1992. Mechanisms underlying induction of homosynaptic long-term depression in area CA1 of the hippocampus. *Neuron* 9: 967–975.

Muller J. 1838. *Handbuch der Physiologie des Menschen für Volesungen,* 2d ed. Coblenz, Germany: Holscher.

Muller W and JA Connor. 1991. Dendritic spines as individual neuronal compartments for synaptic Ca^{2+} responses. *Nature* 354: 73–76.

Murphy TH, JM Baraban, GW Wier, and LA Blatter. 1994. Visualization of quantal synaptic transmission by dendritic calcium imaging. *Science* 263: 529–532.

Murthy VN, F Aoki, and EE Fetz. 1994. Synchronous oscillations in sensory motor cortex of awake monkeys and humans. In *Oscillatory Event-related Brain Dynamics,* ed. C Pantev, T Elbert, and B Lutenhoner. New York: Plenum.

Murthy VN and EE Fetz. 1992. Coherent 25–35 Hz oscillations in the sensorimotor cortex of awake behaving monkeys. *Proc. Natl. Acad. Sci. USA* 89: 5670–5674.

Nakamura K, A Mikani, and K Kubota. 1992. Oscillatory neuronal activity related to visual short-term memory in monkey temporal pole. *Neuroreport* 3: 117–120.

Nakanishi S. 1994. Metabotropic glutamate receptors: Synaptic transmission, modulation and plasticity. *Neuron* 13: 1031–1037.

Natkatsuki M, Y Kodokawa, and H Suemori. 1991. Radial columnar patches in the chimeric cerebral cortex visualized by use of mouse embryonic stem cells expressing β-galactooxidase. *Dev. Growth Differ.* 33: 571–578.

Nehrer E. 1992. Ion channels for communication between and within cells. *Neuron* 8: 605–612.

Nelson JI, PA Salin, MH Munk, M Arzi, and J Bullier. 1992. Spatial and temporal coherence in cortico-cortical connections: A cross-correlation study in areas 17 and 18 in the cat. *Vis. Neurosci.* 9: 21–27.

Nelson S, L Toth, B Sheth, and M Sur. 1994. Orientation selectivity of cortical neurons during intracellular blockade of inhibition. *Science* 265: 774–777.

Neuenschwander S and W Singer. 1996. Long range synchronization of oscillatory light responses in the cat retina and lateral geniculate nucleus. *Nature* 379: 728–733.

Nguyen PV, T Abel, and ER Kandel. 1994. Requirement of a critical period of transcription for induction of the late phase of LTP. *Science* 265: 1104–1107.

Nicoletis, MAL, RCS Lin, DJ Woodward, and JK Chapin. 1993. Dynamic and distributed properties of many-neuron ensembles in the ventral posterior medial thalamus in the awake rat. *Proc. Natl. Acad. Sci. USA* 90: 2212–2216.

Nicoll RA, JA Kauer, and RC Malenka. 1988. The current excitement about long-term potentiation. *Neuron* 1: 97–103.

Nicoll RA and RC Malenka. 1995. Contrasting properties of two forms of long-term potentiation in the hippocampus. *Nature* 377: 115–118.

Nicoll RA, RC Malenka, and JA Kauer. 1990. Functional comparison of neurotransmitter receptor subtypes in mammalian central nervous system. *Physiol. Rev.* 70: 513–565.

Noble A and I Davidson. 1991. The evolutionary emergence of modern human behavior; language and its archeology. *Man* 26: 223–254.

Northcutt RG and Kaas JH. 1995. The emergence and evolution of mammalian neocortex. *Trends Neurosci.* 18: 373–379.

Norwich KH. 1993. *Information, Sensation and Perception.* New York: Academic.

Novak N and J Bolz. 1993. Formation of specific efferent connections in organotypic slice cultures from rat visual cortex co-cultured with lateral geniculate nucleus and superior colliculus. *Eur. J. Neurosci.* 5: 15–24.

Nowak LG, MJH Munk, N Chounlamountri, and J Bullier. 1994. Temporal aspects of information processing in areas V1 and V2 of the macaque monkey. In *Oscillatory Event-Related Brain Dynamics,* ed. C Pantev, T Elbert, and B Lutkenhoner. New York: Plenum.

Nowak LG, MJH Munk, P Girard, and J Bullier. 1995a. Visual latencies in areas V1 and V2 of the macaque monkey. *Vis. Neurosci.* 12: 371–384.

Nowak LG, MJH Munk, JI Nelson, AC James, and J Bullier. 1995b. Structural basis of cortical synchronization. I. Three types of interhemispheric coupling. *J. Neurophysiol.* 74: 2379–2400.

Nunez PL. 1981. *Electrical Fields of the Brain: The Neurophysics of EEG.* Oxford: Oxford U. Press.

—— 1986. The brain's magnetic field: Some effects of multiple sources on localization methods. *Electroencephalogr. Clin. Neurophysiol.* 63: 75–82.

—— 1989. Estimation of large scale neocortical source activity with EEG surface Laplacians. *Brain Topography* 2: 141–154.

—— 1995. *Neocortical Dynamics and Human EEG Rhythms.* Oxford: Oxford U. Press.

Nunez PL and KL Pilgreen. 1991. The spline-Laplacian in clinical neurophysiology: A method to improve EEG spatial resolution. *J. Clin. Neurophysiol.* 8: 397–413.

Nunez PL, KL Pilgreen, AF Westdorp, SK Law, and AV Nelson. 1991. A visual study of surface potentials and Laplacians due to distributed neocortical sources: Computer simulations and evoked potential. *Brain Topography* 4: 151–168.

Nunez PL, RB Silberstein, PJ Cadusch, RS Wijesinghe, AF Westdorp, and R Srinivasan. 1994. A theoretical and experimental study of high resolution EEG based on surface Laplacians and cortical imaging. *Electroencephalogr. Clin. Neurophysiol.* 90: 40–57.

Obermayer K and GG Blasdel. 1993. Geometry of orientation and dominance columns in monkey striate cortex. *J. Neurosci.* 13: 4114–4129.

O'Connor JJ, MJ Rowan, and R Anwyl. 1994. Long-lasting enhancement of NMDA receptor-mediated synaptic transmission by metabotropic glutamate receptor activation. *Nature* 367: 557–559.

O'Dell TJ, PL Huang, TM Dawson, JL Dinerman, SH Snyder, ER Kandel, and MC Fishman. 1994. Endothelial NOS and the blockade of LTP by NOS inhibitors in mice lacking neuronal NOS. *Science* 265: 542–546.

Ogawa M, T Miyata, K Nakajima, Y Yagyu, M Seike, K Ikenaka, H Yamato, and K Mikoshiba. 1995. The *reeler* gene-associated antigen on Cajal-Retzius neurons is a crucial molecule for laminar organization of cortical neurons. *Neuron* 14: 899–912.

Ojima H, CH Honda, and EG Jones. 1991. Patterns of axon collateralization of identified supragranular pyramidal neurons in the cat auditory cortex. *Cerebral Cortex* 1: 80–94.

―――― 1992. Characteristics of intracellularly injected infragranular pyramidal neurons in cat primary auditory cortex. *Cerebral Cortex* 2: 197–216.

O'Kusky J and M Colonnier. 1982. A laminar analysis of the number of neurons, glia and synapses in the visual cortex (area 17) of adult macaque monkeys. *J. Comp. Neurol.* 210: 278–290.

O'Leary DDM. 1989. Do cortical areas emerge from a protocortex? *Trends Neurosci.* 12: 400–406.

O'Leary DDM, AR Bicknese, JA De Carlos, CD Hefner, SE Koestere, LJ Kutka, and T Terashima. 1990. Target selection by cortical axons: Alternative mechanisms to establish axonal connections in the developing brain. *Cold Spring Harbor Symp. Quant. Biol.* 50: 453–468.

O'Leary DDM and SE Koester. 1993. Development of projection neuron types, axon pathways and patterned connections in the mammalian cortex. *Neuron* 10: 991–1006.

O'Leary DDM, NL Ruff, and RH Dyck. 1994. Development, critical period, plasticity, and adult reorganization of mammalian somatosensory systems. *Current Opinion in Neurobiol.* 4: 535–544.

O'Leary DDM, BL Schlaggar, and BB Stanfield. 1992. The specification of sensory cortex: Lesions from cortical transplantation. *Exp. Neurol.* 115: 121–126.

O'Leary DDM, BL Schlagger, and R Tuttle. 1994. Specification of neocortical areas and thalamocortical connections. *Annu. Rev. Neurosci.* 17: 419–439.

Oliver MW, J Larson, and G Lynch. 1990. Activation of the glycine site associated with the NMDA receptor is required for induction of LTP in neonatal hippocampus. *Int. J. Dev. Neurosci.* 8: 417–424.

Olsen CR and AM Graybiel. 1980. Sensory maps in the claustrum of the cat. *Nature* 288: 479–481.

Oppenheim OW. 1991. Cell death during development of the nervous system. *Annu. Rev. Neurosci.* 14: 453–501.

Oram MW and DI Perritt. 1996. Integration of form and motion in the anterior superior polysensory area (STPa) of the macaque monkey. *J. Neurophysiol.* 76: 109–129.

O'Rourke NA, ME Dailey, SJ Smith, and SK McConnell. 1992. Diverse migratory pathways in developing cerebral cortex. *Science* 258: 299–302.

Palm G, AM Aertsen, and GL Gerstein. 1988. On the significance of correlations among neuronal spike trains. *Biol. Cybern.* 59: 1–11.

Pandya DN and B Seltzer. 1982. Intrinsic connections and architectonics of the posterior parietal cortex in the rhesus monkey. *J. Comp. Neurol.* 204: 196–210.

Pantev C, S Makieg, M Hoke, R Galambos, S Hampson, and C Gallen. 1991. Human auditory evoked gamma-band magnetic fields. *Proc. Natl. Acad. Sci. USA* 88: 8996–9000.

Parnavelas JG, JA Barfield, E Franke, and MB Luskin. 1991. Separate progenitor cells give rise to pyramidal and nonpyramidal neurons in the rat telencephalon. *Cerebral Cortex* 1: 463–468.

Parnavelas JG, GC Papadopoulos, and ME Cavanagh. 1988. Changes in neurotransmitters during development. In *Cerebral Cortex, Vol. 7: Development and Maturation of Cerebral Cortex,* ed. A Peters and EG Jones, pp. 177–209. New York: Plenum.

Pasinelli P, GM Ramakers, IJ Urban, JJ Hens, AB Oestreicher, PN deGraan, and WH Gispen. 1995. Long-term potentiation and synaptic protein phosphorylation. *Behav. Brain Res.* 66: 53–59.

Pedley TA and RD Traub. 1990. Physiological basis of the EEG. In *Current Practice of Clinical Electroencephalography,* ed. DD Daly and TA Pedley, pp. 107–137. New York: Raven.

Pei X, TR Vidyasagar, M Volgushev, and OD Creutzfeldt. 1994. Receptive field analysis and orientation selectivity of postsynaptic potentials of simple cells in cat visual cortex. *J. Neurosci.* 14: 2730–2740.

Peinado A, R Yuste, and LC Katz. 1993a. Gap junctional communication and the development of local circuits in neocortex. *Cerebral Cortex* 3: 488–498.

——— 1993b. Extensive dye coupling between rat neocortical neurons during the period of circuit formation. *Neuron* 10: 103–114.

Penfield W and H Jasper. 1954. *Epilepsy and the Functional Anatomy of the Brain*. Boston: Little Brown.

Perl ER and JU Casby. 1954. Localization of cerebral electrical activity in the acoustic cortex of the cat. *J. Neurophysiol.* 17: 429–454.

Perritt DI, JK Hietanen, MW Oran, and PJ Benson. 1992. Organization and function of cells responsive to faces in the temporal cortex. *Phil. Trans. Roy. Soc. Lond.* B335: 31–38.

Perritt DI, PAJ Smith, DD Potter, AJ Mistlin, AS Head, AD Milner, and MA Jeeves. 1985. Visual cells in the temporal cortex sensitive to face view and gaze direction. *Proc. Roy. Soc. Lond.* B223: 293–317.

Peters A. 1994. The organization of the primary visual cortex in the macaque. In *Cerebral Cortex, Vol. 10: Primary Visual Cortex in Primates,* ed. A Peters, EG Jones, and KS Rockland, pp. 1–36. New York: Plenum.

Peters A and EG Jones, eds. 1984–1994. *Cerebral Cortex, Vols. 1–10*. New York: Plenum.

Peters A and BR Payne. 1993. Numerical relationships between geniculocortical afferents and pyramidal cell modules in cat primary visual cortex. *Cerebral Cortex* 3: 69–78.

Peters A and KS Rockland, eds. 1994. *Cerebral Cortex, Vol 10: Primary Visual Cortex in Primates*. New York: Plenum.

Peters A and C Sethares. 1996. Myelinated axons and the pyramidal cell modules in monkey primary visual cortex. *J. Comp. Neurol.* 365: 232–255.

Peters A and TM Walsh. 1972. A study of the organization of apical dendrites in the somatic sensory cortex of the rat. *J. Comp. Neurol.* 144: 253–268.

Peters A and E Yilmaz. 1993. Neuronal organization in area 17 of cat visual cortex. *Cerebral Cortex* 3: 49–68.

Peters S, J Koh, and DW Choi. 1987. Zinc selectively blocks the action of N-methyl-D-aspartate on cortical neurons. *Science* 236: 589–593.

Petit DL, S Perlman, and R Malinow. 1994. Potentiated transmission and prevention of further LTP by increased CaMKII activity in postsynaptic hippocampal slice neurons. *Science* 266: 1881–1885.

Petsche H, H Pockberger, and P Rapplesberger. 1988. Cortical structure and electrogenesis. In *Dynamics of Sensory and Cognitive Processing in the Brain,* ed. E Basar, pp. 123–139. Berlin: Springer-Verlag.

Pfurtscheller G and C Neuper. 1992. Simultaneous EEG 10 Hz desynchronization and 40 Hz synchronization during finger movements. *NeuroReport* 3: 1057–1060.

Pinto-Lord MC, P Evrard, and VS Caviness jr. 1982. Obstructed neuronal migration along radial glial fibers to the neocortex of the reeler mouse: A Golgi-EM analysis. *Brain Res.* 256: 379–393.

Pirlot P. 1987. Contemporary brain morphology in ecological and ethological perspectives. *J. Hirnforsch.* 38: 145–211.

Placzek M, M Tessier-Lavigne, T Yamada, J Dodd, and TM Jessell. 1990. Guidance of developing axons by diffusible chemoattractants. *Cold Spring Harbor Symp. Quant. Biol.* 55: 279–289.

Plateau JAF. 1872. Sur le measure des sensations physiques, et sur la loi qui lie l'intensite de ces sensations to l'intensité de la cause excitant. *Bull de l'Academie Royal des Sciences des Lettres, et des Beaux-Arts de Belgique.* 33: 376–388.

Plutarch. 1937. *Life of Pericles.* From the translation called Dryden's, corrected and revised by AH Clough (1859). *Harvard Classics,* vol. 11. New York: Collier and Son.

Poggio GF and B Fisher. 1977. Binocular interaction and depth sensitivity of striate and prestriate cortical neurons of the behaving rhesus monkey. *J. Neurophysiol.* 40: 1392–1405.

Porter LL, Cedarbaum JM, DDM O'Leary, BB Stanfield, and H Asanuma. 1987. The physiological identification of pyramidal tract neurons within transplants in the rostral cortex taken from the occipital cortex during development. *Brain Res.* 436: 136–142.

Porter R and R Lemon. 1993. *Corticospinal Function and Voluntary Movement.* Oxford: Clarendon.

Povinelli DJ and TM Preuss. 1995. Theory of mind: Evolutionary history of a cognitive specialization. *Trends Neurosci.* 18: 418–424.

Powell TPS. 1981. Certain aspects of the intrinsic organization of the cerebral cortex. In *Brain Mechanisms and Perceptual Awareness,* ed. C Ajmone-Marsan, pp. 1–19. New York: Raven Press.

Powell TPS and AE Hendrikson. 1981. Similarity in number of neurons through the depth of the cortex in the binocular and monocular parts of area 17 of the monkey. *Brain Res.* 216: 409–413.

Powell TPS and VB Mountcastle. 1959. Some aspects of the functional organization of the cortex of the postcentral gyrus of the monkey: A correlation of findings obtained in a single unit analysis with cytoarchitecture. *Bull. Johns Hopkins Hosp.* 105: 133–162.

Preuss TM and PS Goldman-Rakic. 1991. Myelo- and cytoarchitecture of the granular frontal cortex and surrounding regions in the strepsirhine primate *Galago* and the anthropoid primate *Macaca. J. Comp. Neurol.* 310: 429–474.

Price J. 1993. Making sense of cell lineage. *Per. Dev. Neurobiol.* 1: 139–148.

Price J and L Thurlow. 1988. Cell lineage in the rat cerebral cortex. A study using retroviral-mediated gene transfer. *Development* 104: 473.

Price J, D Turner, and C Cepko. 1987. Lineage analysis in the vertebrate nervous system by retrovirus-mediated gene transfer. *Proc. Natl. Acad. Sci. USA* 84: 154.

Price J, B Williams, and E Grove. 1992. The generation of cellular diversity in the cerebral cortex. *Brain Pathology* 2: 23–29.

Price J, B Williams, A Moore, J Read, and E Grove. 1991. Analysis of cell lineage in the rat cerebral cortex. *Ann. NY Acad. Sci.* 633: 56–63.

Prothero JW and JW Sundsten. 1984. Folding of the cerebral cortex in mammals: A scaling model. *Brain Behav. Evol.* 24: 152–167.

Puelles L and JLR Rubenstein. 1993. Expression patterns of homeobox and other putatively regulatory genes in the embryonic mouse forebrain suggest a neuromeric organization. *Trends Neurosci.* 16: 472–479.

Purves D. 1988. *Body and Brain: A Trophic Theory of Neural Connections.* Cambridge, MA: Harvard U. Press.

Rademacher J, VS Caviness jr, H Steinmetz, and AM Galaburda. 1993. Topographical variation of the human primary cortices; implications for neuroimaging, brain mapping, and neurobiology. *Cerebral Cortex* 3: 313–329.

Radons G, JD Becker, B Dullfer, and J Kruger. 1994. Analysis, classification, and coding of multielectrode spike trains with hidden Markov models. *Biol. Cyber.* 71: 359–373.

Raigeul SE, L Lagae, B Gulyas, and GA Orban. 1989. Response latencies of visual cells in macaque areas V1, V2 and V5. *Brain Res.* 493: 155–159.

Rajkowska G and PS Goldman-Rakic. 1995a. Cytoarchitectonic definition of prefrontal areas in the normal human cortex: I. Remapping of areas 9 and 46 using quantitative criteria. *Cerebral Cortex* 5: 307–322.

——— 1995b. Cytoarchitectural definition of prefrontal areas in the normal human cortex: II. Variability in locations of area 9 and 46 and relationship to the Talairach coordinate system. *Cerebral Cortex* 5: 323–338.

Rakic P. 1971. Guidance of neurons migrating to the fetal monkey neocortex. *Brain Res.* 33: 471–476.

——— 1972. Mode of cell migration to the superficial layers of fetal monkey neocortex. *J. Comp. Neurol.* 145: 61–83.

——— 1974. Neurons in the monkey visual cortex: Systematic relation between time of origin and eventual disposition. *Science* 183: 425–427.

——— 1975. Role of cell interaction in development of dendritic patterns. *Adv. Neurol.* 12: 117–134.

——— 1977. Prenatal development of the visual system in rhesus monkey. *Phil. Trans. Roy. Soc. Lond.* B278: 245–260.

——— 1978. Neuronal migration and contact guidance in the primate telencephalon. *Postgrad. Med. J.* 54 Suppl. 1: 25–40.

——— 1982. Early developmental events: Cell lineages, acquisition of neuronal positions, and areal and laminar development. *Neurosci. Res. Prog. Bull.* 20: 439–451.

——— 1985. Contact regulation of neuronal migration. In *The Cell in Con-*

tact: Adhesions and Junctions as Morphological Determinants, ed. GM Edelman and J-P Thiery, pp. 67–41. New York: Wiley.

———— 1988a. Specification of cerebral cortical areas. *Science* 241: 170–176.

———— 1988b. Intrinsic and extrinsic determinants of neocortical parcelation: A radial unit model. In *Neurobiology of Neocortex,* ed. P Rakic and W Singer, pp. 5–28. New York: Wiley.

———— 1990a. Principles of neural cell migration. *Experientia* 46: 170–176.

———— 1990b. Radial unit hypothesis of cerebral cortical evolution. In *The Principles and Design and Operation of the Brain,* ed. JC Eccles and O Creutzfeldt, 78: 25–48. Vatican City: Pontificae Academiae Scripta Varia.

———— 1991. Experimental manipulation of cerebral cortical areas in primates. *Phil. Trans. Roy. Soc. Lond.* B331: 291–294.

———— 1995a. A small step for the cell—a giant leap for mankind: A hypothesis of neocortical expansion during evolution. *Trends Neurosci.* 18: 383–388.

———— 1995b. Radial versus tangential migration of neuronal clones in the developing cerebral cortex. *Proc. Natl. Acad. Sci. USA* 92: 11323–11327.

Rakic P, RS Cameron, and H Komura. 1994. Recognition, adhesion, transmembrane signalling and cell motility in guided neuronal migration. *Current Opinion in Neurobiol.* 4: 63–69.

Rakic P and VS Caviness jr. 1995. Cortical development; view from neurological mutants two decades later. *Neuron* 14: 1101–1104.

Rakic P, PS Goldman-Rakic, and D Galleger. 1988. Quantitative autoradiography of major neurotransmitter receptors in the monkey striate and extrastriate cortex. *J. Neurosci.* 8: 3670–3690.

Rakic P, I Suner, and RW Williams. 1991. A novel cytoarchitectonic area induced experimentally within the primate visual cortex. *Proc. Natl. Acad. Sci. USA* 88: 2083–2087.

Rall W, RE Burke, WR Holmes, JJB Jack, SJ Redman, and I Segev. 1992. Matching dendritic neuron models to experimental data. *Physiol. Rev.* 72: S159–S186.

Rall W, RE Burke, TG Smith, PG Nelson, and K Frank. 1967. Dendritic location of synapses and possible mechanisms for the monosynaptic EPSP in motoneurons. *J. Neurophysiol.* 30: 1169–1193.

Ransom RW and NL Deschenes. 1990. Polyamines regulate glycine interaction with the *N*-methly-D-aspartate receptor. *Synapse* 5: 294–298.

Rausell E and EG Jones. 1991a. Histochemical and immunocytochemical compartments of the thalamic VPM nucleus in monkeys and their relationship to the representational map. *J. Neurosci.* 11: 210–225.

———— 1991b. Chemically distinct compartments of the thalamic VPM nucleus in monkeys relay principal and spinal trigeminal pathways to different layers of the somatosensory cortex. *J. Neurosci.* 11: 226–237.

———— 1995. Extent of intracortical arborization of thalamocortical axons as a determinant of representational plasticity in monkey somatic sensory cortex. *J. Neurosci.* 15: 4270–4278.

Raymond LA, CD Blackstone, and RL Huganir. 1993. Phosphorylation of amino acid neurotransmitter receptors in synaptic plasticity. *Trends Neurosci.* 16: 147–153.

Redman S. 1990. Quantal analysis of postsynaptic potentials in neurons of the central nervous system. *Physiol. Rev.* 70: 165–198.

Regan D. 1989. *Human Brain Electrophysiology: Evoked Potentials and Evoked Magnetic Fields in Science and Medicine.* Amsterdam: Elsevier.

Regehr WG, A Konnerth, and CM Armstrong. 1993. Synaptically triggered action potentials in dendrites. *Neuron* 11: 145–151.

Reid CB, I Liang, and C Walsh. 1995. Systematic widespread clonal organization in cerebral cortex. *Neuron* 15: 299–310.

Reid RC and J-M Alonso. 1995. Specificity of monosynaptic connections from thalamus to visual cortex. *Nature* 378: 281–284.

———— 1996. The processing and encoding of information in the visual cortex. *Current Opinion in Neurobiology* 6: 475–480.

Reitboeck HJ. 1983. A multi-electrode matrix for studies of temporal signal correlations within neural assemblies. In *Synergetics of the Brain,* ed. E Basar et al. Berlin: Springer-Verlag.

Reitboeck HJ, E Eckhorn, and M Pabst. 1987. A model of figure/ground separation based on correlated neural activity in the visual system. In *Synergetics of the Brain,* ed. E Haken, pp. 44–54. Berlin: Springer-Verlag.

Reznikov KY, Z Fulop, and F Hajos. 1984. Mosaicism of the ventricular layer as the developmental basis of autoradiographic study in newborn mice. *Anat. Embryol. (Berlin)* 170: 99–105.

Ribary U, AA Ionnides, KD Siongh, R Hasson, JPR Bolton, F Lado, A Mogilner, and R Llinas. 1991. Magnetic field tomography of coherent thalamocortical 40-Hz oscillations in humans. *Proc. Natl. Acad. Sci. USA* 88: 11037–11041.

Ringach DL, MJ Hawken, and R Shapley. 1997. Dynamics of orientation tuning in macaque primary visual cortex. *Nature* 387: 281–284.

Rio JA del, A Martinez, M Fonseca, C Auladell, and E Soriano. 1995. Glutamate-like immunoreactivity and fate of Cajal-Retzius cells in the murine cortex as identified by calretinin antibody. *Cerebral Cortex* 5: 13–21.

Roche KW, WG Tingley, and RL Huganir. 1994. Glutamate receptor phosphorylation and synaptic plasticity. *Current Opinion in Neurobiol.* 4: 383–388.

Rock I. 1983. *The Logic of Perception.* Cambridge, MA: MIT Press.

———— 1986. The description and analysis of object and event perception. Chapter 33 in *Handbook of Perception and Performance, Vol. II: Cognitive Process and Performance,* ed. KR Boff, L Kaufman, and JP Thomas. New York: Wiley.

Rock I and S Palmer. 1990. The legacy of Gestalt psychology. *Sci. Am.* 263: 84–90.

Rockel AJ, RW Hiorns, and TPS Powell. 1974. Numbers of neurons through the full depth of the neocortex. *Proc. Anat. Soc. Great Britain and Ireland* 118: 371.

—— 1980. The basic uniformity in structure of the neocortex. *Brain* 103: 221–244.

Rockland KS and DN Pandya. 1979. Laminar origins and terminations of cortical connections of the occipital lobe in the rhesus monkey. *Brain Res.* 179: 3–20.

Roelfsema PR, AK Engel, P Konig, and W Singer. 1996. The role of neuronal synchronization in response selection: A biologically plausible theory of structured representation in the visual cortex. *J. Cogn. Neurosci.* 8: 603–625.

—— 1997. Visuomotor integration is associated with zero time-lag synchronization among cortical areas. *Nature* 385: 157–161.

Roelfsema PR, P Konig, AK Engel, R Sireteanu, and W Singer. 1994. Reduced synchronization in the visual cortex of cats with strabismic amblyopia. *Eur. J. Neurosci.* 6: 1645–1655.

Rosen I and A Asanuma. 1972. Peripheral afferent inputs to the forelimb area of the monkey motor cortex. *Brain Res.* 14: 257–273.

Ross EM. 1989. Signal sorting and amplification through G protein coupled receptors. *Neuron* 3: 141–152.

Rougeul A, JJ Bouyer, L Dedet, and O Debray. 1979. Fast fronto-parietal rhythms during combined focal attention and immobility in baboon and squirrel monkey. *Electroencephalogr. Clin. Neurophysiol.* 46: 310–319.

Rougeul-Buser A and P Buser. 1994. Electrocortical rhythms in the attentive cat: Phenomenological data and theoretical issues. In *Oscillatory Events Related to Brain Dynamics,* ed. C Pantev, T Elbert, and B Lutkenhoner. New York: Plenum.

Rubenstein JLR, S Martinez, K Shimamura, and L Puelles. 1994. The embryonic vertebrate forebrain: The prosomeric model. *Science* 266: 578–580.

Sakmann B. 1992. Elementary steps in synaptic transmission revealed by currents through single ion channels. *Neuron* 8: 613–629.

Sanes JR. 1983. Roles of extracellular matrix in neural development. *Annu. Rev. Physiol.* 45: 581–600.

—— 1989a. Extracellular matrix molecules that influence neural development. *Annu. Rev. Neurosci.* 12: 491–516.

—— 1989b. Analyzing cell lineage with a recombinant retrovirus. *Trends Neurosci.* 12: 21–28.

Sanes JN and DP Donaghue. 1993. Oscillations in local field potentials of the primate motor cortex. *Proc. Natl. Acad. Sci. USA* 90: 4470–4474.

Saper CB. 1987. Diffuse cortical projection systems: Anatomical organization and role in cortical function. In *Handbook of Physiology, Section I: The Nervous System, Vol. 5: Higher Functions of the Brain, Part I,* ed. VB Mountcastle, F Plum, and SR Geiger, pp. 169–210. Bethesda, MD: American Physiological Society.

Sarkisov SA, IN Filimonoff, EP Kononowa, IS Preobraschenskaja, and LA Kukuew. 1955. *Atlas of the Cytoarchitectonics of the Human Cerebral Cortex.* Moscow: Medgiz.

Sato M, L Lopezmascaraque, CD Heffner, and DDM O'Leary. 1994. Action of a diffusible target-derived chemoattractant on cortical axon branch induction and directed growth. *Neuron* 13: 791–803.

Sauer FC. 1935. The cellular structure of the neural tube. *J. Comp. Neurol.* 63: 13–23.

Sauer FC and NE Walker. 1959. Radioautographic study of interkinetic nuclear migration in the neural tube. *Proc. Soc. Exp. Biol. Med.* 102: 557–560.

Scannell JW, C Blakemore, and MP Young. 1995. Analysis of connectivity in the cat cerebral cortex. *J. Neurosci.* 15: 1463–1483.

Scannell JW and MP Young. 1993. The connectional organization of neural systems in the cat cerebral cortex. *Current Biol.* 3: 191–200.

Scanziani M, RC Malenka, and RA Nicoll. 1996. Role of intercellular interactions in heterosynaptic long-term depression. *Nature* 380: 446–450.

Schall JD, DJ Vitek, and AG Levanthal. 1986. Retinal constraints on orientation specificity in cat visual cortex. *J. Neurosci.* 6: 823–836.

Schlaggar BL and DDM O'Leary. 1991. Potential of visual cortex to develop an array of functional units unique to somatosensory cortex. *Science* 252: 1556–1560.

Schlaggar BL and DDM O'Leary. 1993. Patterning of the barrel field in somatosensory cortex with implications for the specification of neocortical areas. *Perspectives Dev. Neurobiol.* 1: 82–92.

—— 1994. Early development of the somatosensory map and barrel patterning in rat somatosensory cortex. *J. Comp. Neurol.* 346: 80–96.

Schlenska. 1969. Messungen der Oberflache und der Volumenanteile des Gehirns meschlicher Erwachsenser mit neuen Methoden. *Z. Anat. Entw. Gesch.* 128: 47–59.

Schmechel DE and P Rakic. 1973. Evolution of fetal radial glial cells in rhesus monkey telencephalon. *Anat. Rec.* 175: 436–450.

—— 1979a. A Golgi study of radial glial cells in developing monkey telencephalon: Morphogenesis and transformation into astrocytes. *Anat. Embryo.* 156: 115–152.

—— 1979b. Arrested proliferation of radial glial cells during midgestation in rhesus monkey. *Nature* 277: 303–305.

Schneider J, R Eckhorn, and H Reitboeck. 1983. Evaluation of neuronal coupling dynamics. *Biol. Cybern.* 46: 129–134.

Schreiner CE, JR Mendelson, and ML Sutter. 1992. Functional topography of cat primary auditory cortex: Representation of tone intensity. *Exp. Brain Res.* 92: 105–122.

Schreiner CE and ML Sutter. 1992. Topography of excitatory bandwidth in cat primary auditory cortex: Single-neuron versus multiple-neuron recordings. *J. Neurophysiol.* 68: 1482–1502.

Schuman EM and DV Madison. 1994. Nitric oxide and synaptic function. *Annu. Rev. Neurosci.* 176: 153–183.

Schwab ME, JP Kapfhammer, and CE Bandtlow. 1993. Inhibitors of neurite growth. *Annu. Rev. Neurosci.* 16: 565–595.

Schwartz ML and PS Goldman-Rakic. 1984. Callosal and intrahemispheric connectivity of the prefrontal association cortex in the rhesus monkey: Relation between intraparietal and principal sulcal cortex. *J. Comp. Neurol.* 226: 403–420.

Schwartz ML, P Rakic, and PS Goldman-Rakic. 1991. Early phenotype expression of cortical neurons: Evidence that a subclass of migrating neurons have callosal axons. *Proc. Natl. Acad. Sci. USA* 88: 1354–1358.

Seeburg PH. 1993. The TINNS\TIPS lecture: The molecular biology of mammalian glutamate receptor channels. *Trends Neurosci.* 16: 359–364.

Seeburg PH, W Wisden, TA Verdoon, DB Pritchett, P Werner, A Hero, H Sprengel, and B Sakmann. 1990. The GABA$_A$ receptor family: Molecular and functional diversity. *Cold Spring Harbor Symp. Quant. Biol.* 55: 29–40.

Seidemann E, T Meilijson, M Abeles, H Bergman, and E Vaadia. 1996. Simultaneously recorded single units in the frontal cortex go through sequences of discrete and stable states in monkeys performing a delayed localization task. *J. Neurosci.* 16: 752–768.

Selemon LD and PS Goldman-Rakic. 1985. Longitudinal topography and interdigitation of corticostriatal projections in the rhesus monkey. *J. Neurosci.* 5: 776–794.

——— 1988. Common cortical and subcortical targets of the dorsolateral prefrontal and posterior parietal cortices in the rhesus monkey: Evidence for a distributed neural network subserving spatially guided behavior. *J. Neurosci.* 8:449–468.

Seltzer B and DN Pandya. 1980. Posterior parietal projections to the intraparietal sulcus in the rhesus monkey. *Exp. Brain Res.* 62: 459–469.

Selverston AI. 1993. Neuromodulatory control of rhythmic behaviors in invertebrates. *Int. Rev. Cytology* 147: 1–24.

Selverston AI and M Moulins. 1985. Oscillatory neural networks. *Annu. Rev. Physiol.* 47: 29–48.

Senft SL and TA Woolsey. 1991a. Growth of thalamic afferents into mouse barrel cortex. *Cerebral Cortex* 1: 308–335.

——— 1991b. Computer-aided analyses of thalamocortical afferent ingrowth. *Cerebral Cortex* 1: 336–347.

———— 1991c. Mouse barrel cortex viewed as Dirichlet domains. *Cerebral Cortex* 1: 348–363.

Shanks MF, AJ Rockel, and TPS Powell. 1975. The commissural fibre connections of the primary somatic sensory cortex. *Brain Res.* 98: 166–171.

Shatz CJ. 1990. Impulse activity and the patterning of connections during CNS development. *Neuron* 5: 745–756.

Shatz CJ, JJ Chun, and MB Luskin. 1988. The role of the subplate in the development of the mammalian telencephalon. In *Cerebral Cortex, Vol. 7: Development and Maturation of the Cerebral Cortex,* ed. A Peters and EG Jones, pp. 35–58. New York: Plenum.

Shatz CJ, A Ghosh, SK McConnell, KL Allendorfer, E Friauf, and A Antonini. 1990. Pioneer neurons and target selection in cerebral cortical development. *Cold Spring Harbor Symp. Quant. Biol.* 55: 469–480.

Shatz CJ and MB Luskin. 1986. The relationship between the geniculocortical afferents and their cortical target cells during development of the cat's primary visual cortex. *J. Neurosci.* 6: 3655–3668.

Shaw G, J Kruger, DJ Silverman, AMJH Aertsen, F Aiple, and HC Liu. 1993. Rhythmic and patterned neuronal firing in the visual cortex. *Neurol. Res.* 15: 46–60.

Sheer DE. 1989. Sensory and cognitive 40-Hz event-related potentials: Behavioral correlates, brain function, and clinical application. In *Springer Series in Brain Dynamics 2,* ed. E Basar and TH Bullock, pp. 339–374. Berlin and New York: Springer-Verlag.

Sheetz MP, DB Wayne, and AL Pearlman. 1992. Extension of filopodia by motor-dependent actin assembly. *Cell. Motl. Cytoskeleton* 22: 160–169.

Shepard RN. 1962. The analysis of proximities: Multi-dimensional scaling with an unknown distance function. *Psychometrika* 27: 125–140.

———— 1980. Multidimensional scaling, tree fitting and clustering. *Science* 210: 390–398.

Sheppard AM, SK Hamilton, and AL Pearlman. 1991. Changes in the distribution of extracellular matrix components accompany early morphogenetic events in mammalian cortical development. *J. Neurosci.* 11: 3928–3942.

Sherk H. 1986. The claustrum and the cerebral cortex. In *Cerebral Cortex, Vol. 5: Sensory-motor Areas and Aspects of Cortical Connectivity,* ed. EG Jones and A Peters, pp. 467–500. New York: Plenum.

Sherk H and S LeVay. 1981. The visual claustrum in the cat. III. Receptive field properties. *J. Neurosci.* 1: 993–1002.

———— 1983. Contribution of the cortico-claustral loop to receptive field properties in area 17 of the cat. *J. Neurosci.* 3: 2121–2127.

Shipp A and S Zeki. 1985. Segregation of pathways leading from area V2 to areas V4 and V5 of macaque monkey visual cortex. *Nature* 315: 322–325.

———— 1989. The organization of connections between V5 and V2 in macaque monkey visual cortex. *Eur. J. Neurosci.* 1: 333–354.

Shou T and AG Levanthal. 1989. Organized arrangement of orientation selective relay cells in cat's dorsal lateral geniculate nucleus. *J. Neurosci.* 9: 4287–4302.

Sidman RL and P Rakic. 1973. Neuronal migration, with special reference to developing human brain: A review. *Brain Res.* 62: 1–35.

Sillito AM, JA Kemp, JA Milson, and N Berardi. 1980. A re-evaluation of the mechanisms underlying simple cell orientation selectivity. *Brain Res.* 194: 517–520.

Silva AJ, CF Stevens, S Tonegawa, and Y Wang. 1992. Deficient hippocampal long-term potentiation in alpha-CA-Calmodulin Kinase II mutant mice. *Science* 257: 201–206.

Silver RB, M Sugimori, EJ Lang, and R Llinas. 1994. Time-resolved imaging of Ca(2+)-dependent aequorin luminescence of microdomains and QEDs in synaptic preterminals. *Biol. Bull.* 1887: 293–299.

Simmons PA, V Lemmon, and AL Pearlman. 1982. Afferent and efferent connections of the striate and extrastriate visual cortex of the normal and reeler mouse. *J. Comp. Neurol.* 211: 295–308.

Simmons PA and AL Pearlman. 1983. Receptive field properties of transcallosal visual cortical neurons in the normal and reeler mouse. *J. Neurophysiol.* 50: 838–848.

Simons DJ. 1978. Response properties of vibrissa units in rat SI somatosensory neocortex. *J. Neurophysiol.* 41: 798–820.

Simons DJ and TA Woolsey. 1984. Morphology of Golgi-Cox-impregnated barrel neurons in rat SmI cortex. *J. Comp. Neurol.* 230: 119–132.

Simons EL. 1981. Man's immediate prerunners. *Phil. Trans. Roy. Soc. Lond.* B292: 21–41.

Singer W. 1995. Development and plasticity of cortical processing. *Science* 270: 758–764.

Singer W, AK Engel, AK Kreiter, MJH Munk, S Neunschwander, and PR Roelfsema. 1997. Neuronal assemblies: Necessity, signature and detectability. *Trends Cog. Sci.* 1: 252–259.

Singer W and CM Gray. 1995. Visual feature integration and the temporal correlation hypothesis. *Annu. Rev. Neurosci.* 18: 555–586.

Slimp JC and AL Towe. 1990. Spatial distribution of modalities and receptive fields in sensorimotor cortex of awake cats. *Exp. Neurol.* 107: 78–96.

Sloper JJ. 1973. An electron microscopic study of neurons of the primate motor and somatic sensory cortices. *J. Neurophysiol.* 2: 351–359.

Sloper JJ, RW Hiorns, and TPS Powell. 1979. A qualitative and quantitative electron microscopic study of the neurons in the primate motor and somatic sensory cortices. *Phil. Trans. Roy. Soc. Lond.* B285: 141–171.

Smith FH and F Spencer, eds. 1984. *The Origins of Modern Humans: A World Survey of the Fossil Evidence.* New York: Alan R. Liss.

Snell O. 1891. Die Anhangigkeit des Hirngewichtes von dem Körperwicht und den geistigen Fähigkeiten. *Arch. Psychiat. Nervkrankh.* 23: 436–446.

Somers DC, SB Nelson, and M Sur. 1995. An emergent model of orientation selectivity in cat visual cortical single cells. *J. Neurosci.* 15: 5446–5465.

Somoygi P. 1977. A specific axo-axonal neuron in the visual cortex of the rat. *Brain Res.* 136: 345–350.

Somoygi P and A Cowey. 1981. Combined Golgi and electron microscopic study on the synapses formed by double bouquet cells in the visual cortex of the cat and monkey. *J. Comp. Neurol.* 191: 547–566.

Somoygi P, TF Freund, AJ Hodgson, J Somoygi, D Beroukas, and IW Chubb. 1985. Identified axo-axonic cells are immunoreactive for GABA in the hippocampus and visual cortex of cats. *Brain Res.* 332: 143–149.

Soodak RE, RM Shapley, and E Kaplan. 1987. Linear mechanism of orientation. *J. Neurophysiol.* 58: 267–275.

Soriano E, N Dumensnil, C Auladell, M Cohen-Tannoudji, and C Sotelo. 1995. Molecular heterogeneity of progenitors and radial migration in the developing cerebral cortex revealed by transgene expression. *Proc. Natl. Acad. Sci. USA* 92: 11676–11680.

Spatz WB. 1977. Topographically organized connections between areas 17 and MT (visual area of superior temporal sulcus) in the marmoset *Callithrix jacchus. Exp. Brain Res.* 27: 559–572.

Spatz WB, J Tigges, and M Tigges. 1970. Subcortical projections, cortical associations, and some intrinsic interlaminar connections of the striate cortex of the squirrel monkey *(Saimiri). J. Comp. Neurol.* 140: 155–174.

Spencer WA and ER Kandel. 1961. Electrophysiology of hippocampal neurons. IV. Fast prepotentials. *J. Neurophysiol.* 24: 272–285.

Sperry RW. 1963. Chemoaffinity in the orderly growth of nerve fiber patterns and connections. *Proc. Natl. Acad. Sci. USA* 60: 703–710.

Spoor F, B Wood, and F Zonneveld. 1994. Implications of early hominid labyrinthine morphology for evaluation of human bipedal locomotion. *Nature* 369: 645–648.

Sporns O, JA Gally, GN Reeke jr, and GM Edelman. 1989. Re-entrant signalling among simulated neuronal groups leads to coherency of their oscillatory activity. *Proc. Natl. Acad. Sci. USA* 86: 7265–7269.

———— 1991. Modeling perceptual grouping and figure-ground segregation by means of active re-entrant connections. *Proc. Natl. Acad. Sci. USA* 88: 129–133.

Sporns O, G Tononi, and GM Edelman. 1994. Reentry and dynamical interactions of cortical networks. In *Models of Neural Networks II,* ed. JL van Hemmen and L Schulten, pp. 315–341. Berlin and New York: Springer.

Spuhler JN. 1988. Evolution of mitochondrial DNA in monkeys, apes and humans. *Yearbook of Physical Anthropology* 31: 15–48.

Spurzheim JG. 1925. *Phrenology, or the Doctrine of the Mind*, 3d ed. London: Knight.

Sretavan D and RW Dykes. 1983. The organization of two cutaneous submodalities in the forearm region of area 3b of cat somatosensory cortex. *J. Comp. Neurol.* 213: 281–398.

Stanley MS. 1975. A theory of evolution above the species level. *Proc. Natl. Acad. Sci. USA* 72: 646–650.

———— 1979. *Macroevolution.* San Francisco: Freeman.

Stebbins GL. 1982. *From Darwin to DNA, Molecules to Humanity.* San Francisco: Freeman.

Stebbins WC, ed. 1970. *Animal Psychophysics; The Design and Conduct of Sensory Experiments.* New York: Plenum.

Stebbins WC, CH Brown, and MR Peterson. 1984. Sensory function in animals. In *Handbook of Physiology, Section I: The Nervous System, Volume III: Sensory Processes, Part 1,* ed. I Darian-Smith, JM Brookhart, VB Mountcastle, and SR Geiger. Bethesda, MD: American Physiological Society.

Steinmetz MA, BC Motter, CJ Duffy, and VB Mountcastle. 1987. Functional properties of parietal visual neurons: Radial organization of directionalities within the visual field. *J. Neurosci.* 7: 177–191.

Stemple DL and DJ Anderson. 1991. Isolation of a stem cell for neurons and glia from the mammalian neural crest. *Cell* 71: 973–985.

Stent GS. 1973. A physiological mechanism for Hebb's postulate of learning. *Proc. Natl. Acad. Sci. USA* 70: 997–1001.

Stephan H, G Baron, and HD Frahm. 1988. Comparative size of brains and brain components. In *Comparative Primate Biology, Vol. 4: Neurosciences,* pp. 1–38. New York: Alan R. Liss.

———— eds. 1991. *Comparative Brain Research in Mammals, Vol. 1: Insectivora.* Berlin: Springer.

Steriade M. 1991. Alertness, quiet sleep, dreaming. In *Cerebral Cortex, Vol. 9: Normal and Altered States of Function,* ed. A Peters and EG Jones. New York: Plenum.

———— 1993. Central core modulation of spontaneous oscillations and sensory transmission in thalamocortical systems. *Current Opinion in Neurobiol.* 3: 619–625.

Steriade M and F Amzica. 1996. Intracortical and corticothalamic coherency of fast spontaneous oscillations. *Proc. Natl. Acad. Sci. USA* 93: 2533–2538.

Steriade M, F Amzica, and D Contreras. 1996a. Synchronization of fast (30–40 Hz) spontaneous cortical rhythms during brain activation. *J. Neurosci.* 16: 392–417.

Steriade M and G Buzsaki. 1989. Parallel activation of thalamic and cortical neurons by brainstem and basal forebrain cholinergic systems. In *Brain Cholinergic Systems,* ed. M Steriade and D Biesold. Oxford: Oxford U. Press.

Steriade M, D Contreras, and F Amzica. 1994. Synchronized sleep oscillations and their paroxysmal developments. *Trends Neurosci.* 17: 199–207.

Steriade M, D Contreras, F Amzica, and I Timofeev. 1996b. Synchronization of fast (30–40) spontaneous oscillations in intrathalamic and thalamo-cortical networks. *J. Neurosci.* 16: 2788–2808.

Steriade M, D Contreras, R Curro Dossi, and A Nunez. 1993. The slow (<1Hz) oscillation in reticular thalamic and thalamocortical neurons: Scenario of sleep rhythm generation in interacting thalamic and neocortical networks. *J. Neurosci.* 13: 324–329.

Steriade M and M Deschenes. 1984. The thalamus as a neuronal oscillator. *Brain Res. Rev.* 8: 1–63.

Steriade M, DA McCormick, and TJ Sejnowski. 1996c. Thalamocortical oscillations in the sleeping brain. *Science* 262: 679–685.

Steriade M, A Nunez, and F Amzica. 1993a. A novel slow (<1 Hz) oscillation of neocortical neurons *in vivo:* Depolarizing and hyperpolarizing components. *J. Neurosci.* 13: 3252–3265.

——— 1993b. Intracellular analysis of relations between the slow (<1 Hz) neocortical oscillation and other sleep rhythms of the electroencephalogram. *J. Neurosci.* 13: 3266–3283.

Stevens CF. 1993. Quantal release of neurotransmitters and long term potentiation. *Cell,* vol. 72 *Neuron,* vol. 10: 55–63.

Stevens CF, S Tonegawa, and Y Wang. 1994. The role of calcium-calmodulin kinase II in three forms of synaptic plasticity. *Curr. Biol.* 4: 687–693.

Stevens SS. 1957. On the psychophysical law. *Psychol. Rev.* 64: 153–161.

——— 1959. Measurement, psychophysics, and utility. In *Measurement: Definitions and Theories,* ed. CW Churchman. New York: Wiley.

——— 1960. Psychophysics of sensory perception. In *Sensory Communication,* ed. WR Rosenblith, pp. 1–34. Cambridge, MA: MIT Press.

——— 1961. To honor Fechner and repeal his law. *Science* 133: 80–86.

——— 1970. Neural events and the psychophysical law. *Science* 170: 1043–1050.

Stevens SS and E Galanter. 1957. Ratio scales and category scales on a dozen perceptual continua. *J. Acoust. Soc. Am.* 51: 575–593.

Stitt TN, UE Gasser, and ME Hatten. 1991. Molecular mechanisms of glial-guided neuronal migration. *Ann. NY Acad. Sci.* 633: 113–121.

Storm-Mathiesen J and OP Ottersen. 1990. Immunocytochemistry of glutamate at the synaptic level. *J. Histochem. Cytochem.* 38: 1733–1743.

Streit P. 1984. Glutamate and aspartate as transmitter candidates for systems of the cerebral cortex. In *Cerebral Cortex, vol. 2: Functional Properties of Cortical Cells,* ed. EG Jones and A Peters, pp. 119–143. New York: Plenum.

Stringer C and C Gamble. 1993. *In Search of the Neanderthals.* New York: Thames and Hudson.

Stringer CB, JS Harlow, and B Vandermeersch. 1984. Origin of anatomically modern humans in Western Europe. In *The Origins of Modern Humans,* ed. FH Smith and H Spencer, pp. 57–135. New York: Alan R. Liss.

Stryker MP, B Chapman, KD Miller, and KR Zahs. 1990. Experimental and theoretical studies of the organization of afferents to single orientation columns in the visual cortex. *Cold Spring Harbor Symp. Quant. Biol.* 55: 515–527.

Stuart GJ and SJ Redman. 1991. Mechanisms of presynaptic inhibition studied using paired-pulse facilitation. *Neurosci. Lett.* 126: 179–183.

Stuart GJ and B Sakmann. 1994. Active propagation of somatic action potentials into neocortical pyramidal cell dendrites. *Nature* 367: 69–72.

Sudhof TC. 1995. The synaptic vesicle cycle: A cascade of protein-protein interactions. *Nature* 375: 645–653.

Sugimori M, EWJ Lang, RB Silver, and R Llinas. 1994. High-resolution measurement of the time course of calcium-concentration microdomains at squid presynaptic terminals. *Biol. Bull.* 187: 300–303.

Sur M, JT Wall, and JH Kaas. 1984. Modular distribution of neurons with slowly adapting and rapidly adapting responses in area 3b of somatosensory cortex in monkeys. *J. Neurophysiol.* 51: 724–744.

Susman RL. 1994. Fossil evidence for early hominid tool use. *Science* 265: 1570–1573.

Swisher CC, SC Anton, HP Schwarcz, GH Curtis, A Suprijo, and Widiasmoro. 1996. Latest *Homo erectus* in Java; potential contemporaneity with *Homo sapiens* in southeast Asia. *Science* 275: 1870–1874.

Swisher CC, GH Curtis, T Jacob, AG Getty, A Suprijo, and Widiasmoro. 1994. Age of the earliest known hominids in Java, Indonesia. *Science* 263: 1118–1121.

Tagaris GA, S-G Kim, JR Strupp, P Andersen, K Ugurbil, and AP Georgopoulis. 1997. Mental rotation studied by functional magnetic resonance imaging at high field (4 Tesla): Performance and cortical activation. *J. Cog. Neurosci.* 9: 419–432.

Takahashi T, RS Nowakowski, and VE Caviness jr. 1996a. Interkinetic and migratory behavior of a cohort of neocortical neurons arising in the early embryonic murine cerebral wall. *J. Neurosci.* 16: 5762–5776.

———— 1996b. The leaving or Q fraction of the murine cerebral proliferative epithelium: A general model of neocortical neurogenesis. *J. Neurosci.* 16: 6183–6196.

Tan SS and S Breen. 1993. Radial mosaicism and tangential cell dispersion both contribute to mouse neocortical development. *Nature* 362: 638–640.

Tanaka K. 1983. Cross-correlation analysis of geniculostriate neuronal relationships in the cat. *J. Neurophysiol.* 49: 1303–1318.

———— 1992. Inferotemporal cortex and higher visual functions. *Current Opinion in Neurobiology* 2: 502–505.

———— 1996. Inferotemporal cortex and object vision. *Annu. Rev. Neurosci.* 19: 109–139.

Tanaka K, I Fujita, E Kobatake, K Cheng, and M Ito. 1992. Serial processing of visual object features in the posterior and anterior parts of inferotemporal cortex. In *Brain Mechanisms of Perception and Memory: From Neuron to Behavior,* ed. T Ono, L Squire, RE Raichle, D Perrett, and M Fukada. Oxford: Oxford U. Press.

Tattersall I. 1995. *The Fossil Trail: How We Know What We Think We Know about Human Evolution.* Oxford: Oxford U. Press.

Teyler T, V Aroniadou, RL Berry, A Borroni, P DiScenna, L Grover, and N Lambert. 1990. LTP in neocortex. *Sem. Neurosci.* 2: 365–379.

Thompson KG, AG Levanthal, Y Zhou, and D Liu. 1994. Stimulus dependence of orientation and directional sensitivity of cat LGNd relay cells without cortical inputs: A comparison with area 17 cells. *Vis. Neurosci.* 11: 939–951.

Thomson AM. 1989. Glycine modulation of the NMDA receptor/channel complex. *Trends Neurosci.* 112: 349–353.

Thomson AM and J Deuchars. 1994. Temporal and spatial properties of local circuits in neocortex. *Trends Neurosci.* 17: 119–126.

Thomson AM, J Deuchars, and DC West. 1993a. Large, deep layer pyramid-pyramid single axon EPSPs in slices of rat motor cortex display paired pulse and frequency dependent depression, mediated presynaptically and self-facilitation, mediated postsynaptically. *J. Neurophysiol.* 79: 2354–2369.

———— 1993b. Single axon excitatory postsynaptic potentials in neocortical interneurons exhibit pronounced paired pulse facilitation. *Neurosci.* 54: 347–360.

Thorne AG and MH Wolpoff. 1992. The multiregional evolution of humans. *Sci. Am.* 266: 76–83.

Tiemei C, Y Quan, and W En. 1994. Antiquity of *Homo sapiens* in China. *Nature* 368: 55–56.

Tigges J, WB Spatz, and M Tigges. 1973. Reciprocal point to point connections between parastriate and striate cortex in the squirrel monkey *(Saimiri). J. Comp. Neurol.* 148: 481–492.

Tigges J, M Tigges, S Anschel, N Cross, WD Ledbetter, and RL McBride. 1981.

Areal and laminar distribution of neurons interconnecting the central visual cortical areas 17, 18, 19 and MT in squirrel monkey *(Saimiri)*. *J. Comp. Neurol.* 202: 539–252.

Tishkoff SA, E Dietzsch, et al. 1996. Global patterns of linkage disequilibrium at the CD4 locus and modern human origins. *Science* 271: 1380–1387.

Tobias PV. 1981a. Brain-size, grey matter and race—fact or fiction? *Am. J. Phys. Anthrop.* 32: 3–26.

——— 1981b. The emergence of man in Africa and beyond. *Phil. Trans. Roy. Soc. Lond.* B292: 43–56.

——— 1982. Hominid evolution in Africa. *Canad. J. Anthrop.* 3: 162–190.

——— 1983. Recent advances in the evolution of the hominids with special reference to brain and speech. In *Recent Advances in the Evolution of Primates,* ed. C Chagas, 50: 85–140. Vatican City: Pontificiae Academiae Scientiarum Scripta Varia.

——— 1987. The brain of *Homo habilis:* A new level of organization in cerebral evolution. *J. Hum. Evol.* 16: 741–761.

——— 1990. Some critical steps in the evolution of the hominid brain. In *The Principles of Design and Operation of the Brain,* ed. JC Eccles and O Creutzfeldt, 78: 1–23. Vatican City: Pontificiae Academiae Scientiarum Scripta Varia.

——— 1991. *Olduvai Gorge,* vol. 4. Cambridge and New York: Cambridge U. Press.

Tobias PV. 1997. Evolution of brain size, morphological restructuring and longevity in early hominids. In SU Dani, AJ Pro, and GF Walter, eds., *Principles of Neural Aging,* pp. 153–174. Amsterdam: Elsevier.

Todd PH. 1982. A geometric model for the cortical folding of simple folded brains. *J. Theor. Biol.* 97: 529–538.

Tomasiewicz H, K Ono, D Yee, C Thompson, C Corildis, U Rutishauser, and T Magnuson. 1993. Genetic deletion of a neural cell adhesion molecule variant (N-CAM-180) produces distinct defects in the central nervous system. *Neuron* 11: 1163–1174.

Tommerdahl M, O Favorow, BL Whitsel, B Nakhle, and YA Gonchar. 1993. Minicolumnar activation patterns in cat and monkey S1 cortex. *Cerebral Cortex* 3: 399–411.

Tonnies JFG. 1933. Naturwissenschaften. *22 Jahrg.* 22/24, 411.

Tononi G, O Sporns, and GM Edelman. 1992a. Reentry and the problem of integrating multiple cortical areas: Simulation of dynamic integration in the visual cortex. *Cerebral Cortex* 2: 310–335.

——— 1992b. The problem of neural integration: Induced rhythms and short-term correlations. In *Induced Rhythms in the Brain,* ed. E Basar and TH Bullock. Boston: Birkhauser.

Tootell RB, MS Silverman, SL Hamilton, E Switkes, and RL DeValois. 1991. Spatial frequency tuning of single units in macaque supragranular striate cortex. *Proc. Natl. Acad. Sci. USA* 88: 7066–7088.

Toyama K, M Kimura, and K Tanaka. 1981. Cross-correlation analysis of interneuronal connectivity in cat visual cortex. *J. Neurophysiol.* 46: 191–201.

Traub RD, MA Whittington, IM Stanford, and JGR Jeffreys. 1996. A mechanism for generation of long-range synchronous fast oscillations in the cortex. *Nature* 383: 621–624.

Tsien JZ, DF Chen, D Gerber, C Tom, EH Mercer, DJ Anderson, M Mayford, ER Kandel, and S Tonegawa. 1996a. Subregion- and cell type-restricted gene knockout in mouse brain. *Cell* 87: 1317–1326.

Tsien JZ, PY Huerta, and S Tonegawa. 1996b. The essential role of hippocampal receptor-dependent synaptic plasticity in spatial memory. *Cell* 87: 1327–1338.

T'so DY, CD Gilbert, and TN Wiesel. 1986. Relationship between horizontal interactions and functional architecture in cat striate cortex as revealed by cross-correlation analysis. *J. Neurosci.* 6: 1160–1170.

Tsumoto T. 1992. Long-term potentiation and long-term depression in the neocortex. *Prog. Neurobiol.* 39: 209–226.

Tunturi AR. 1950. Physiological determination of the arrangement of the afferent connections to the middle ectosylvian auditory area in the dog. *Am. J. Physiol.* 162: 489–502.

Uchizona K. 1965. Characteristics of excitatory and inhibitory synapses in the central nervous system of the cat. *Nature* 207: 642–643.

——— 1967. Synaptic organization of the Purkinje cells in the cerebellum of the cat. *Exp. Brain Res.* 4: 97–113.

Vaadia E, I Haalman, M Abeles, H Bergman, Y Prut, H Slovin, and A Aertsen. 1995. Dynamics of neuronal interactions in monkey cortex in relation to behavioral events. *Nature* 373: 513–518.

Valtorta F, F Benfenati, and P Greengard. 1992. Structure and function of the synapsins. *J. Biol. Chem.* 267: 7195–7198.

Valtshanoff JG, RJ Weinberg, and A Rustioni. 1993. Amino acid immunoreactivity in corticospinal terminals. *Brain Res.* 93: 95–103.

Valverde F, L Lopez-Moscaraque, M Santana, and JA DeCarlos. 1995. Persistence of early-generated neurons in the rodent subplate; assessment of cell death in neocortex during the early postnatal period. *J. Neurosci.* 15: 5014–5024.

Van Brederode JFM, KA Mulligan, and AE Hendrickson. 1990. Calcium-binding proteins as markers for subpopulations of GABAergic neurons in monkey striate cortex. *J. Comp. Neurol.* 298: 1–22.

Van Essen DC, DJ Felleman, EA DeYoe, J Olavarria, and JU Knierim. 1990.

Modular and hierarchical organization of extrastriate visual cortex in the macaque monkey. *Cold Spring Harbor Symp. Quant. Biol.* 55: 679–696.

Van Essen DC and JM Maunsell. 1980. Two-dimensional maps of the cerebral cortex. *J. Comp. Neurol.* 191: 255–281.

Vidyasagar TR. 1984. Contribution of inhibitory mechanisms to the orientation sensitivity of cat dLGN neurones. *Exp. Brain Res.* 55: 192–195.

Vidyasagar TR and W Heide. 1984. Geniculate orientation biases seen with moving sine wave gratings: Implications for a model of a simple cell afferent connectivity. *Exp. Brain Res.* 57: 176–200.

Vidyasagar TR, X Pei, and M Volgushev. 1996. Multiple mechanisms underlying the orientation selectivity of visual cortical neurons. *Trends Neurosci.* 19: 272–277.

Vidyasagar TR and JV Urbas. 1982. Orientation sensitivity of cat LGN neurones with and without inputs from visual cortical areas 17 and 18. *Exp. Brain Res.* 46: 257–169.

Viebahn C. 1990. Correlation between differences in structure of dendritic bundles and cytoarchitectonic pattern in the cerebral cortex of the rabbit. *J. Hirnforsch.* 5: 645–652.

Vogt BA. 1991. The role of layer I in cortical function. In *Cerebral Cortex, Vol. 9: Normal and Altered States of Function,* ed. A Peters and EG Jones, pp. 49–90. New York: Plenum.

Vogt O and C Vogt. 1919. Ergebnisse unserer Hirnforschung. *J. Psychol. Neurol. Lpz.* 25: 277–462.

Voight T. 1989. Development of glial cells in the cerebral wall of ferrets: Direct tracing of their transformation from radial glia to astrocytes. *J. Comp. Neurol.* 289: 74–88.

Von der Malsberg C. 1995. Binding in models of perception and brain function. *Current Opinion in Neurobiol.* 5: 520–526.

Von der Malsberg and CW Schneider. 1986. A neural cocktail-party processor. *Biol. Cybern.* 54: 29–40.

———— 1992. Sensory segmentation with coupled neural oscillators. *Biol. Cybern.* 67: 233–242.

Von Krosigk M, T Bal, and DA McCormick. 1993. Cellular mechanisms of a synchronized oscillation in the thalamus. *Science* 261: 361–364.

Voronin LL. 1994. Quantal analysis of hippocampal long-term potentiation. *Rev. Neurosci.* 5: 141–170.

Waddle DM. 1994. Matrix correlation tests support a single origin for modern humans. *Nature* 368: 452–454.

Wahle P. 1993. Differential regulation of substance P and somatostatin in Martinotti cells of the developing cat visual cortex. *J. Comp. Neurol.* 329: 519–538.

Walker A and R Leakey. 1993. *The Nariokotome Homo erectus Skeleton.* Cambridge, MA: Harvard U. Press.

Wallace MN, LM Kitzes, and EG Jones. 1991. Intrinsic inter- and intralaminar connections and their relationship to the tonotopic map in cat primary auditory cortex. *Exp. Brain Res.* 86: 527–544.

Walsh C and CL Cepko. 1988. Clonally related cortical cells show several migration patterns. *Science* 241: 1342–1345.

——— 1992. Widespread dispersion of neuronal clones across functional regions in the cerebral cortex. *Science* 255: 434–440.

——— 1993. Clonal dispersion in proliferative layers of developing cerebral cortex. *Nature* 362: 632–635.

Wanpo H, R Ciochon, G Yumin, R Larrick, F Qiren, H Schwarcz, C Yonge, J de Vos, and W Rink. 1995. Early *Homo* and associated artefacts from Asia. *Nature* 378: 275–278.

Weilikey M, K Kandler, D Fitzpatrick, and LC Katz. 1995. Patterns of excitation and inhibition evoked by horizontal connections in visual cortex share a common relationship to orientation columns. *Neuron* 15: 541–552.

Weiss S, BA Reynolds, AL Vescovi, C Morshead, CC Craig, and D Van der Kooy. 1996. Is there a stem cell in the mammalian forebrain? *Trends Neurosci.* 19: 387–393.

Weisskopf MG, PE Castillo, RA Zalutsky, and RA Nicoll. 1994. Mediation of hippocampal mossy fiber long-term potentiation by cyclic AMP. *Science* 265: 1878–1883.

Welker C. 1971. Microelectrode delineation of fine grain somatotopic organization of SmI cerebral neocortex in albino rat. *Brain Res.* 26: 259–275.

Welker E, M Armstrong-James, H Van der Loos, and R Kraftsik. 1993. The mode of activation of a barrel column: Response properties of single units in the somatosensory cortex of the mouse upon whisker deflection. *Eur. J. Neurosci.* 5: 691–712.

Welker W. 1990. Why does the cerebral cortex fissure and fold? A review of determinants of gyri and sulci. In *Cerebral Cortex, Vol. 8B: Comparative Structure and Evolution of Cerebral Cortex, Part II,* ed. EG Jones and A Peters. New York: Plenum.

Wentland BW, FE Schweizer, TA Ryan, M Nakane, F Murad, RH Scheller, and RW Tsien. 1994. Existence of nitric oxide synthase in rat hippocampal pyramidal cells. *Proc. Natl. Acad. Sci. USA* 91: 2151–2155.

West MJ. 1993. New stereological methods for counting neurons. *Neurobiol. Aging* 14: 275–285.

Wheal HV and AM Thomson, eds. 1991. *Excitatory Amino Acids and Synaptic Transmission.* New York: Academic Press.

White EL and A Peters. 1993. Cortical modules in the posteromedial barrel field (SM1) of the mouse. *J. Comp. Neurol.* 334: 86–96.

White TD, DC Johanson, and W Kimbel. 1981. *Australopithecus africanus:* Its phylogenetic position reconsidered. *South African J. Sci.* 077: 445–470.

White TD, G Suwa, and B Asfaw. 1994. *Australopithecus ramidus,* a new species of hominid from Aramis, Ethiopia. *Nature* 371: 306–312.

Whitsel BL, LM Petrucelli, and G Werner. 1969. Symmetry and connectivity in the map of the body surface in the somatosensory area II of primates. *J. Neurophysiol.* 32: 170–183.

Whittaker VP. 1993. Thirty years of synaptosome research. *J. Neurocytol.* 22: 735–742.

Whittaker VP, IA Michaelson, and RJA Kirkland. 1964. The separation of synaptic vesicles from nerve-ending particles ("synapsomes"). *Biochem. J.* 90: 293–303.

Williams JH, ML Errington, Y-G Li, MA Lynch, and TVP Bliss. 1989. Arachidonic acid induces a long-term activity-dependent enhancement of synaptic transmission in the hippocampus. *Nature* 341: 739–742.

Williams RW, K Ryder, and P Rakic. 1987. Emergence of cytoarchitectonic differences between area 17 and 18 in the developing rhesus. *Soc. Neurosci. Abstr.* 13: 1044.

Williams SM, PS Goldman-Rakic, and C Leranth. 1992. The synaptology of parvalbumin-immunoreactive neurons in the primate prefrontal cortex. *J. Comp. Neurol.* 320: 353–369.

Wilson AC and RL Cann. 1992. The recent African genesis of humans. *Sci. Am.* 266: 66–70.

Wilson EO. 1992. *The Diversity of Life.* Cambridge, MA: Harvard U. Press.

Wilson MA and ME Molliver. 1991a. The organization of serotonergic projections to cerebral cortex in primates; regional distribution of axon terminals. *Neurosci.* 44: 537–553.

———— 1991b. The organization of serotonergic projections to cerebral cortex in primates: Retrograde transport studies. *Neurosci.* 44: 555–570.

Wilson MA and S Tonegawa. 1997. Synaptic plasticity, place cells, and spatial memory: Study with second generation knockouts. *Trends Neurosci.* 20: 102–106.

Winfield DA, KC Gatter, and TPS Powell. 1980. An electron microscopic study of the types and proportions of neurons in the cortex of the motor and visual areas of the cat and rat. *Brain* 103: 245–258.

Wiser AK and EM Callaway. 1996. Contributions of individual layer VI pyramidal neurons to local circuitry in primary visual cortex. *J. Neurosci.* 16: 2724–2739.

Witelson SF, DL Kigar, and TS Harvey. 1997. The exceptional brain of Albert Einstein. Pers. comm.

Wolman BB, ed. 1968. *Historical Roots of Contemporary Psychology.* New York: Harper Row.

Wolpoff MH. 1989. Multi-regional evolution: The fossil alternative to Eden. In *The Human Revolution: Behavioral and Biological Perspectives on the Origin of Modern Humans,* ed. P Mellors and C Stringer, pp. 62–108. Princeton: Princeton U. Press.

Wolpoff MH, WZ Zhi, and AG Thorne. 1984. Modern *Homo sapiens* origins: A general theory of hominid evolution involving the fossil evidence from east Asia. In *The Origins of Modern Humans: A World Survey of the Fossil Evidence,* ed. FH Smith and F Spencer, pp. 411–484. New York: Alan R. Liss.

Wong D. 1991. Cellular organization of the cat's auditory cortex. In *The Neurobiology of Hearing,* ed. RA Altschuler et al., pp. 367–387. New York: Raven.

Wong-Riley M. 1978. Reciprocal connections between striate and prestriate cortex in squirrel monkey as demonstrated by combined peroxidase histochemistry and autoradiography. *Brain Res.* 147: 159–164.

——— 1979. Changes in the visual system of monocularly sutured or enucleated kittens demonstrable with cytochrome oxidase histochemistry. *Brain Res.* 171: 11–26.

Woolsey CN and EM Walzl. 1942. Topical projection of nerve fibers from local regions of the cochlea to the cerebral cortex of the cat. *Bull. Johns Hopkins Hosp.* 71: 315–344.

Woolsey TA. 1967. Somatosensory, auditory, and visual cortical areas in the mouse. *Johns Hopkins Med. J.* 121: 91–112.

——— 1990. Peripheral alteration and somatosensory development. In *Development of Sensory Systems in Mammals,* ed. JR Coleman, pp. 461–516. New York: Wiley.

Woolsey TA and H Van der Loos. 1970. The structural organization of layer IV in the somatosensory region (SI) of the mouse cerebral cortex. *Brain Res.* 17: 205–242.

Worgotter F and C Koch. 1991. A detailed model of the primary visual pathway in the cat: A comparison of afferent excitatory and intracortical inhibitory connections schemes for orientation selectivity. *J. Neurosci.* 11: 1958–1979.

Worley PF, AJ Cole, TH Murphy, BA Christy, Y Nakabeppu, and JM Baraban. 1990. Synaptic regulation of immediate-early genes in brain. *Cold Spring Harbor Symp. Quant. Biol.* 55: 213–223.

Yamamoto Y, T Kurotani, and K Toyama. 1989. Neural connections between the lateral geniculate nucleus and visual cortex in vitro. *Science* 245: 192–194.

Yamamoto Y, K Yamada, T Kurotani, and K Toyama. 1992. Laminar specificity of extrinsic cortical connections studied in coculture preparations. *Neuron* 2: 217–228.

Young MP. 1992. Objective analysis of the topological organization of the primate visual cortex. *Nature* 358: 152–155.

——— 1993. The organization of neural systems in the primate cerebral cortex. *Proc. Roy. Soc. Lond.* B252: 113–118.

Young MP, JW Scannell, and G Burns. 1995a. *The Analysis of Cortical Connectivity.* Austin, TX: RG Landes; New York: Springer.

Young MP, JW Scannell, MA O'Neill, GC Hilgetag, G Burns, and C Blakemore. 1995b. Non-metric multidimensional scaling in the analysis of neuroanatomical connection data and the organization of the primate cortical visual system. *Phil. Trans. Roy. Soc. Lond.* B348: 281–308.

Young MP, K Tanaka, and S Yamane. 1992. On oscillating neuronal responses in the visual cortex of the monkey. *J. Neurophysiol.* 67: 1464–1474.

Yuste R, MJ Gutnick, D Saar, KR Delaney, and TW Tank. 1994. Ca^{2+} accumulations in dendrites of neocortical pyramidal neurons: An apical band and evidence for two functional compartments. *Neuron* 13: 23–43.

Yuste R and LC Katz. 1991. Control of postsynaptic Ca^{2+} in developing neocortex by excitatory and inhibitory neurotransmitters. *Neuron* 6: 333–344.

Yuste R, DA Nelson, WW Rubin, and LC Katz. 1995. Neuronal domains in developing neocortex: Mechanisms of coactivation. *Neuron* 14: 7–17.

Yuste R, A Peinado, and LC Katz. 1992. Neuronal domains in developing neocortex. *Science* 257: 665–669.

Yuste R and DW Tank. 1966. Dendritic integration in mammalian neurons, a century after Cajal. *Neuron* 16: 701–716.

Zacco A, V Cooper, PD Chandler, S Fishere-Hyland, HL Horton, and P Levitt. 1990. Isolation, biochemical characterization and ultrastructural analysis of the limbic system-associated membrane protein (LAMP), a protein expressed by neruons comprising functional neural circuits. *J. Neurosci.* 10: 7–90.

Zecevic N, JP Bourgeois, and P Rakic. 1989. Changes in synaptic density in motor cortex of rhesus monkey during fetal and postnatal life. *Dev. Brain Res.* 50: 11–32.

Zecevic N and P Rakic. 1991. Synaptogenesis in monkey somatosensory cortex. *Cerebral Cortex* 1: 510–523.

Zeki S. 1974. Functional organization of a visual area of the posterior bank of the superior temporal sulcus of the rhesus monkey. *J. Physiol. Lond.* 236: 549–573.

——— 1993. *A Vision of the Brain.* Oxford: Blackwell.

Zeki S, JDG Watson, CJ Lueck, KJ Friston, C Kennard, and RSJ Frackowiak.

1991. A direct demonstration of functional specialization in the human visual cortex. *J. Neurosci.* 11: 641–649.

Zihl J, D von Cramon, and N Mai. 1983. Selective disturbance of movement vision after bilateral brain damage. *Brain* 106: 313–340.

Zilles K, E Armstrong, KH Moser, A Schleicher, and H Stephan. 1989. Gyrification in the cerebral cortex of primates. *Brain Behav. Evol.* 34: 143–150.

Zimmerman H. 1993. *Synaptic Transmission: Cellular and Molecular Basis.* New York: Thieme/Oxford.

Zola-Morgan SM and LR Squire. 1990. The primate hippocampal formation: Evidence for a time-limited role in memory storage. *Science* 250: 288–290.

Zola-Morgan S, LR Squire, and DG Amaral. 1986. Human amnesia and the medial temporal region: Enduring memory impairment following a bilateral lesion limited to field CA1 of the hippocampus. *J. Neurosci.* 6: 2950–2967.

Credits

Chapter 2

Table 2.1: Reprinted from G. L. Stebbins, *Darwin to DNA, Molecules to Humanity,* © 1982 by W. H. Freeman and Company. Used with permission.

Table 2.2: Reprinted from P. A. Filapek et al., "The young adult human brain: An MRI-based morphometric analysis," *Cerebral Cortex* 4 (1994): 344–361, with permission of Oxford University Press.

Figures 2.1, 2.2, 2.4, 2.6, 2.7, 2.8: Reproduced with permission of S. Karger AG, Basel.

Figure 2.5: Reprinted from M. A. Hofman, *Progress in Neurobiology,* © 1989, 32: 137–158, with kind permission from Elsevier Science Ltd., The Boulevard, Langford Lane, Kidlington OX5 1GB, UK.

Figure 2.9: Courtesy I. Tattersall.

Figure 2.10: Reprinted from D. Johanson and L. Johanson, *Ancestors: In Search of Human Origins* (New York: Villard Books, Random House, 1994), unnumbered illustration on page 67, with permission from The Royal Society, London.

Figure 2.11: Reprinted from C. Stringer and C. Gamble, *In Search of the Neanderthal,* © Christopher Stringer and Clive Gamble, by permission of the publisher, Thames and Hudson.

Figure 2.12: Used with permission of *Canadian Journal of Anthropology.*

Chapter 3

Figure 3.1: Used with permission of Plenum Press.

Figures 3.2, 3.3: Reprinted from J. DeFelipe and I. Farinas, *Progress in Neurobiology,* © 1992, 39: 563–607, with kind permission from Elsevier Press Ltd., The Boulevard, Langford Lane, Kidlington OX5 1GB, UK.

Figure 3.4:   Reprinted from E. G. Jones, "GABAergic neurons and their role in cortical plasticity in primates," *Cerebral Cortex* 3 (1993): 361–372, with permission of Oxford University Press.

Figure 3.5:   Used with permission of Plenum Press.

Figure 3.6:   Reprinted from M. A. Wilson and M. E. Molliver, *Neuroscience,* © 1991, 44: 537–553, with kind permission from Elsevier Press Ltd., The Boulevard, Langford Lane, Kidlington OX5 1GB, UK.

Chapter 4

Table 4.2:   Reprinted from T. P. Powell, "Brain mechanisms of perceptual awareness," *Brain* 103 (1981): 1–19, with permission of Oxford University Press.

Figures 4.4, 4.5:   Reprinted from G. Rajkowska and P. S. Goldman-Rakic, "Cytoarchitectural definition of prefrontal areas in the normal human cortex," *Cerebral Cortex* 5 (1993): 323–338, with permission of Oxford University Press.

Figures 4.8, 4.9:   Used with permission of Springer-Verlag.

Figure 4.10:   Reprinted from A. J. Rockel et al., "The basic uniformity in structure of the neocortex," *Brain* 103 (1980): 221–244, with permission of Oxford University Press.

Chapter 5

Figure 5.1:   Used with permission of The Physiological Society, London.

Figures 5.3, 5.5:   Used with permission of The American Physiological Society.

Figures 5.4a, 5.4b: Used with permission of The Physiology Society.

Figure 5.6:   Reprinted with permission from *Nature* 375: 645–653, © 1995 by Macmillan Magazines Ltd.

Figure 5.7:   Reprinted from D. A. McCormick et al., "Neurotransmitter control of neocortical neuronea activity and excitability," *Cerebral Cortex* 3 (1993): 387–398, with permission of Oxford University Press.

Figure 5.8:   Used with permission of The Physiology Society.

Figure 5.9:   Reprinted from *Neural Notes* II: (2) 3–7 (1996), Promega Corporation.

Figure 5.10:   Reprinted from Z. W. Hall, *An Introduction to Molecular Neurobiology,* 1992, by permission of Sinauer Associates, Inc.

Chapter 6

Figure 6.1:   Reprinted from Z. W. Hall, *An Introduction to Molecular Neurobiology,* 1992, by permission of Sinauer Associates, Inc.

Figure 6.2: Reprinted with permission from the *Annual Review of Neuroscience,* vol. 13, © 1990 by Annual Reviews Inc.

Figure 6.3: Reprinted with permission from *Neuron* 6: 53–60, © 1991 by Cell Press.

Figure 6.4: Reprinted with permission from Current Biology Ltd.

Figure 6.5: O. Hvalby et al., "Specificity of protein kinase inhibitor peptide and induction of long-term potentiation," Proc. Nat'l Acad. Science, U.S.A. 91: 4761–4765, © 1995, National Academy of Sciences, U.S.A.

Figure 6.6: P-M Lledo et al., "Calcium/calmodulin-dependent kinase II and long-term potentiation enhance synaptic transmission by the same mechanism," *Proc. Nat'l Acad. Science U.S.A.* 92: 11175–11179, © 1995, National Academy of Sciences, U.S.A.

Figure 6.7: S. M. Dudek and Bear, "Homosynaptic long-term depression in area CA1, of hippocampus and effects of N-methyl 1-D-aspartate receptor blockade," *Proc. Nat'l Acad. Science U.S.A.* 89: 4363–4367, © 1992, National Academy of Sciences, U.S.A.

Figure 6.8: Reprinted with permission from Current Biology Ltd.

Figure 6.9: Reprinted with permission from *Neuron* 15: 1–4, © 1995 by Cell Press.

Figures 6.10, 6.11: W. R. Chen et al., "Long-term modification of synaptic efficiency in the human inferior and middle temporal cortex," *Proc. Nat'l. Acad. Sci. U.S.A.* 93: 8011–8015, © 1996, National Academy of Sciences, U.S.A.

Chapter 7

Figures 7.1, 7.2: Used with permission of The Johns Hopkins University Press.

Figures 7.4, 7.5, and 7.6: Courtesy O. V. Favorov.

Figure 7.7: Reprinted from F. Schmitt et al., eds., *The Organization of the Cerebral Cortex: Proceedings of a Colloquium Held at Woods Hole, Mass.* (Cambridge, Mass.: MIT Press, 1981).

Figures 7.8, 7.12, 7.14, 7.17: Used with permission of The American Physiological Society.

Figure 7.11: Used with permission of Humana Press.

Figure 7.15: Reprinted with permission from the *Annual Review of Neuroscience,* vol. 13, © 1990 by Annual Reviews, Inc.

Chapter 8

Figure 8.2: Reprinted from P. Rakic, *Trends in Neuroscience* 18: 383–388, © 1995, with kind permission from Elsevier Science Ltd., The Boulevard, Langford Lane, Kidlington OX5 1GB, UK.

Figure 8.3: Used with permission of W. B. Saunders Company.

Figure 8.5: Used with permission of The Neuroscience Institute.

Chapter 9

Figures 9.1, 9.2: Reprinted from A. Peinado et al., "Gap junctional communication and the development of local circuits in neocortex," *Cerebral Cortex* 3 (1993): 488–498.

Chapter 10

Figures 10.1, 10.2, 10.5: Reprinted from D. J. Felleman and D. C. Van Essen, "Distributed hierarchical processing in the primate cerebral cortex," *Cerebral Cortex* 1 (1991): 1–47, with permission of Oxford University Press.

Figures 10.3, 10.4: Reprinted from M. P. Young, "The organization of neural systems in the primate cerebral cortex," Proceedings of the Royal Society of London B252: 113–118, © 1993, with permission from The Royal Society.

Figure 10.6: Used with permission of Cold Spring Harbor Laboratory Press.

Figure 10.7: Reprinted from P. Goldman and W. Nauta, "Columnar distribution of cortico-cortical fibers in the frontal association, limbic and motor cortex of the developing rhesus monkey," *Brain Research* 122: 393–413, © 1977, with kind permission from Elsevier Science-NL, Sara Burgerhartstraat 25, 1055 KV Amsterdam, The Netherlands.

Figure 10.8: Reprinted with permission from the *Annual Review of Neuroscience,* vol. 13, © 1990 by Annual Reviews Inc.

Figure 10.9: L. D. Selemon and P. S. Goldman-Rakic, "Common cortical and subcortical targets of the dorsolateral prefrontal and posterior parietal cortices in the rhesus monkey," *Journal of Neuroscience* 8 (11): 4065 (1988).

Chapter 11

Figure 11.1a: T. A. Cleland and A. I. Selverston, "Glutamate-gated inhibitory currents of central pattern generator neurons in the lobster stomatogastric ganglion," *Journal of Neuroscience* 15 (10): 6632 (1995).

Figure 11.1b: Reprinted from P. S. Katz and R. M. Harris-Warwick, *TINNS* 13: 367–373, © 1990, with kind permission from Elsevier Science Ltd., The Boulevard, Langford Lane, Kidlington OX5 1GB, UK.

Figures 11.2a, 11.2b: Used with permission of The American Physiological Society.

Figure 11.3: Used with permission of Plenum Press.

Figure 11.4: Reprinted from A. M. Thomson and J. Deuchars, *TINNS* 17: 119, © 1994, with kind permission from Elsevier Science Ltd., The Boulevard, Langford Lane, Kidlington OX5 1GB, UK.

Figure 11.5: Used with permission of The Physiology Society.

Figures 11.6, 11.8:   Reprinted from T. R. Vidyasagar et al., *TINNS* 19: 272, © 1996, with kind permission from Elsevier Science Ltd., The Boulevard, Langford Lane, Kidlington OX5 1GB, UK.

Figure 11.7:   Reprinted with permission from Current Biology Ltd.

Figure 11.10:   Used with permission of the Neurosciences Research Foundation.

Figure 11.11:   Used with permission of the Society for Neuroscience.

Chapter 12

Figures 12.1, 12.2, 12.9:   F. A. Gibbs and E. L. Gibbs, *Atlas of Electroencephalography: I. Methodology and Controls,* 2nd ed. (Cambridge, Mass.: Addison-Wesley, 1950).

Figure 12.3:   Reprinted from Paul Nunez, *Electrical Fields in the Brain: The Neurophysics of EEG,* © 1981 by Oxford University Press. Used by permission of Oxford University Press, Inc.

Figures 12.7, 12.8:   Used with permission of Lippincott-Raven Publishers.

Figure 12.11:   Reprinted from M. Steriade et al., *TINNS* 17: 199, © 1994, with kind permission from Elsevier Science Ltd., The Boulevard, Langford Lane, Kidlington OX5 1GB, UK.

Figure 12.12:   Courtesy R. Galambos.

Figure 12.13:   Reprinted from J. E. Desmedt and C. Tomberg, *Neuroscience Letters* 168: 126–129, © 1994, with kind permission from Elsevier Science Ltd., The Boulevard, Langford Lane, Kidlington OX5 1GB, UK.

Figure 12.14a: R. Eckhorn et al., "Coherent oscillations: A mechanism for feature linking in the visual cortex? Multiple electrode and correlation analysis in the cat," *Biological Cybernetics* 60: 121–130, © 1988. Reprinted with permission of Springer-Verlag.

Figures 12.14b, 12.15:   Reprinted from C. M. Gray et al., "Stimulus-dependent neuronal oscillations in cat visual cortex: Receptive field properties and feature dependence," *European Journal of Neuroscience* 2 (1990): 607–619, with permission of Oxford University Press.

Figure 12.16:   Reprinted from A. K. Engel et al., *TINNS* 15: 218–226, © 1992, with kind permission from Elsevier Science Ltd., The Boulevard, Langford Lane, Kidlington OX 5 1GB, UK.

Figure 12.17:   Reprinted from Eckhorn et al., "Biological cybernetics," *Network* 2: 293–307, Figure 9, © 1990 by Springer-Verlag GmbH & Co.

Figure 12.18:   Used with permission of Birkhauser Books.

Figure 12.19:   Reprinted from C. M. Gray and D. A. McCormick, "Chattering cells: Superficial pyramidal neurons contributing to generation of synchronous oscillations in the visual cortex," *Science* 274: 109–113, © 1996, with permission from the American Association for the Advancement of Science.

Index

Brain-body relation, 20–23, 47
Brain clocks, 276
Brain-derived neurotrophin factor, 232, 233, 234
Brain function: in human evolution, 46
Brain pathology: EEG rhythms and, 323. *See also* Lesions; Psychosis
Brain size: limits of, 30; of australopithecines, 35; in *Homo habilis,* 38, 49; in *Homo erectus,* 39, 49; human, 41–42, 49, 95–97; in assessing brain evolution, 46–47; intelligence and, 96–97; in human evolution, 364, 365
Brain states: fast oscillations in, 333–335. *See also* Sleep; Waking state
Brain volume: cortical volume and, 23–25; cortical surface area and, 26; evolutionary increases in, 44–45; in assessing brain evolution, 46–47; relationship with cortical columns, 46–47; measuring, 95
Brain waves. *See* Electroencephalographic rhythms
Broca's area, 38, 45
Brodmann, Korbinian, 80
Brodmann areas, 80–83, 87, 259, 260
Bunge, Mario, 14–15
Bursting neurons: in supragranular layers, 107; pyramidal cells as, 107, 314, 354–355; oscillations and, 283 284, 318, 354–355, 377; membrane potential of, 284; stomatogastric nervous system and, 285; in layer V, 313, 314; in oscillatory synchronization, 347, 348; middle temporal area, variability in, 360; EEG rhythms and, 375

CA1 synapses: long-term potentiation and, 143–150, 163; short-term potentiation and, 158
CA3 synapses: long-term potentiation and, 158–159
Cadherins, 229, 230
Cajal, Santiago. *See* Ramón y Cajal, Santiago
Cajal-Retzius cells: in layer I circuitry, 70, 79; minicolumns and, 165; intrinsic connectivity and, 193; in neo-

cortical ontogenesis, 205; neuronal migration and, 225–226
Calbindin, 56, 61
Calcineurin, 155
Calcitonin-gene-related peptide, 236
Calcium binding proteins: in pyramidal cells, 56. *See also specific proteins*
Calcium ion: in exocytosis, 113; in direct synaptic transmission, 120; in second messenger systems, 129–130; postsynaptic, dendritic spines and, 134; in post-tetanic potentiation, 141; in long-term depression, 143, 153, 155, 161; in long-term potentiation, 155, 159, 161, 163; short-term potentiation and, 158; sliding threshold hypothesis and, 161–162
Calcium ion/calmodulin-dependent protein kinase II (CaM-KII): in vesicle exocytosis, 117; second messenger systems and, 130; long-term potentiation and, 146, 147–148; long-term depression and, 147; post-tetanic potentiation and, 147
Calmodulin, 56, 130
Calpain, 130
CaM-KII. *See* Calcium ion/calmodulin-dependent protein kinase II
cAMP. *See* Cyclic adenosine monophosphate
cAMP-dependent protein kinases, 129
Carbon monoxide, 150
CAT 301 (extracellular proteoglycan), 95
Cat 301 (monoclonal antibody), 235
Cats: horizontal intracortical connections in, 69; claustrocortical projection system and, 77; neurophysiological experiments in, 346; visual cortex, synchronization in, 347–354, 357–358, 359
Cell adhesion molecules, 216, 229
Cell assemblies concept, 312–313
Cell cycle: germinal, 209
Cell death, 238–239
Cell density: neocortical, 97–98
Cell developmental potential: concept of, 208; *vs.* presumptive fate, 222
Cell ensembles: temporal-correlation hypothesis and, 345–346; oscillations and, 361

Cortical neurons *(continued)* cytoarchitectural studies and, 79–90; intrinsic, 90, 236; number of, 98, 101, 366, 378; presynaptic terminals and, 102; biophysical properties of, 104–109; regular-spiking, 105–107, 298, 313; fast-spiking, 107–109, 294, 298; synaptic endings of, 115–116; cell-layer position and, 221, 224–226; development of, 236; projection, 236; gap junctions and, 242–245; hierarchical analysis of, 269; modulatory systems and, 310–312; comparative studies and, 364–365; organization of, 366–367. *See also* Bursting neurons

Cortical operations: neural mechanisms in, 2–6; overview of, 314–316; imaging methods and, 370–371; models of, 380

Cortical plasticity: synaptic changes and, 233; neuronal overproduction and, 239–240; forms of, 316

Cortical plate: formation of, 205, 209; neuronal migration in, 213; innervation of, 251–252

Cortical slice preparations: synaptic transmission and, 104, 369; microcircuits and, 288–289; overview of, 295–296; double intracellular recording methods and, 296; results from, 296–298

Cortical surface area: evolutionary enlargement in, 25–26, 48; brain volume and, 26; ontogenetic units and, 27, 28

Cortical thickness: evolutionary trends in, 25–26, 48; in models of fissurization, 30; variations in, 97–98

Cortical volume: brain volume and, 23–25

Corticocortical afferents: classes of, 72; distributive properties of, 271–275; in linkages between separate cortical columns, 354

Corticospinal system: collateral pruning in, 242; distributive properties of, 276–277

Corticothalamic fibers: reticular thalamic nucleus innervation, 330

Corticotrophin releasing factor, 59

Crustaceans. *See* Decapod crustaceans

Culture: in human evolution, 45, 49

Cutaneous afferents, 174

Cyclic adenosine monophosphate (cAMP), 129

Cyclic guanosine monophosphate (cGMP), 129

Cytoarchitecture, 79–90, 102, 245–249, 252

Cytochrome oxidase method, 87, 179

Cytology: Golgi method and, 51

Cytoskeleton: in vesicle transport, 117

Cytotactin, 219

DAG. *See* Diacylglycerol

Dating methods: in paleoanthropology, 32, 39, 42

Decapod crustaceans: stomatogastric nervous system in, 285–287, 309

Declarative memory: characteristics of, 137–138; hippocampus and, 139–141

Decoding: neuronal, 288

Democritus, 1

Dendrites: of pyramidal cells, 55; excitatory synapses and, 102; inhibitory synapses and, 102; functions of, 132–134, 136; minicolumn structure and, 194–196; neurotrophins and, 232–233; gap junctions and, 243

Dendritic clusters, 194–196

Dendritic spines. *See* Spines

Dentate gyrus, 141, 143, 221

2-Deoxyglucose labeling method: cortical columns and, 175–176; ocular-dominance columns and, 179; barrels and, 200–201

Derivative function, 287

Descending connections, 263, 264–265, 266, 269

Desynchronization: in alpha waves, 322

Diacylglycerol (DAG), 129

Diesterase, 130

Dipoles: EEG rhythms and, 326

Direct synaptic transmission, 112–113, 119–126, 136

Dirichlet domains, 201

Dissociative anesthetics, 124

Distributed-representation hypothesis, 318–320

Distributed systems, 380; defined, 254; requirements of, 254–255, 276; time factors and, 254–255, 276; nodes in, 255, 282, 370; neural activities within, 255–256; evidence for, 256–261; cortical columns and, 271–275; neocortical networks and, 275–278; effects of lesions in, 277; emergent properties and, 278, 381; conservation of topology in, 278–279; error compensation in, 279; microcircuit operations and, 282; perception and, 318–320, 367–368, 375–376; synchronization and, 319, 360–361; recognition-unit model and, 344; temporal-correlation hypothesis and, 344, 345–346; composition of, 367–368; experimental methods and, 370–371; binding hypothesis and, 376–378

Distribution function, 287–288

DNA technology: human evolution and, 42

Dopamine, 73, 122, 309

Dorsal thalamus: subplate neurons and, 237, 238; EEG rhythms and, 327–328, 375; neuronal oscillations and, 328–333; innervation by modulatory systems, 332; cortical columns and, 367

Dorsolateral frontal cortex, 69

Double bouquet cells: described, 61; in intrinsic connectivity, 62–63, 193; in layer III, 79; motor cortex and, 182; dendritic clusters and, 196; in barrels, 197; in cortical microcircuits, 294

Double intracellular recording methods: technique of, 296; results from, 296–298, 369

Dreaming, 333

Dryopithecus, 34

D-Serine, 124

Dualism, 14

Eccles, J. C., 103–104, 109

Edelman, Gerald, 318, 358

EEG rhythms. *See* Electroencephalographic rhythms

Efferent fibers/systems: spiny pyramidal cells as, 54–58; callosal, 72; myelination and, 90; number of, 101; of cortical columns, 166; growth of, 230–231

Eidola, 1

Einstein, Albert: brain size of, 96–97

Electrical activity. *See* Electroencephalographic rhythms; Oscillations

Electroconvulsive shock, 153

Electroencephalograms, 12–13

Electroencephalographic rhythms (EEG rhythms): human, general properties of, 317, 320–328; mechanisms producing, 317–318, 375; discovery of, 320–321, 374; behavioral correlations and, 321; neuronal activity and, 321, 379; brain pathology and, 323; biological origins of, 325–328; in sleep, dorsal thalamus and, 328–333; micro-analysis of, 335–338; high-density recording of, 336–337; spatial and temporal analysis of, 336–338; magnetic field tomography and, 338; induced, 338–343; scanning function and, 377

Electroencephalography, 323, 337–338

Electrophysiological methods/studies: in systems neurophysiology, 11; cytoarchitectural studies and, 90; of long-term potentiation, 152; somatic sensory cortex and, 166–169; barrels and, 198–199; of microcircuit operations, 280; of sleep, 328

Emergent materialism, 14–15

Emergent properties: defined, 6; distributed systems and, 278, 381; in cortical microcircuits, 280, 371

Encephalization index, 21–23, 39, 47

Endocasts, 32, 365

Endocranial volume: evolutionary trends in, 32–33

Endogenous bursting neurons, 285, 318

Endothelial relaxing factor, 150. *See also* Nitric oxide

End-plate potentials, 114–115

Ensemble coding, 255

Entorhinal complex, 140

Environmental factors: in neuronal migration, 224

Epilepsy, 321, 341

EPSPs. *See* Excitatory postsynaptic potentials

Equivalent recognition units, 344

Errors: in distributed systems, compensation for, 279
Evolution: brain, 6, 23–49, 211–212, 363–365; cortical enlargement and, 28; ontogenetic units and, 28, 47, 211–212; human, 37, 40–41, 42–43, 45–46; race and, 43, 49; theories in, 43–45; role of culture in, 45; use of allometric studies in, 46; assessing through measurements of brain size, 46–47; neocortical expansion and, 211–212
Excitatory interneurons: glutaminergic, description of, 58; in intrinsic connectivity, 192–194; in cortical microcircuits, 293; feed-forward circuits and, 315. *See also* Spiny, nonpyramidal cells
Excitatory loops: in orientation selectivity, 304
Excitatory neurons: terminals of, 101; specific axonal growth in, 241
Excitatory postsynaptic potentials (EPSPs): in single-trigger-zone model, 109; induction of, 113–114; in direct synaptic transmission, 119–120; in dendrites, 132–133; pyramidal cell linkages and, 296
Excitatory synapses, 53, 54
Excitatory transmission, 115, 116
Excitatory transmitters, 56–57
Exocytosis, 118, 134
External capsule, 202
Extracellular matrix: neuronal migration and, 219; axonal growth and, 229; in synaptic stabilization, 235
Extracellular space: current flow in, 325
Extrinsic gene expression, 246

Family: human evolution and, 49
Fast oscillations: alpha blocking and, 322; brain states and, 333–335; induced, 338–343, 376–377; synchronization and, 339, 342–343, 377
Fast-spiking neurons, 107–109, 294, 298
Fast synaptic transmission, 112–113. *See also* Direct synaptic transmission
Feature convergence, 287, 306–307, 374
"Feature detection," 2

Feature-detector model, 343
Fechner, Gustav, 8–9
Feedback loops, 56. *See also* Descending connections
Feed-forward loops, 315. *See also* Ascending connections
Fibroblast growth factor, 236
Fibronectin, 219
First somatic sensory cortex. *See* Primary somatic sensory cortex
Fissurization: brain volume and, 26; in cortical enlargement, 28–29; models of, 29–32
Fissurization index, 30
Fluorescent-cytochemistry, 93
Focused attention: induced fast oscillations and, 339, 341; synchronization and, 344–345
Folding. *See* Fissurization
Forebrain: presynaptic inhibition in, 131; segmentation, models of, 248
Fractures, 179
Frequency: in synchronization, role of, 361
Frontal association cortex, 188
Frontal lobe projections: distributive properties of, 273–274
Fronto-parietal system, 271
Fusion pores, 118
Fusion protein, 118

GABA. *See* Gamma-aminobutyric acid
GABAergic interneurons, 120. *See also* Inhibitory interneurons; Nonspiny, nonpyramidal cells
GABA receptors: in direct synaptic transmission, 120; synaptic inhibition and, 126–127; second-messenger systems and, 127–128; in presynaptic inhibition, 131–132
Gamma-aminobutyric acid (GABA), 117; inhibitory interneurons and, 59; in mediation of direct synaptic transmission, 121; inhibitory neurons and, 126–127, 136; neuroactive peptides and, 130, 136; in presynaptic inhibition, 131–132
Ganglionic layer. *See* Layer V
Gap junctions: in central neurons, 122; in interneuronal signaling, 135; in dendritic clusters, 194; cortical circuits and, 242–245

Gene expression: effects of synaptic potentiation and depression on, 161; in cerebral development, 246, 368

Genetic studies: on human evolution, 42

Gene transcription: G proteins and, 128

Geniculate neurons: activity-dependent competition and, 233–234; subplate innervation and, 237

Geniculocortical fibers, 373

Germinal cell cycle, 209

Germinal epithelium, 379; ontogenetic units and, 367; in cerebral ontogenesis, 368. *See also* Neuroepithelium

Gestalt psychology: perception and, 7–8; synchronization and, 319

Glial cells: glia-to-neuron ratio, 101; in cortical ontogenesis, 204; generation of, 209; radial unit hypothesis and, 211, 213–214; neuronal migration and, 213–214, 217–219; *reeler* mutation and, 225; number in cerebral cortex, 366

Glutamate, 117; as excitatory transmitter, 56–57; in single-trigger-zone model, 109; in mediation of direct synaptic transmission, 121; NMDA receptors and, 124, 125; in long-term potentiation, 143, 150; stomatogastric neurons and, 285

Glutamate receptors: pharmacological agonists, 122; subunits of, 123; in long-term potentiation, 145–146, 149. *See also* Metabotropic receptors; NMDA receptors; Non-NMDA receptors

Glycine: in single-trigger-zone model, 109; in mediation of direct synaptic transmission, 121–122; NMDA receptors and, 124, 156

Glycoproteins, 95, 229

Golgi, Camillo, 51

Golgi apparatus: vesicle synthesis and, 117

Golgi method, 51, 92

G-protein-linked receptors, 128

G proteins: indirect synaptic transmission and, 113; metabotropic receptors and, 126; structure and actions of, 128

Gradualism: in evolution, 43–45

Granular layer. *See* Layer IV

Granular vesicles, 117

Gray matter: phylogenetic changes and, 26

Growth cones: chemotropic molecules and, 229–231; in neuromuscular junction formation, 236. *See also* Axonal growth

Guanosine diphosphate: indirect synaptic transmission and, 113

Gyri: patterning of, 30, 32; endocasts and, 32; as functional entities, 32

Gyrification: brain volume and, 26; in cortical enlargement, 28–29; models of, 30–32

Hand. *See* Manipulative skills

Hebb, Donald, 234

Helmholtz, Hermann von, 2, 6–7

Heterotypical cortex: cytoarchitectural studies on, 83, 87; thalamic nuclei and, 88; afferent innervation patterns in, 102; cortical columns and, 176–185, 367

Hierarchical processing model, 254, 263–271, 375

High-density EEG recording, 336–337

Hippocampus: declarative memories and, 139–141; neocortical connections, 140; long-term potentiation in, 141–153, 158–159; long-term depression in, 153–155; short-term potentiation in, 158

Histamine, 73, 122, 332

Hominids: evolution of brain in, 32–43, 363–364, 365; bipedalism and, 35–36; evolution in, 37, 39–40, 45, 48–49; language ability and, 46

Homo erectus, 37, 44; labyrinthine morphology of, 36; brain size of, 39; evolution of, 39–40; transition to *Homo sapiens* and, 41, 42–43, 45, 49

Homo ergaster. See Homo erectus

Homo habilis, 37–39, 45, 49

Homo sapiens. See Humans

Homo sapiens neanderthalensis, 40–41

Homotypical cortex: interpretation of behavior and, 43; thalamocortical afferents and, 66; cytoarchitectural studies on, 83, 87; afferent innerva-

Homotypical cortex *(continued)*
tion patterns in, 102; cortical columns and, 185–188, 367; distributive properties of, 276; transformations in, 306–307, 374; synchronized neural activity in, 360–361
Horizontal cells, 70
Horizontal intracortical connections, 68–69, 353–354
Hubel, David, 176, 177
Human brain: microstructural uniqueness of, 4–5; size of, 41–42, 45, 49, 95–97; changes in function of, 46, 49; sexual dimorphism in, 95–96; surface area of, 97; EEG rhythms in, 320–328; induced rhythms in, 338–343
Human neurophysiology, 338
Humans: evolution of, 37, 40–41, 42–43, 45–46; transition from *Homo erectus* and, 41, 42–43, 45, 49; changes in brain function and, 46, 49

Ideas: innate, 362
Imaging methods, 370–371
Immunocytochemistry, 93, 366
Immunoglobulins: axonal growth and, 229
Indirect synaptic transmission, 113, 127–131, 136
Induced rhythms, 338–343, 376
Inferotemporal cortex, 187–188, 359–360
Information: types of, 3
Infragranular layers: regular-spiking neurons and, 107; neuronal migration and, 213; in hierarchical connections, 263
Inhibitory circuits: in intrinsic circuitry, 67–68
Inhibitory interneurons: neuropeptides and, 59–60; classes of, 60–64; thalamocortical afferents and, 67; in intrinsic connectivity, 193; in cortical microcircuits, 293–294; pyramidal cells as, 315. *See also* Nonspiny, nonpyramidal cells
Inhibitory mechanisms: in orientation selectivity, 304–305
Inhibitory neurons: as fast-spiking

neurons, 108; GABA and, 126–127, 136; specific axonal growth in, 241
Inhibitory postsynaptic potentials (IPSPs): in single-trigger-zone model, 109; induction of, 114; in direct synaptic transmission, 120; in pyramidal cells, 298
Inhibitory synapses, 53–54
Inhibitory terminals, 101, 102
Inhibitory transmission: quantal nature of, 115; cell types generating, 116; presynaptic, 131–132
Inhibitory transmitters, 59
Innate ideas, 362
Innervation: transitions in, 102; neurotrophins and, 231–233; subplate neurons and, 236–238. *See also* Axonal growth
Inositol triphosphate (IP$_3$), 129
Insectivores: brain evolution in, 23–25
Integration: perceptual, temporal correlation and, 343–356; cortical, modeling experiments in, 358–359
Integrins, 229, 230
Intelligence: brain convolutedness and, 29, 48; brain size and, 42, 96–97
Interhemispheric projections, 273
Interneuronal signaling: volume transmission and, 134–135; gap junctions and, 135. *See also* Synaptic transmission
Interneurons: intrinsic, in neocortical ontogenesis, 206; pyramidal cells and, 282, 298, 313; in cortical microcircuits, 293–294. *See also* Excitatory interneurons; Inhibitory interneurons
Interstitial cells, 64
Intracortical circuits. *See* Intrinsic circuits
Intracortical microstimulation methods, 183
Intracortical neurons. *See* Intrinsic cortical neurons
Intracortical transformations: experimental methods and, 280–281; visual cortex and, 299–306; orientation selectivity and, 373. *See also* Cortical microcircuits
Intralaminar thalamocortical afferents, 71–72
Intraparietal sulcus, 88

Intrinsically bursting neurons, 107, 313

Intrinsic circuits: identification of, 64–65; thalamocortical afferents and, 65–67; role of inhibition in, 67–68; horizontal intracortical connections in, 68–69; of layer I, 70–71; columniation and, 192–194; in cortical histogenesis, 192–194; barrels and, 197; specific axonal growth in, 241; extrinsic connections and, 282; prototypical, 292–295; EEG rhythms and, 328. *See also* Cortical circuits; Re-entrant circuits

Intrinsic cortical neurons: myelination and, 90; development of, 236

Intrinsic gene expression, 246

Invertebrates: neural operations in, 282–287, 309

Ion channels: in synaptic transmissions, 112, 113, 114; GABA receptors and, 126; G proteins and, 128

Ionic hypothesis, 103, 369

Ions: movement in channels, 122

IP$_3$. *See* Inositol triphosphate

Ipsilateral corticocortical system, 72, 191

Isocortex. *See* Neocortex

Isofrequency bands, 180–181

JNDs. *See* Just noticeable differences

Joint afferents, 174

Just noticeable differences (JNDs), 9

Kainate receptors, 122, 124. *See also* Non-NMDA receptors

"Kernels," 284

Ketamine, 124

Koniocortex, 168

Label-and-reconstruct method, 289–292, 295–296, 300

lacZ gene: neuronal migration studies and, 214, 215; in cell labeling experiments, 222

Laminar packing density, 83

Laminar relations: irreciprocity and, 260, 263; hierarchical properties of, 263–271

Laminations: neocortical, 79–80. *See also entries under* Layer

Laminin, 219, 230

Language: in hominid evolution, 38, 46

L-AP4, 126

Large basket cells: described, 60–61; thalamocortical afferents and, 66; in layer III, 79; in intrinsic connectivity, 193; in cortical microcircuits, 293, 294

Large nonpyramidal cells, 101

Large pyramidal cells, 80

Lateral connections, 263–264

Lateral geniculate body: ocular-dominance columns and, 179; oscillatory activity and, 355–356

Lateral geniculate nucleus: size of, impact of afferents on, 248; in orientation selectivity, 300–303

Lateral ventricle: stem-like cells in, 221

Layer I (neocortical): intrinsic circuit of, 70–71; described, 79; intrinsic connectivity and, 193–194; formation of, 205

Layer II (neocortical), 79

Layer III (neocortical), 79

Layer IV (neocortical): described, 80; barrels and, 197, 199, 200–201; in hierarchical connections, 263; ascending connections and, 266; excitatory loops in, 304

Layer V (neocortical): described, 80; collateral pruning in, 242; neocortical functioning and, 313–314

Layer VI (neocortical): described, 80; in sleep oscillations, 330

Learning: synaptic plasticity and, 137, 138; nitrous oxide and, 150; long-term potentiation and, 152–153; homotypical cortical areas and, 185; cortical plasticity and, 316

Lemniscus, 66, 191

Lesions: effects on distributive systems, 277; degradation of cerebral activity and, 379–380

LFP. *See* Local field potentials (LFP)

Ligand-gated channels: subfamilies of, 122; in indirect synaptic transmission, 127; modulatory systems and, 286

Limbic-associated membrane protein, 95

Limbic cortex, 95

Migration. *See* Neuronal migration

Mind: in emergent materialism, 14–15; theory of, 43

Miniature end-plate potentials, 114–115

Minicolumns: formation of, 27, 165, 215, 216; cortical columns and, 27–28, 165, 171, 173, 176, 367, 378; dendritic clusters and, 194–196; in barrels, 201. *See also* Ontogenetic units

Mitochondria: human evolution and, 42

Modality specificity: in cortical columns, 167, 173–175

Modulatory systems: afferent, 73–75; qualitative effects of, 286; stomatogastric nervous system and, 286, 309; intrinsic neocortical operations and, 307, 308–312; in cortical plasticity, 316; in transitions from sleep to waking, 331–332

Modulatory transmitters, 309, 310, 332

Modules: in nervous system organization, 203. *See also* Cortical columns

"Molecular clocks," 32

Molecular layer. *See* Layer I

Monaminergic afferents: barrel development and, 201–202

Monamines, 117, 122, 201–202

Monkeys: in paradigmatic experiments, 13; horizontal intracortical connections in, 69; cytoarchitectural maps and, 80, 82–83; brain values for, 97; homotypical cortex, transformations in, 306–307; neurophysiological experiments in, 346–347; visual cortex, synchronization in, 349, 354. *See also* Macaque monkeys; Primates

Mossy fiber synapses, 143, 150, 158

Motivation: perception and, 17

Motor cortex: horizontal intracortical connections and, 69; columnar organization of, 182–185; afferent projections and, 192; synchronized oscillations in, 356–357

Motor learning: long-term depression and, 153

Movement: initiation of, 17; motor cortex and, 182–185; perception of,

homotypical areas and, 186–187; induced fast oscillations and, 341

MT. *See* Medial temporal area

"Multiform" layer. *See* Layer VI

Multiple-microelectrode analysis, 5, 13

Multipolar cells, 70

Multi-unit activity, 346

mu rhythms, 323

Muscarinic receptors, 310

Muscle afferents, 174

Muscles: motor cortex and, 182–185

Mutants: *reeler*, neuronal phenotype determination and, 224–226

Mutation: in cortical evolution, 28

myc proto-oncogene family, 223

Myelination, 90

Myeloarchitecture, 79, 90–92

Mystacial vibrissae, 159, 196, 197, 198–199, 298–299

Naloxone, 159

Nauta's techniques, 260

N-CAM, 219, 229

Neanderthals, 40–41

Neighborhood relations: conservation of, 278

Neocortex: neuronal populations and, 5, 315–316; higher-order processing in, 5–6; function of, 6; uniformity and diversity in, 50–51; cell types in, 54–64; intrinsic circuitry of, 64–71; afferent systems and, 71–75; central core afferent systems and, 73–75; claustrocortical projection system and, 75, 77; reductionist analysis of, 78; defined, 79; cytoarchitecture of, 79–90; myeloarchitecture of, 90–92; chemoarchitecture of, 92–95; numerical parameters of, 97–98; thickness of, 97–98; neurons in, number of, 98, 101; synapses in, number and types of, 101–102; synaptic transmission in, 119–121, 127–131; synaptic inhibition in, 126–127; memory consolidation in, 139, 140; hippocampal connections and, 140; synaptic change and, 159–162, 228, 233; organization of, 165–166, 366–367; evolution of, 211–212; ontogenetic units and, 211–214; histogenesis in, 227–228; innervation of, 236–238; cell death and, 238–239;

104–109; central, channels in, 122; binaural, 180; in cortical ontogenesis, 204, 205; generation of, 208–210; phenotypic properties of, 221; cell-layer position and, 221, 224–226; cell lineage and, 221–224; *trk* protein kinases and, 232; cell death and, 238–239; overproduction of, 239–240; collateral pruning in, 240–242; "cell assemblies" and, 312–313. *See also* Neuronal migration; Neuronogenesis; *specific neuron types*

Neuropeptides: in nonspiny, nonpyramidal cells, 59–60; in central core systems, 73; storage in vesicles, 115; granular vesicles and, 117; types and actions of, 130–131; blood flow and, 131

Neuropeptide Y (NPY), 59, 130

Neuropeptide Y receptors, 130–131

Neurophysiology: in perceptual neuroscience, 12; temporal-correlation hypothesis and, 346–347. *See also* Systems neurophysiology

Neurotrophins (NT), 231–233, 234, 239

Ng-CAM, 217, 219

Nicotinic receptor family, 122

Nissl staining: in cytoarchitectural studies, 79, 87, 90; in pigmentoarchitectural studies, 92

Nitric oxide: in long-term potentiation, 150–151, 152

Nitric oxide synthase, 130, 151

NMDA-mediated long-term depression, 153–155, 160–161

NMDA receptors: in horizontal intracortical connections, 68; in direct synaptic transmission, 120; agonists of, 122; characteristics of, 124–126; second-messenger systems and, 127; in long-term potentiation, 145, 149, 155, 156, 158, 160–161; in long-term depression, 153, 155; post-tetanic potentiation and, 158; short-term potentiation and, 158; in synaptic connections between pyramidal cells, 296

N-Methyl-D-aspartic ion receptors. *See* NMDA receptors

N-myc proto-oncogene, 223

Nodes: in distributed systems, 255,

282, 370; recognition-unit model and, 344; connections between, temporal-correlation hypothesis and, 346

Noncolumnar organizations, 202–203

Nonmetric multidimensional scaling, 261–263, 269

Non-NMDA receptors: in horizontal intracortical connections, 68; members of, 123; in long-term potentiation, 150; in connections between pyramidal cells, 296; in connections between pyramidal cells and interneurons, 298

Nonpyramidal cells: pigmentation of, 92; relative proportions of, 101; motor cortex and, 182; in barrels, 197; gap junctions and, 243. *See also* Nonspiny, nonpyramidal cells; Spiny, nonpyramidal cells

Nonspiny, nonpyramidal cells: description of, 59; neuropeptides and, 59–60; classes of, 60–64; in cortical circuits, 62–63; thalamocortical afferents and, 67; claustral, 77; in layer III, 79; as fast-spiking neurons, 107–108; inhibitory synapses and, 116; nitrous oxide synthase and, 151; in barrels, 197

Nonsynaptic terminals, 134–135

Norepinephrine, 73, 122, 156, 309, 332

NO-synthase. *See* Nitric oxide synthase

NPY. *See* Neuropeptide Y

NPY receptors, 130–131

NT. *See* Neurotrophins

Nucleus caudalis, 67

Object vision: inferotemporal cortex and, 187

Occipital lobe: cytoarchitectural studies in, 87

Ocular-dominance columns, 177–179, 234

Oligodendrocytes, 90

Oncogenes, 212

Ontogenetic units: overview of, 27; brain evolution and, 28, 47, 211–212; in formation of minicolumns, 165, 367, 379; dendritic clusters and, 194; radial unit hypothesis and, 211–214. *See also* Minicolumns

Subplate *(continued)*
  in cortical development, 251–252, 368
Substance K, 59
Substance P, 59
Substantia nigra, 73
Substrate adhesion molecules, 216
Subsynaptic cleft, 115–116
Subthalamus, 202
Subventricular epithelium, 204, 205
Sulci: cortical boundaries and, 30; modeling of, 30; central, 30, 341; endocasts and, 32; magnetoencephalography and, 338. *See also* Fissurization
Supragranular layers: intrinsically bursting neurons and, 107; regular-spiking neurons and, 107; neuronal migration and, 213; in hierarchical connections, 263; cortical columns and, 272
Surface area. *See* Cortical surface area
Sylvian fissure: in Einstein's brain, 97
Synapses: dynamism and, 4; types of, 53–54; of pyramidal cells, characteristics of, 58; of thalamocortical afferents and spiny, nonpyramidal interneurons, 66; in horizontal intracortical connections, 68; ultrastructure of, 115–116; regulation of, 118; plasticity and, 137–139, 233, 239–240, 316; overproduction of, 239–240; cortical, number of, 366, 378
Synapsins, 117, 130
Synaptic plasticity, 137–139
Synaptic stabilization, 368, 379; activity-based mechanisms of, 228, 233–235; proteoglycans and, 235; neuromuscular junction model of, 235–236
Synaptic strength: post-tetanic potentiation and, 141; long-term potentiation and, 141–153, 159–162, 233; long-term depression and, 143, 153–155, 159, 160–162, 233; short-term potentiation and, 158; long-term changes in, 159–162, 380
Synaptic transmission: basic principles of, 103–104, 135–136; experimental methods in, 104; biophysical properties and, 104–109; single-trigger-zone model of, 109–113; principal modes of, 112–113; direct, 112–113, 119–126, 136; indirect, 113, 127–131, 136; transmitter storage and release in, 113–116; vesicle dynamics in, 116–119; regulation of, 118; mediation of, 121–126; GABA receptors and, 126–127; presynaptic inhibition and, 131–132; volume transmission and, 134–135; synaptic plasticity and, 137–139; between pyramidal cells, 296; double intracellular recording methods and, 296; cortical microcircuits and, 369
Synaptogenesis: neurotrophins and, 231–233; time course of, 239
Synaptosomes, 117
Synchronization, 288; layer V pyramid cells and, 313; distributed-representation hypothesis and, 319; perception and, 319, 339, 343; alpha blocking as, 322; fast oscillations and, 339, 342–343, 377; temporal-correlation hypothesis and, 344–346; oscillatory, 347–348, 356–357; between cortical columns, 348–354; mechanisms of, 354–356; sensory-motor performance and, 356–358; variabilities in, 359; in distributed systems, 360–361; representation and, 361; binding hypothesis and, 376–378; in and between cortical columns, 377
Systems neurophysiology: development of, 11–12

Tachykinins, 59, 61
Tegmental area, 73
Temporal-correlation hypothesis, 319, 320; overview of, 343–346; predictions of, 345–346; experimental observations in, 346–347; oscillatory synchronizations and, 347–348; synchronization between cortical columns and, 348–354; mechanisms of oscillation and synchronization in, 354–356; cortical integration modeling experiments and, 358–359; evidence against, 359–360. *See also* Binding hypothesis
Temporal lobe projections, 273
Tenascin, 219

Visual cortex *(continued)*
180; *reeler* mutation and, 225; axonal competition in, 233–234; simultaneous processing in, 270; microcircuits in, 299–306; orientation selectivity in, 300–306; dynamic operations in, 305–306; synchronization in, 347–354, 357–358; cortical microcircuit transformations in, 372–373

Visual discrimination, 187

Visual neurons: number of, 101; feature construction and, 306–307

Voltage-gated channels: in central neurons, 122; G proteins and, 128; on dendrites, 132–133, 136; stomatogastric neurons and, 285; modulatory systems and, 286

Volume. *See* Brain volume; Cortical volume

Volume transmission, 132, 134–135

Waking state: transitions to, 331–332; induced fast oscillations and, 341

Weber's law, 9

Whiskers. *See* Mystacial vibrissae

White matter: phylogenetic changes and, 26; subplate neurons and, 237

Wiesel, Torsten, 176, 177

Zinc: NMDA receptors and, 124